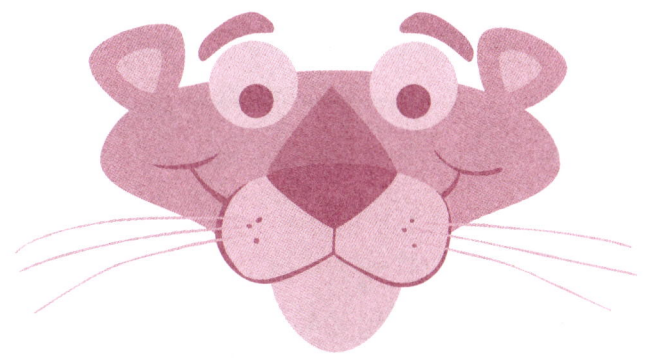

OTHER BOOKS IN THE SERIES

A First Book for Understanding Diabetes
(with translations in Spanish, Chinese, Hebrew, Syrian & Ukrainian)

Un Primer Libro Para Entender La Diabetes

Understanding Insulin Pumps, Continuous Glucose Monitors and the Artificial Pancreas

Management of Diabetes in Adults

Diabetes: A History of a Center and a Patient

DIABETES EDUCATIONAL NOVELS

A Cure – by H. Peter Chase, MD

A Second Cure – by H. Peter Chase, MD

Look in the back of the book for how to order.

UNDERSTANDING DIABETES

A handbook for people who are living with diabetes

14th Edition

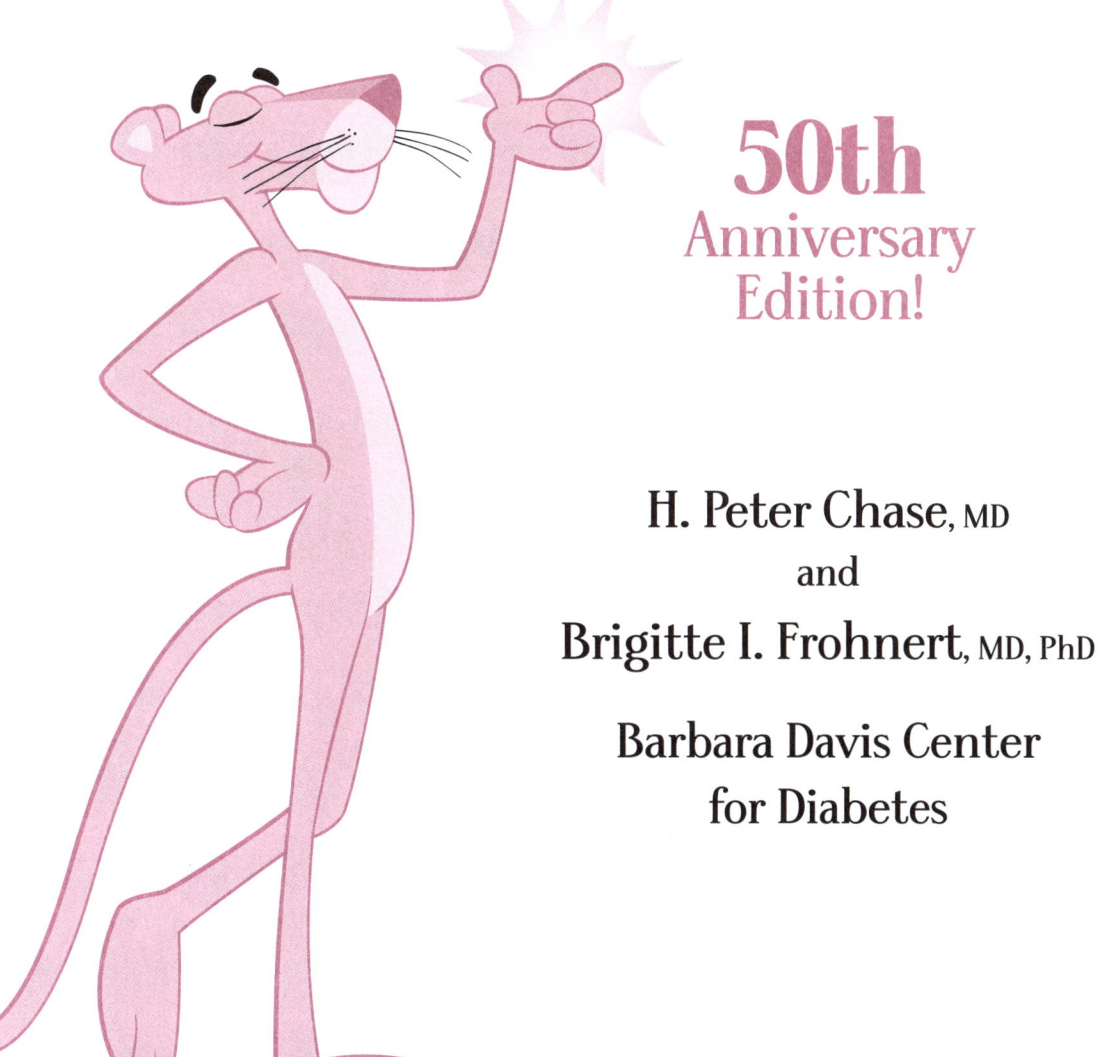

50th Anniversary Edition!

H. Peter Chase, MD
and
Brigitte I. Frohnert, MD, PhD

Barbara Davis Center
for Diabetes

Copyright © 2020
by H. Peter Chase and Brigitte I. Frohnert

THE PINK PANTHER™ & ©1964-2020
Metro-Goldwyn-Mayer Studios Inc.
All Rights Reserved.

All "Pink Panther" and "The Inspector" (the "Characters") images
are not to be reproduced without permission from
Metro-Goldwyn-Mayer Studios, Inc.

All rights reserved.
No part of this book may be reproduced
in any form or by any means without permission in writing,
with the exception of those pages expressly noted.

For information, contact the publisher:

Children's Diabetes Foundation
4380 South Syracuse Street, Suite 430
Denver, CO 80237
303-863-1200
www.childrensdiabetesfoundation.org

Library of Congress Control Number 2020914140

ISBN 978-1-7320485-2-2

Book designed by Scott Johnson

Printed in the United States of America
by Publication Printers, Denver, Colorado

Table of Contents

1. The Importance of Education in Diabetes 9
2. What is Diabetes? 17
3. Type 1 Diabetes 25
4. Type 2 Diabetes 31
5. Checking Ketones 43
6. Low Blood Sugar (Hypoglycemia or Insulin Reaction) 49
7. Blood/CGM Sugar Monitoring ... 63
8. Insulin: Types and Activity 75
9. Drawing Up and Giving Insulin .. 85
10. Feelings/Emotional Adjustment at Diabetes Onset 101
11. Normal Nutrition 107
12. Food Management and Diabetes 125
13. Exercise and Diabetes 141
14. Monitoring Diabetes 157
15. Ketones and Diabetic Ketoacidosis (KDA) 167
16. Sick Day and Surgery Management 177
17. Family and Behavioral Concerns 189
18. Care of Children at Different Ages 197
19. Diabetes Management in the Toddler/ Preschooler 209
20. Challenges of the Teen Years 215
21. Outpatient Management, Education, Support Groups, and Standards of Care 225
22. Adjusting the Insulin Dosage and "Thinking" Scales 231
23. Long-Term Complications of Diabetes 243
24. Associated Autoimmune Conditions of Type 1 Diabetes... 255
25. The School and Diabetes: A Standard of Care 261
26. Child-Sitters, Grandparents and Diabetes 283
27. Vacations and Camp 289
28. Insulin Pumps 295
29. Continuous Glucose Monitors (CGM) 313
30. The Artificial Pancreas (AP) 323
31. Pregnancy and Diabetes 327
32. Research and Diabetes 333

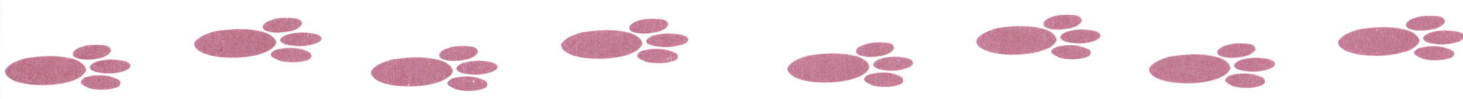

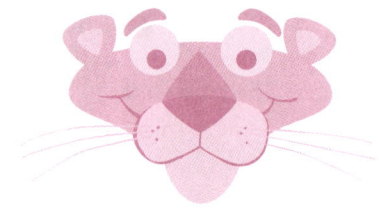

SPECIAL THANKS TO...

Regina Reece for manuscript preparation and editing.

Emily Fose for manuscript preparation and editing.

Scott Johnson for book design and graphics.

The staff of the Children's Diabetes Foundation.

MGM Consumer Products
for allowing the use of THE PINK PANTHER™.
www.mgm.com/franchise/pinkpanther

Additional copies of
this publication may be purchased from
the Children's Diabetes Foundation.
See available publications at the end of this book.

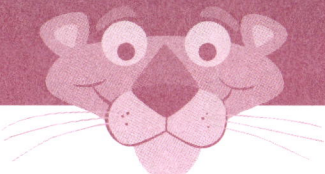

Topics for the Recommended ADA Curriculum With Their Related Chapters

Topic	Chapter Location
Diabetes disease process	1-4
Goal setting and problem solving	10, 13, 14 and 18-21
Medications	4, 8, 9, 22 and 28
Monitoring	1, 4, 5, 7, 14, 21-26, 29 and 30
Nutritional management	4, 11 and 12
Physical activity	4, 13 and 27
Preconception care, management during pregnancy and gestational management	19, 23 and 30
Prevent, detect and treat acute complications	4-6, 15, 16, 25, 26 and 30
Prevent, detect and treat chronic complications	4, 14, 23, 24 and 31
Psychosocial adjustment	10, 17-27
Research	32

TEACHING OBJECTIVES: These are provided with each chapter to assist the person(s) doing the teaching.

LEARNING OBJECTIVES: These are provided with each chapter to help the learners (parents, child, relatives or self) know the important points.

Dedicated to

Regina Reece,

a friend and outstanding coordinator

at the Barbara Davis Center,

who has now helped with our educational

books over the past 25 years.

Thank you, Regina!

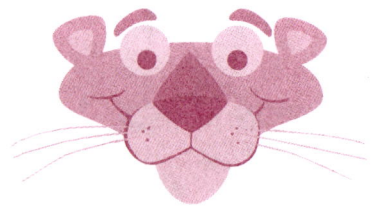

CHAPTER 1

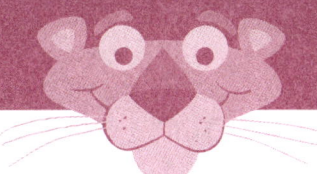

The Importance of Education in Diabetes

INTRODUCTION

Families and children need to understand as much as possible about diabetes. A shorter book, *A First Book for Understanding Diabetes* is also available. It provides a synopsis of each of the chapters in this book, and may be easier for a family with a newly-diagnosed child to read in the first week after diagnosis. The knowledge provided in this book and the skills learned will help people with diabetes and their families feel more secure about managing diabetes. It will help them manage problems when no doctor or nurse is available. It will also help them minimize hospitalizations for diabetes problems.

This book is written for families when diabetes is a new condition to them. It is also for those who have had the condition for a long time. It may serve as a reference that can be used with the doctor and diabetes team. It may also be used alone as a "refresher" course. Some of the chapters are written to provide very basic information. Other chapters are for readers wanting more in-depth information. Advances are taking place at such a rapid rate that new editions are needed about every three years.

One of the major changes currently occurring in diabetes management involves the availability of the start of the artificial pancreas. The readers should also be aware that when referring to glucose levels, the words "blood/**CGM** glucose (sugar) levels" may be used. This indicates that the glucose value may be from a blood finger stick or a continuous glucose monitor (**CGM**) value (or both). Also be aware that "glucose" and "sugar" are used interchangeably in this book.

> **TOPICS:**
> **Diabetes Disease Process**
>
> **TEACHING OBJECTIVES:**
> The teacher will:
> 1. Design a care plan that reflects the family's lifestyle and the person's educational level/developmental stage (also see Chapters 17-20).
> 2. Design a care plan that allows the person/family to become skilled in the management of diabetes.
>
> **LEARNING OBJECTIVES:**
> Learner (parents, child, relative or self) will be able to:
> 1. Identify basic management routines.
> 2. Assist the healthcare-provider in developing a diabetes care plan.
> 3. Begin the process of understanding management through charting and recording blood/CGM sugars or using electronic downloads.
> 4. Know how/when to communicate blood/CGM sugars to the healthcare-provider (including concerns about high or low values)

OUTLINE FOR INITIAL EDUCATION (see Table 1)

Initial education is variable based on:

- how sick the person is
- the emotional and physical readiness of the person and family to learn
- hospitalization versus outpatient care
- the availability of appropriately-trained educators and healthcare team

It is **essential for all parents, guardians or other care-providers** to be present for the initial education. Families initially come to the clinic for four to eight hours per day for the first few days. Other programs do education while in the hospital.

Initial teaching (survival skills) often includes:

✔ What diabetes is and what causes it
✔ Urine and/or blood ketone checking
✔ Blood/CGM sugar checking
✔ Recognizing a low blood sugar and how to treat it
✔ Insulin types and actions
✔ Drawing up insulin
✔ Giving shots
✔ Food survival skills

In addition to survival skills, other areas often covered are:

✔ A school plan
✔ When to call your diabetes care-provider
✔ Details of treatment (including "thinking" scales)
✔ Education about food (dietitian)
✔ Feelings (psych-social team)
✔ Plans for the next few days

Special instructions for the first night are summarized in Table 2.

Possible insulin dosages for day 2 are outlined in Table 3.

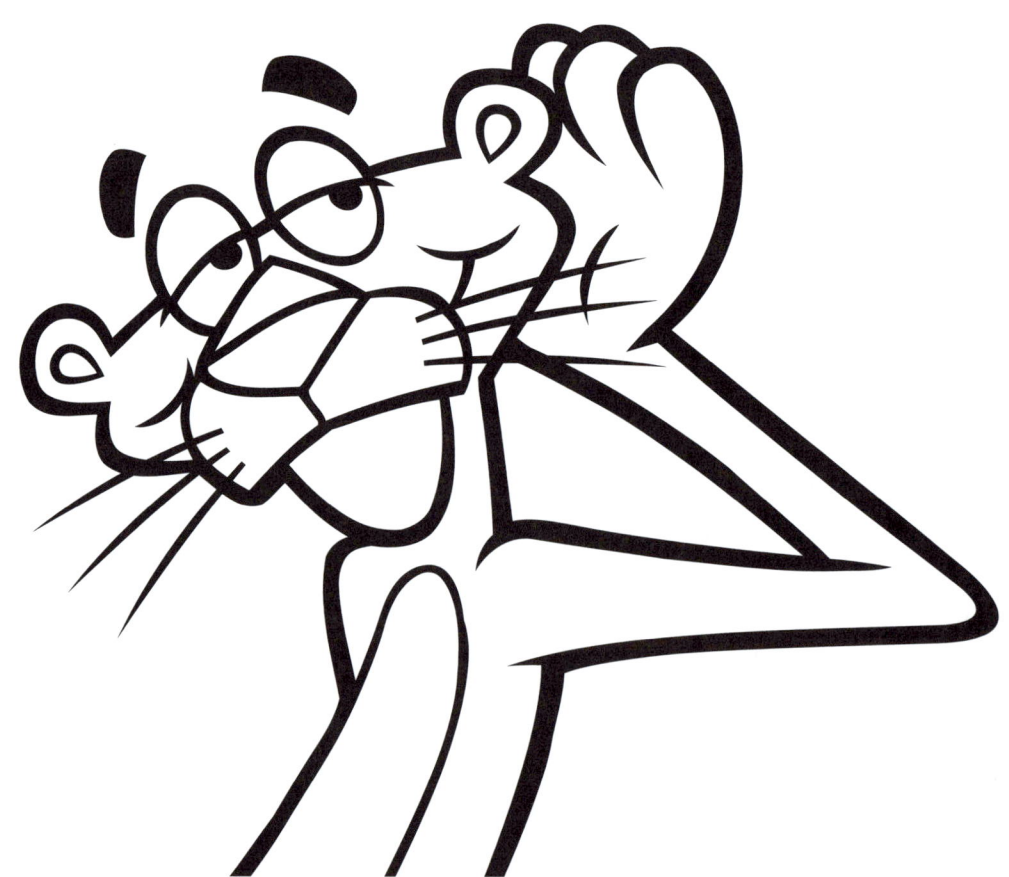

THE IMPORTANCE OF EDUCATION IN DIABETES

ONE WEEK FOLLOW-UP

Usually at one week the family and child return for group education with other families. The content includes teaching done by the dietitian and nurse and a clinic visit with the physician, a nurse practitioner or physician assistant. Areas covered include:

- ✔ Details of food management with diabetes
- ✔ Review of HbA1c: what it is and why it is important
- ✔ Insulin actions and different insulin regimens
- ✔ Pattern management of blood/CGM sugars: how to identify trends and when to fax or email numbers (all families are given fax sheets to send in weekly until blood sugars and insulin doses stabilize)
- ✔ The importance of blood/CGM sugar "time in range"
- ✔ Low blood sugar care: causes, signs and treatment of mild to severe low blood sugar levels, including a review of the use of glucose tablets and gel and the administration of glucagon
- ✔ High blood sugar care and avoiding diabetic ketoacidosis (causes, signs and treatment)
- ✔ Sick day management: how often to check blood/CGM sugars and ketones; fluid replacement, what type and how much; and when to make a call for assistance

Topics are covered in the order of urgency. How much is covered the first day depends on the family's emotional state and readiness to learn. Additional teaching may require more than one day.

It is essential that families know how to recognize and handle low blood sugar from day one. Anyone who has received insulin has the potential to have low blood sugar. Families must understand the causes, signs and treatment of mild to severe low blood sugar, including treatment with gel or glucagon. The educator will discuss this with you (Chapter 6).

CONTINUING EDUCATION

Following initial education, the family usually returns to the clinic:

- in one week
- after one month
- after three months
- then every three months

This may vary for different families and different clinics. Clinic visits every three months should include an evaluation of the family's current diabetes management. Modifications to care are made with feedback from the person and family. Children who were too young to learn self-care when diagnosed with diabetes will need age-appropriate ongoing education. Clinic visits every three months with the healthcare team can assist in their learning process.

Children who develop diabetes prior to age 10-13 will need to learn specifics about the disease as they are ready. A science project on diabetes is one way to encourage learning and self-discovery. This book can provide information for such a report.

The diabetes nurse educator may gradually start working on chapters in the book with the child alone. This can encourage the child to ask and answer questions. Education from all the diabetes team members should continue with the every-three-month clinic visits as needed. A solid educational foundation and the development of correct habits will help the person to manage the diabetes throughout life. With a supportive family and appropriate habits, the risk for later diabetes-related hospitalizations or problems is reduced.

Helpful ways to continue learning are:

- writing down questions and making notes
- websites: www.ChildrenWithDiabetes.com or www.BarbaraDavisCenter.org (please see the back of the book for additional website addresses)

- video tapes and library books
- parent and child educational group meetings

The topics considered important for initial diabetes education by the American Diabetes Association (ADA) are outlined at the beginning of this book. The chapters where each of these topics is covered are also shown. Please let your diabetes healthcare-provider know if there are topics which apply to you/your child that are unclear or ones which you would like to spend more time discussing.

FAMILY RESPONSIBILITIES

Diabetes is a unique disease. It requires ongoing communication and assistance between the person and significant others in all areas of the day-to-day care. **A knowledgeable and supportive family is very important for optimal diabetes care.** This is discussed in more detail in Chapter 17, Family Concerns.

Families must assume responsibility for:

- consistency in meals, snacks and shots
- blood/CGM sugar checks as directed
- insulin injections or insulin pump (type 1), oral medicines and/or insulin (type 2)
- regular exercise
- blood or urine ketone checks
- ordering and having supplies available
- communication with daycare/school or work
- knowing when to contact healthcare-providers for insulin adjustments between routine visits when blood sugar numbers are out of the desired range
- maintaining knowledge for treating high and low blood sugars and learning about new developments in diabetes treatment

It should be apparent that the family does 95 percent of the diabetes management.

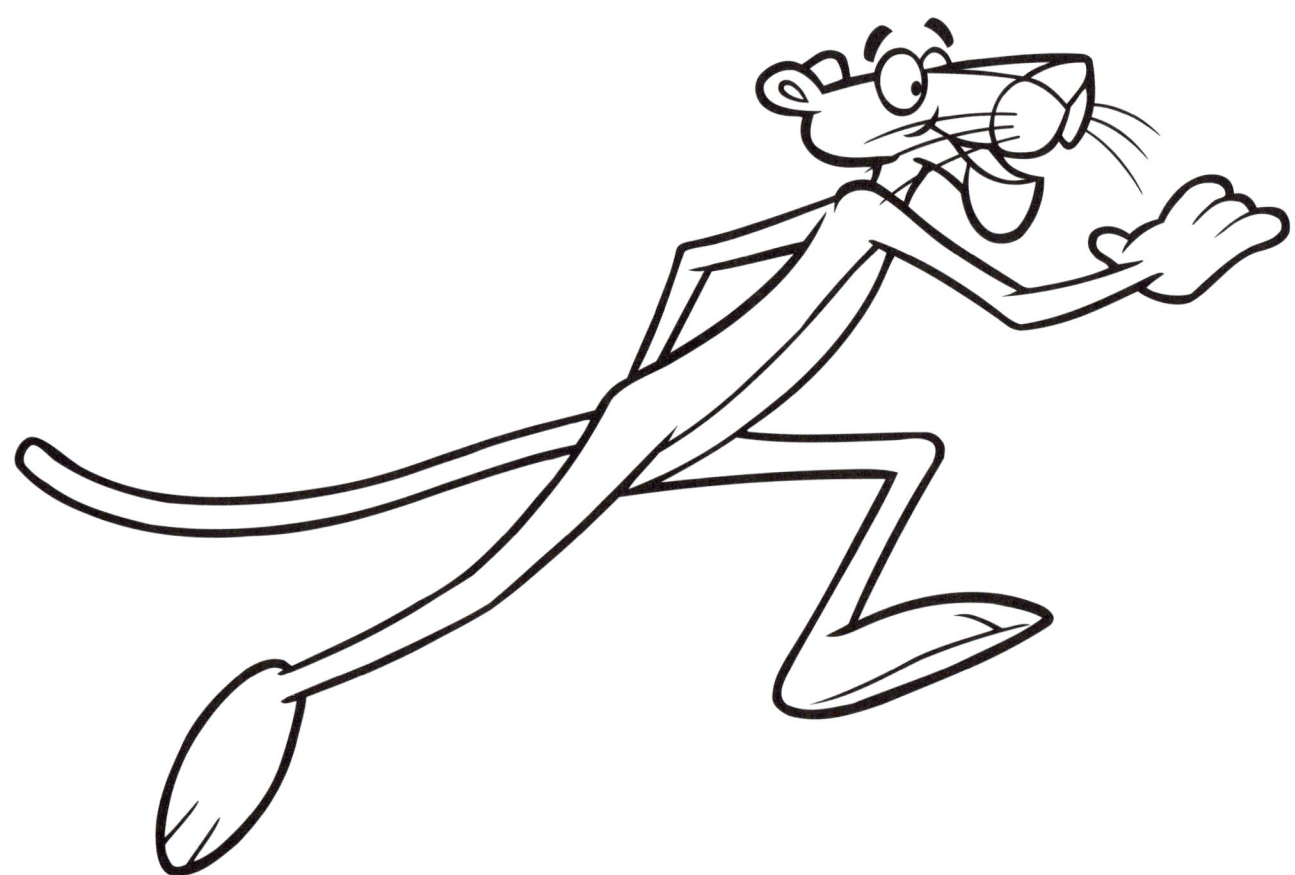

TABLE 1:
Topics Covered After New Diagnosis

Survival Skills in Hospital or Clinic

Different clinics have different schedules for education of newly-diagnosed families. Education may be done primarily in the clinic setting (after discharge if hospitalization was necessary). Day one usually involves learning survival skills needed for care in the home setting.

These include:
- ☐ Blood sugar checking on a specific meter (Chapter 7)
- ☐ Learning about insulin (Chapter 8)
- ☐ How to draw up and administer insulin (Chapter 9)
- ☐ Urine or blood ketone measurements (Chapter 5)
- ☐ Recognizing the signs of low blood sugar and how to treat (Chapter 6)

We write specific instructions (see Table 2) for the family. These relate to: meals, snacks, when to check blood sugar or urine ketone levels and how to record results, and when to phone your healthcare provider. The dietitian may discuss ideas for meals and snacks.

Any of the following may be covered:
- ☐ The Importance of Education in Diabetes (Chapter 1)
- ☐ What is Diabetes? (Chapter 2)
- ☐ What Causes Diabetes? (Type 1: Chapter 3; Type 2: Chapter 4)
- ☐ Blood/CGM Sugar Checking (Chapter 7)
- ☐ Insulin (Chapter 8)
- ☐ Insulin Injections (Chapter 9)
- ☐ Practice injection technique
- ☐ Urine or Blood Ketone Checking (Chapter 5)
- ☐ Low Blood Sugar (Chapter 6)

Additional Initial Education

- ☐ Review above concepts and answer questions
- ☐ Review insulin and insulin injection technique
- ☐ Review Low Blood Sugar (Chapter 6)
- ☐ Normal Nutrition (Chapter 11) and meet with dietitian
- ☐ Food Management and Diabetes (Chapter 12)
- ☐ Prescriptions for supplies
- ☐ Communication plan for the next week
- ☐ Grief-Adjustment Issues (Chapter 10) and meet social worker
- ☐ Review of specific routines and recommendations for exercise (Chapter 13)
- ☐ Monitoring Blood/CGM Sugar Levels (Chapter 14)
- ☐ Complete the care plan for school/daycare (Chapter 25)
- ☐ Adjusting insulin (Chapter 22; if appropriate)
- ☐ Review the two emergencies of diabetes (Chapters 6 and 15)

Additional Initial Education (variable with 1 Week Visit)

- ☐ Review above concepts and answer questions
- ☐ Family Concerns (Chapter 17) and reducing fears of shots and pokes
- ☐ The Outpatient Management of Diabetes (Chapter 21)
- ☐ Long-Term Complications of Diabetes - if questions (Chapters 23 and 24)

At One-Week/ 1 Month Visit

- ☐ Research and Diabetes (Chapter 32)
- ☐ Review all of the above
- ☐ Review Ketonuria, Ketones and Acidosis (Ketoacidosis; Chapter 15)
- ☐ Sick Day Management (Chapter 16)
- ☐ Problem solving and/or quiz
- ☐ Child-sitters and Diabetes (Chapter 26)
- ☐ Vacations and Camp (Chapter 27)
- ☐ Long-Term Complications of Diabetes - if questions (Chapters 23 and 24)
- ☐ Pregnancy and Diabetes if appropriate (Chapter 31)
- ☐ Problem solving and/or quiz

This is a general plan. The timing is varied and may change if the person is hospitalized versus when treated only in the clinic. A trend in recent years has been to teach survival skills in the first one to two days, and to make the visit at one week (when stress is lower) a longer and more in-depth visit.

TABLE 2:
Special Instructions for the First Night Are Summarized Below:

A. The diabetes supplies you will need the first night include (your nurse will mark which you need):

___ Blood glucose meter   ___ Meter glucose strips   ___ Alcohol swabs
___ Ketone check strips   ___ Glucose gel & tabs   ___ Log book
___ Insulin   ___ Syringes   ___ Phone card

The first night you will either get your insulin injection at our clinic, or you will give the shot at home or where you are staying.

B. If the insulin is given while at the clinic:
1. If Humalog®/NovoLog® or Apidra® insulin has been given, eat in 15-20 minutes (or have a snack if blood sugar below 100 mg/dL [<5.5 mmol/L]).
2. If Regular insulin has been given, try to eat your meal in 30 minutes – or have a snack containing carbohydrates if it will be more than 30 minutes.
3. Eat until the appetite is satisfied, avoiding high sugar foods (especially regular sugar pop [soda], other sweetened drinks, juice and sweet desserts).

C. If the dinner insulin is to be given at home:
1. Check the blood/CGM sugar right before the injection. Enter the result into the log book.
2. Check for urine ketones.
3. Call _____ at _____ or page at _____ for an insulin dose, or you may have been instructed to give a dose based on an insulin plan (see Table 3).
4. Draw up and give the insulin injection 15-20 minutes before the meal (give at mealtime if below 100 mg/dL [<5.5 mmol/L]). If you are not very hungry, or are too tired to eat, call the diabetes care team with any dose questions.

D. Before Bed:
1. Check the blood/CGM sugar. Enter the result into the log book.
2. Check for urine or blood ketones.
3. Call your physician at the numbers listed above if the sugar level is below _____ or above _____, or if urine ketones are "moderate" or "large" or if blood ketones are >0.6 mmol/L. If urine ketones are "trace" or "small," drink 8-12 oz of water before going to bed.
4. Give an insulin injection if your diabetes care team instructs you to do so (dose, if ordered = _____).
5. Eat a bedtime snack. This will not always be needed in the future, but the insulin dose is still being adjusted. Some ideas for this snack include: cereal and milk, toast and peanut butter, a slice of pizza, yogurt and graham crackers, or cheese and crackers. (See Chapter 12 for additional suggestions.)

E. The next morning:
1. Check the blood/CGM sugar and the urine ketones upon awakening (if sugar level is less than 70 mg/dL [3.9 mmol/L], drink 4-6 oz of juice promptly).
2. If your physician has instructed you to give the morning insulin at home, then follow your insulin dosing plan (see Table 3). Follow the steps listed above (see letter "C") for last night's meal dose if you have questions.
3. If you have been instructed to wait to give the morning dose until after coming to the clinic, check the blood sugar and the urine ketones upon awakening (if sugar level is less than 70 mg/dL [3.9 mmol/L], drink 4-6 oz of juice promptly).
4. If you are coming/returning to the clinic the next day, you may be asked to do any of the options below:
   - ☐ Take your insulin shot at home (as above) and eat breakfast before coming.
   - ☐ Eat breakfast at home and then come to the clinic for your insulin injection.
   - ☐ Bring your breakfast to the clinic and eat it after the insulin has been given.
   - ☐ Bring all blood checking supplies and materials you received the first day back to the clinic (including your log book, Pink Panther book, insulin and supplies).

TABLE 3: Insulin Injection Dosing – Onset Day 2*

	Blood Sugar mg/dL (mmol/L)	A.M.	Lunch	P.M.	Dinner	Bedtime
A) Long-Acting Insulin						
B) Intermediate-Acting Insulin (NPH)						
C) Rapid-Acting Insulin dose if:	70-150 (3.9-8.3)					
	150-250 (8.3-13.9)					
	250-350 (13.9-19.4)					
	350-450 (19.4-25.0)					
	>450 (>25.0)					

This Table will be filled out by your diabetes care-provider if he or she has instructed. Above 300 mg/dL or 16.7 mmol/L, call diabetes care-provider after ketones checked.

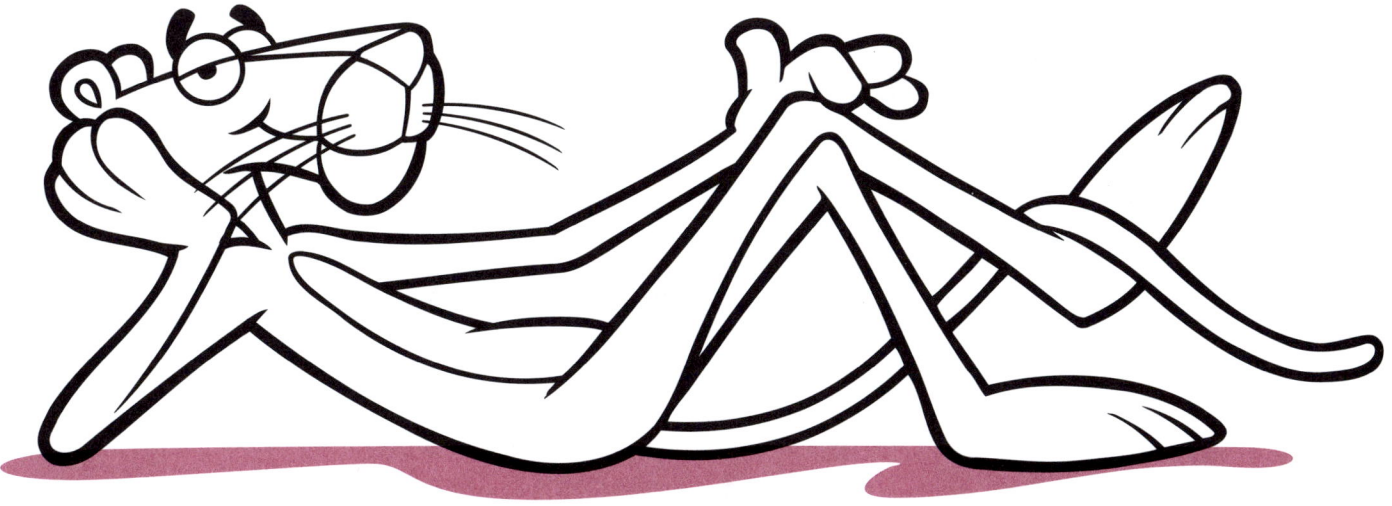

THE IMPORTANCE OF EDUCATION IN DIABETES

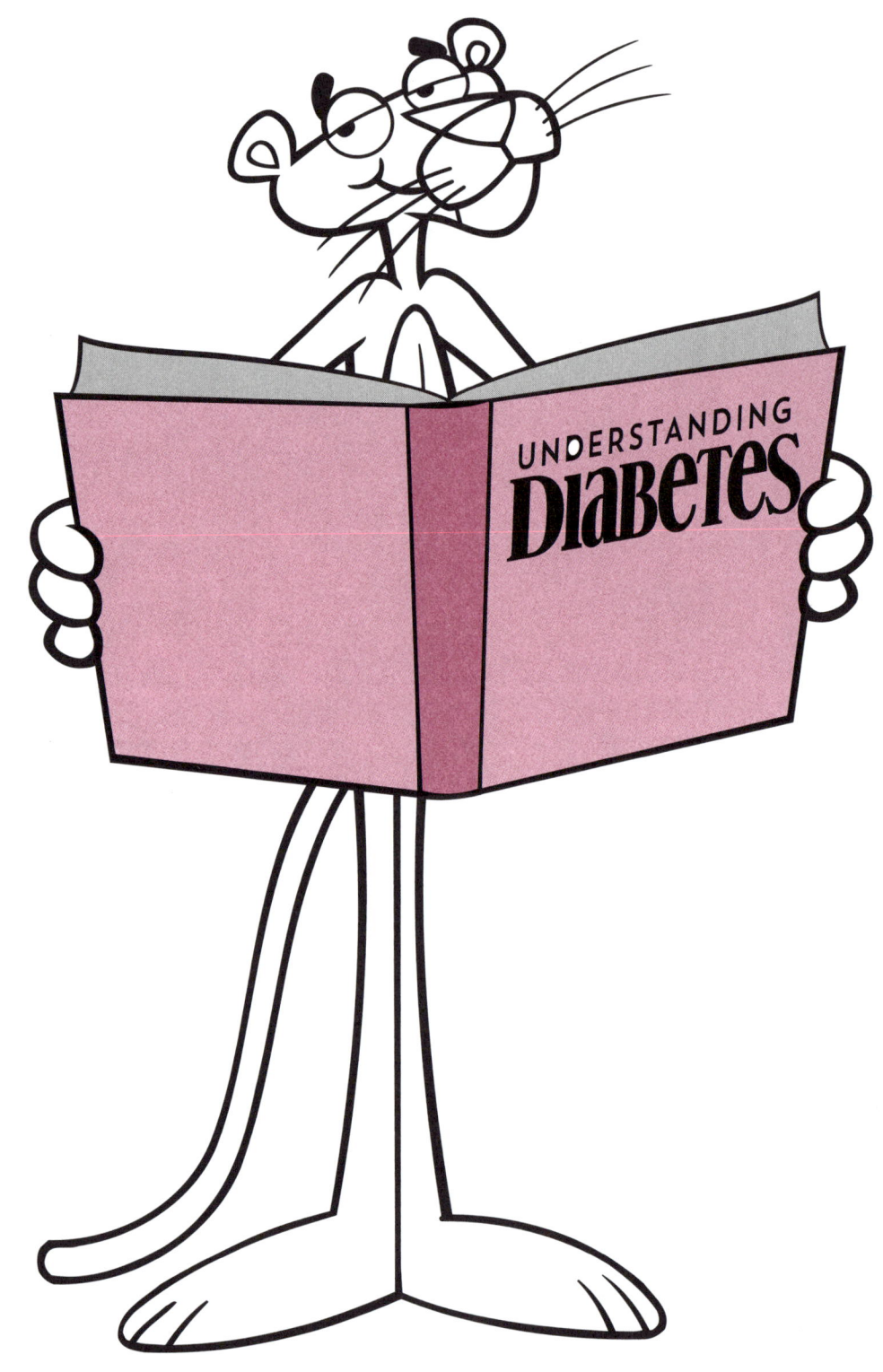

Education is key to
optimal diabetes management.

CHAPTER 2

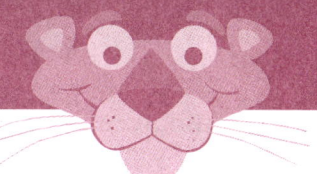

What Is Diabetes?

TYPE 1 (INSULIN-DEPENDENT) DIABETES

Type 1 (also known as insulin-dependent diabetes mellitus [IDDM] or juvenile or childhood diabetes) is the most common type found in children and young adults. **This condition occurs when the pancreas (see Figure 1) doesn't make enough insulin.** Thus, insulin injections are always required. Insulin cannot be taken in pill form because the acid in the stomach would break it down. As explained in Chapter 3, type 1 diabetes is in part due to autoimmunity (a "self-allergy"). Thus, most people with type 1 diabetes have islet-cell antibodies, which reflect an allergy against the islet cells (where insulin is made) in the pancreas.

TYPE 2 DIABETES

Another kind of diabetes is sometimes found in overweight preteens and teenagers, and is also the most common type of diabetes in adults over age 40 years. It is called **type 2 diabetes**, or sometimes **adult-onset** or **non-insulin-dependent diabetes mellitus (NIDDM)**. In type 2 diabetes, **insulin is still made** in normal or increased amounts (at least initially), but it doesn't work very well in helping the body use sugar.

In type 2 diabetes, if ketones are present, or the HbA1c is very high, insulin shots may be started. At a later time, if the islet-cell antibodies (Chapter 3) are negative and the blood sugars and HbA1c levels have decreased to near normal, then oral medications may be tried. If lifestyle modifications (weight loss and exercise)

> **TOPICS:**
> **Diabetes Disease Process**
>
> **TEACHING OBJECTIVES:**
> The teacher will:
> Design informational sessions for families in all chapters with consideration for their:
> - educational level
> - primary language
> - culture and ethnicity
> - family structure
> - learning style
> - previous experience with the medical community
>
> **LEARNING OBJECTIVES:**
> Learner (parents, child, relative or self) will be able to:
> 1. Define the basic disease process of type 1 and type 2 diabetes (also see Chapters 3 and 4).
> 2. Define normal and abnormal blood sugars along with HbA1c as part of the diagnosis of diabetes.
> 3. Define symptoms of type 1 or type 2 diabetes and compare with your symptoms experienced at diagnosis.

do not occur, insulin injections may be needed at a later time. Type 2 diabetes is discussed in more detail in Chapter 4.

MODY DIABETES

Maturity Onset Diabetes of the Young (MODY) accounts for one to three percent of cases of childhood diabetes. It may resemble type 1 diabetes in symptoms and onset. It results from a single gene defect (with at least 13 different defects now described). It is not autoimmune, and the islet cell antibodies (Chapter 3) are negative. If a parent has MODY, the offspring have a 50 percent chance of inheriting the gene and a high risk of developing MODY.

With MODY, as in all types of diabetes, ketones (Chapter 5) may be present at diagnosis, as well as high blood sugars (Chapter 7) and an elevated HbA1c level (Chapter 14).

WHY WE NEED INSULIN:

- **Insulin allows sugar to pass into our cells so that it can be "burned" for our energy.** The cells are like a furnace, which burn fuel to make energy. Our bodies constantly need energy for all of our body functions, such as allowing our heart to beat and our lungs to breathe. Sugar comes from two places (see Figure 2 in this chapter). **"Internal"** sugar comes from our body's own ongoing production in the liver or from the release of stored sugar from the liver. This sugar is released into the blood stream. **"External"** sugar comes from the food we eat (Figure 2). It enters the stomach and then moves into the intestine where it is absorbed. When people **do not** have diabetes, the pancreas makes insulin to allow both internal and external sugar to move into the body's cells.

- **A second function of insulin is to shut off the body's "internal" production of sugar** (Figure 2). Internal sugar comes mostly from the liver. When the insulin level is too low, internal sugar is made in excess by the liver. There is not enough insulin to "turn off" the liver's sugar production.

FIGURE 1
Body Parts

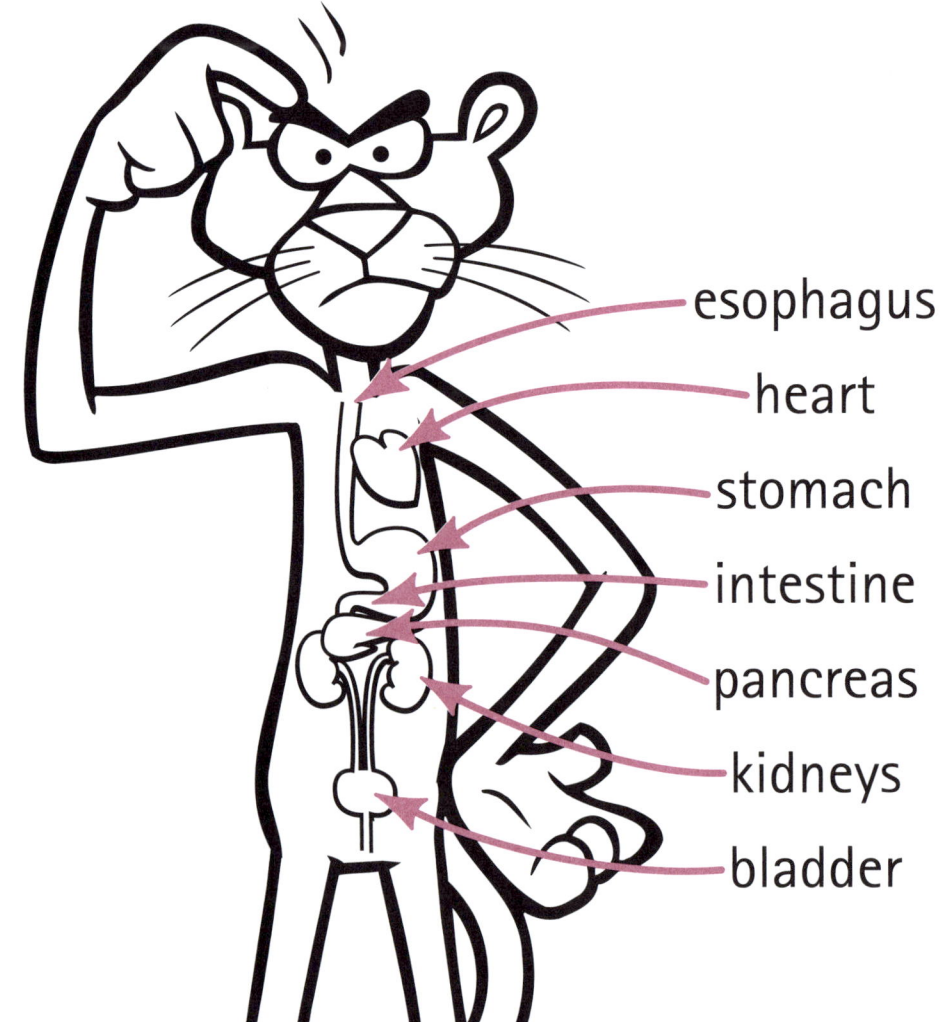

WHAT IS DIABETES?

When there is not enough insulin, or when the insulin is not working correctly (as in type 2 diabetes) the blood sugar level can be high for two reasons:

- too much internal sugar being made (not enough insulin to "turn off" the liver's sugar production).
- the sugar (from internal production and from external food) cannot pass into the cells due to lack of insulin action.

SYMPTOMS OF DIABETES

When people have type 1 diabetes, the pancreas does not make enough insulin. With type 2 diabetes, the insulin is usually not working correctly (Chapter 4). With both types of diabetes, the sugar in the blood cannot pass into the body's cells to be burned for energy. Instead, the blood sugar rises to a high level and overflows through the kidneys into the urine. When sugar enters the urine, water is pulled from all over the body to go out with the sugar. *The results are the usual symptoms of diabetes, as outlined in the following:*

1. **Frequent passing of urine (polyuria):** This happens because blood sugar levels are high and as the sugar passes through the kidney, water is needed to carry the sugar into the urine.

2. **Frequent drinking of liquids (polydipsia):** This happens to make up for the increased water lost from the frequent passing of urine.

3. **Weight loss:** This happens when the body can't get sugar into the cells. The body burns its own fat and protein for energy, resulting in weight loss. Dehydration is another contributing factor in weight loss.

4. **Frequent eating of food:** This happens because the body can't use the food it takes in and is hungry for the energy it isn't getting. This hunger is not always present in children. Sometimes the appetite may even decrease, possibly due to ketones (see Chapter 5) which can cause an upset stomach.

5. **Changes in behavior:** If the person is getting up frequently at night to pass urine, sound sleep will not occur. This and other factors can result in behavioral changes such as irritability.

Some people with type 2 diabetes have no symptoms and are diagnosed because of high blood sugar levels.

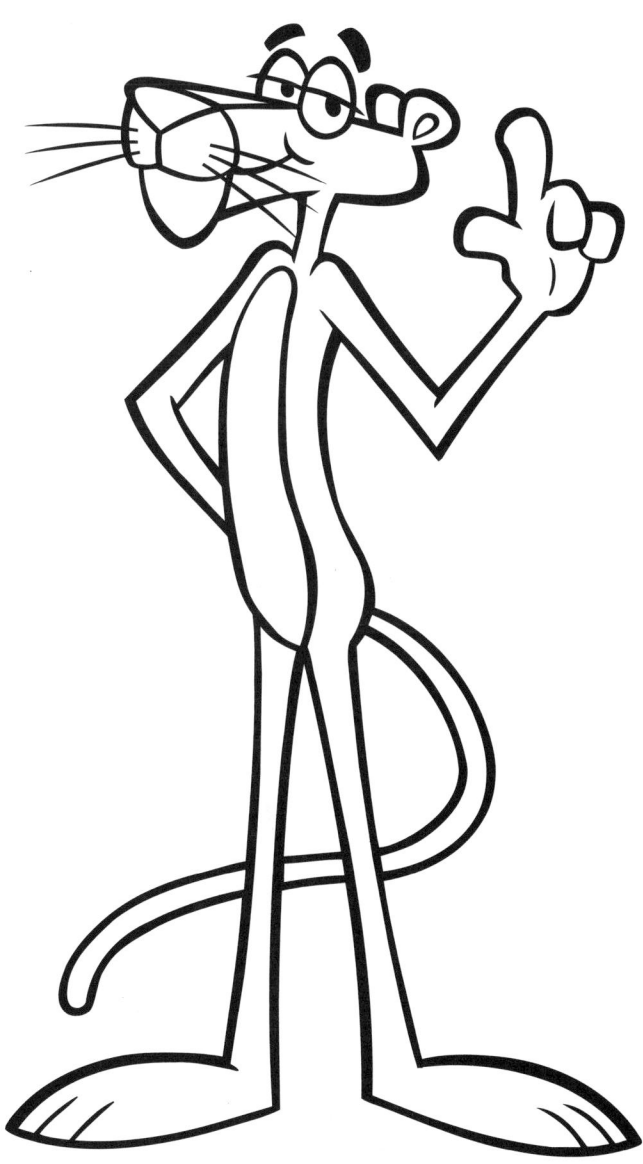

FIGURE 2
Sugar Metabolism

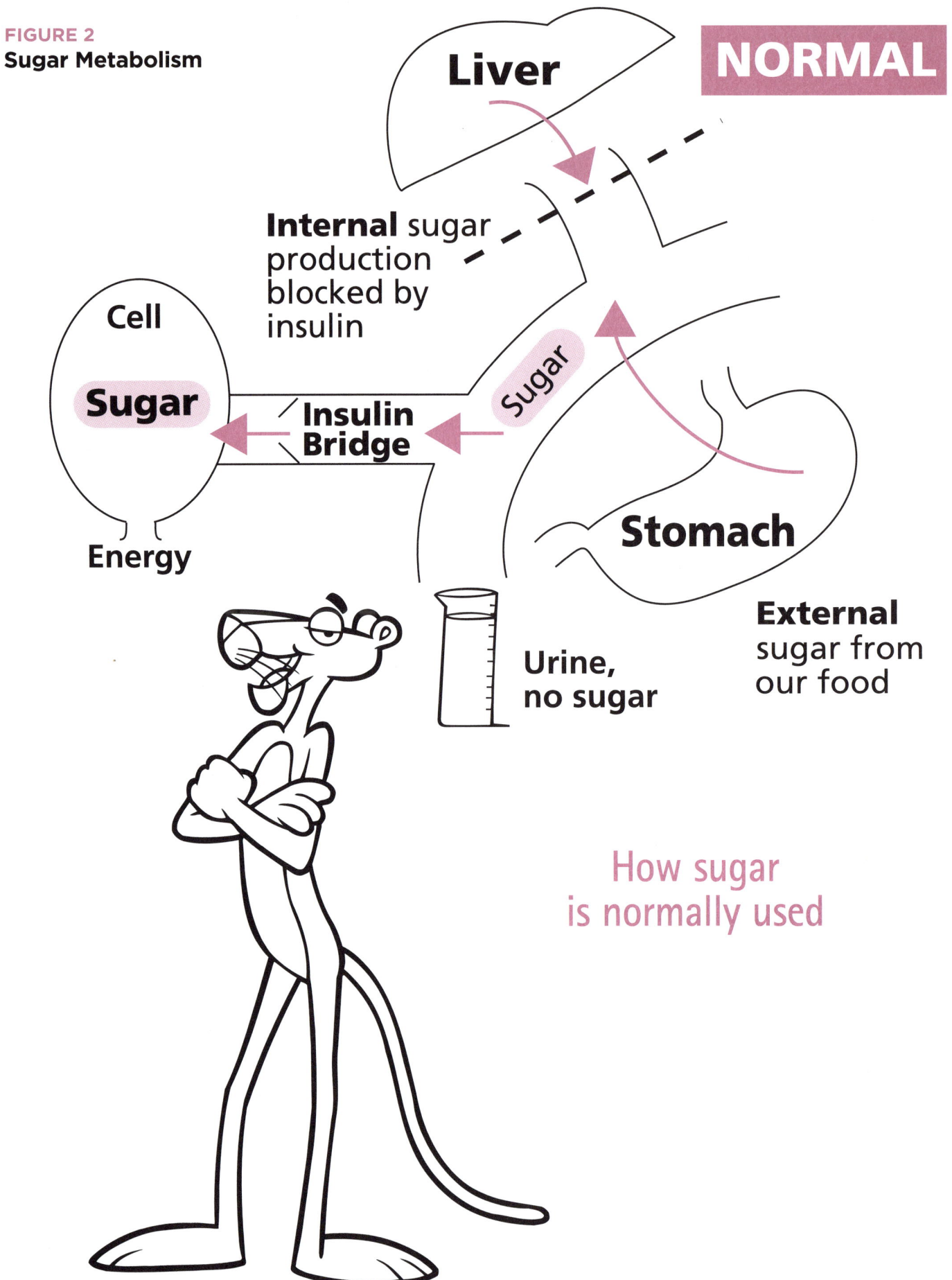

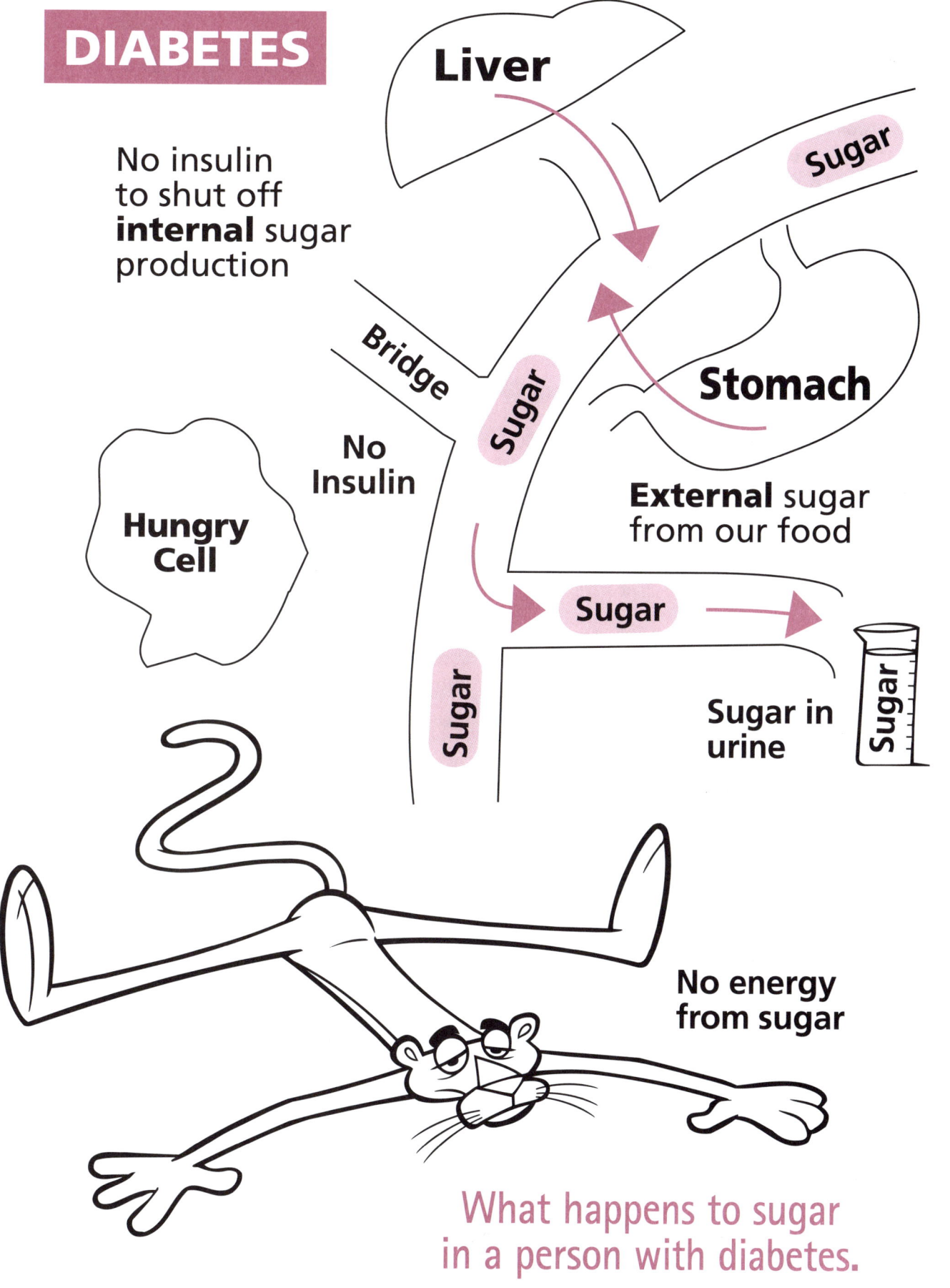

What happens to sugar in a person with diabetes.

WHAT IS DIABETES?

HONEYMOON (GRACE) PERIOD

Often there is a honeymoon or grace period that may occur a short time after the onset of diabetes. It commonly starts within two to four weeks, although not all people have this honeymoon period. Prior to the honeymoon period, there has not been adequate insulin to turn off the overnight production of sugar by the liver. During the honeymoon, sugar production is turned off in the liver and often, a fair bit of insulin is still being made in the pancreas. During this time, the body may not need much extra insulin. People may think they don't have diabetes. They may be attracted to miracle cures. The honeymoon period may last a few weeks to a few years. After this period, the body will again need more insulin, although small amounts of insulin are still made. We advise our patients to continue their insulin during the grace period, even though the dose may be small. Usually with growth, illness or stress there will again be a need for more insulin. This need may be evident when the morning blood sugars start to be above the desired range. It can be hard emotionally to restart insulin shots again if the shots were discontinued.

Similarly, some people with type 2 diabetes who lose weight may be able to discontinue all diabetes medicines. Unfortunately, if the weight is regained, medications will again be needed (Chapter 4).

PRE-DIABETES

Pre-diabetes refers to the period before developing diabetes. It is usually found in people who will develop type 1 diabetes because they have had the blood test to detect islet cell antibodies (see Chapters 3 and 32).

Pre-type 2 diabetes is very common. It is usually diagnosed in people who are overweight and who have borderline blood sugar and/or HbAlc levels (see Table 1 in Chapter 4). Weight loss and exercise can help delay or prevent the onset of type 2 diabetes (but not type 1 diabetes).

DEFINITIONS

Bladder: The organ (sac) that collects the water from the kidneys and holds it until it is passed as urine (see Figure 1).

Bloodstream: The flow of blood within the blood vessels to and from the different parts of the body.

Cells: Very small units of the body. You can only see them with a microscope.

Enzymes: Proteins in liver, muscle and intestine that help make sugar. (There are many enzymes that have other functions.)

Esophagus: The swallowing tube (see Figure 1).

External sugar: The sugar taken in from food. Insulin allows the external sugar to pass into the body's cells to be used for energy.

Insulin: The substance (hormone) made by the pancreas that allows sugar to pass into cells.

Internal sugar: The sugar made by the body (or sugar released from stored sugar in the liver). Insulin shuts off the excess production of internal sugar.

Intestine: The part of the GI tract (gut) below the stomach where most sugar (and other food) is actually absorbed into our blood stream (see Figure 1).

Islet cells (pronounced eye-let): The groups of cells within the pancreas that make insulin.

Islet cell antibody: The material we measure in the person's blood to show that they have had an allergy against the cells in the pancreas (the islet cells) that make insulin. They are usually present in the blood of people with type 1 diabetes. People with type 2 diabetes do not have these antibodies.

Kidneys: The two organs in the body that remove waste products and water from the bloodstream and make urine (see Figure 1).

Pancreas: The organ where insulin is normally made (see Figure 1). People who have type 1 diabetes cannot make enough insulin and are thus insulin-dependent.

Stomach: Where the food is collected and processed after it is swallowed (see Figure 1).

Type 1 diabetes (Also called juvenile diabetes or childhood diabetes or insulin-dependent diabetes mellitus [IDDM]): This condition results when the body cannot make enough insulin. This is the most common type of diabetes in persons under age 40 and results in the need for insulin that must be taken by shots. This type of diabetes is discussed in detail in Chapter 3.

Type 2 diabetes (Also called adult-onset diabetes or non-insulin-dependent diabetes mellitus [NIDDM]): The condition in which the body still makes insulin but is unable to use it. This is the most common type in adults over age 40. It also occurs in overweight preteens and teenagers. Pills may be able to stimulate the pancreas to make more insulin or help the person to use the insulin better. The pills are not insulin. People with type 2 diabetes do not have islet cell antibodies. This type of diabetes is discussed in detail in Chapter 4.

Urine: Water with waste passed from the body by the kidneys.

Questions and Answers from NewsNotes

Q When our son was diagnosed with diabetes, he had been vomiting and had kept no food down for over 24 hours. Yet his blood sugar was over 1,000 mg/dL (55 mmol/L). How could that be when he had not eaten any sugar?

a Insulin has several actions in the body. One is to allow all (or any) sugar to pass from the blood stream into cells where it can be burned for energy. A second function is to shut off the body's own production of sugar (primarily from the liver). When insulin is not available, as in your son at the time of diagnosis, the liver production of sugar can be enormous. This likely accounted for the high blood sugar, even though no sugar had been eaten. The vomiting was likely secondary to ketones being present (see Chapter 15).

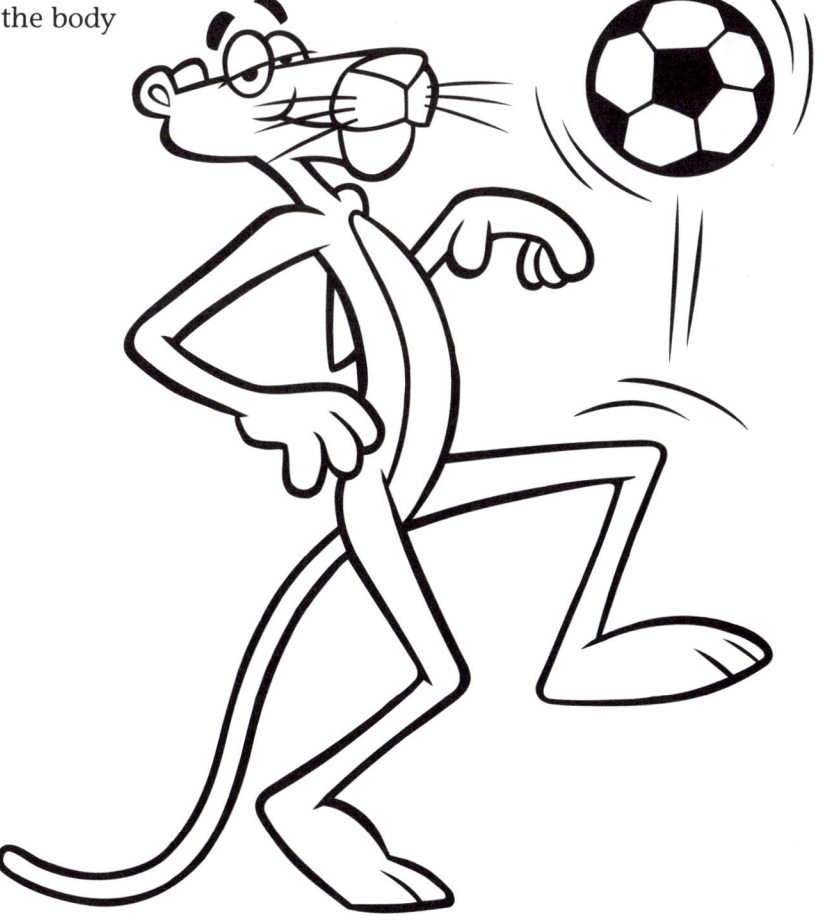

WHAT IS DIABETES?

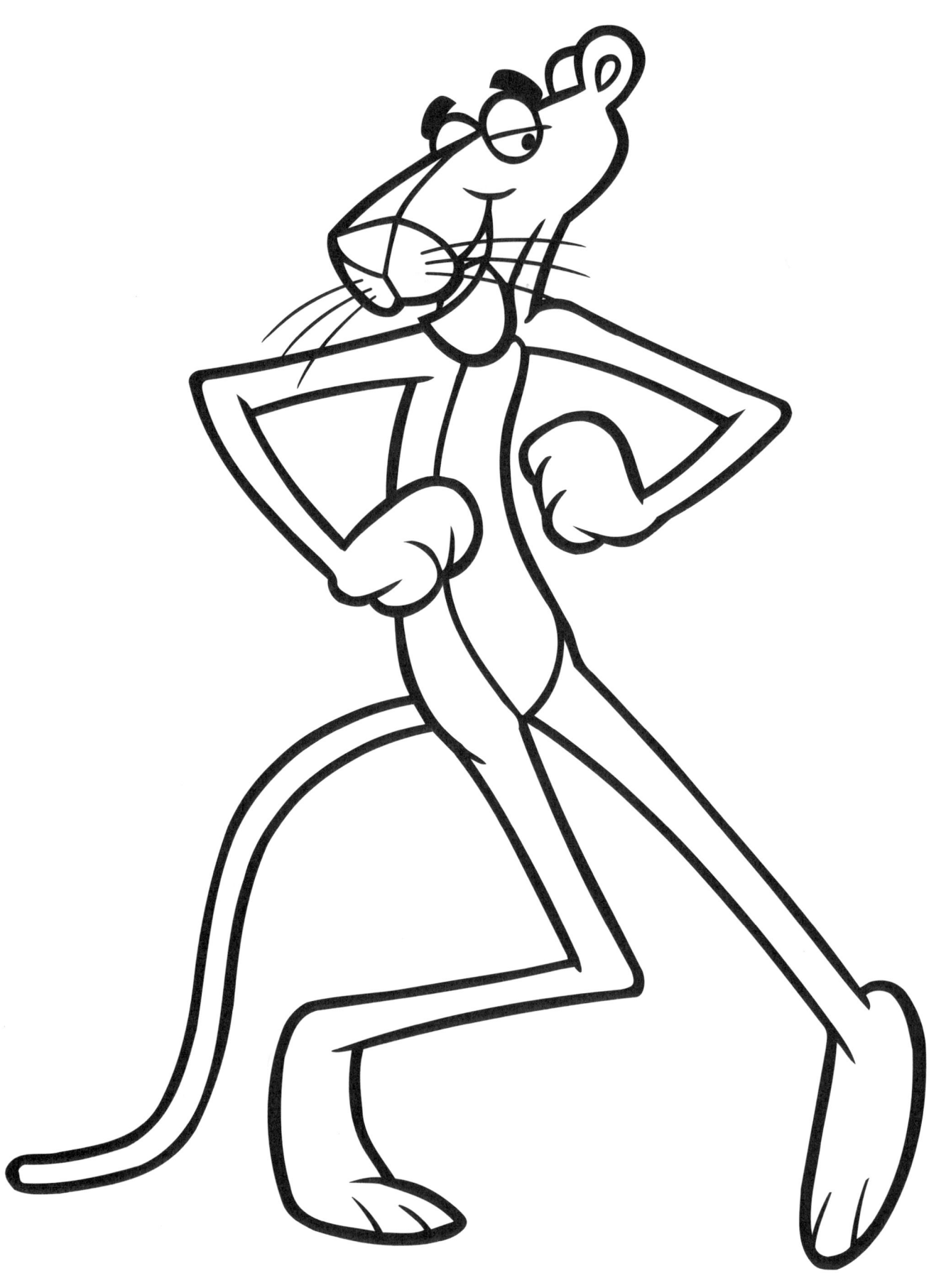

WHAT IS DIABETES?

CHAPTER 3

Type 1 Diabetes

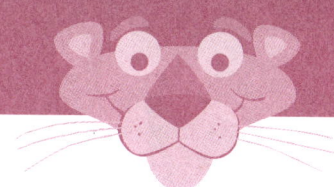

Type 1 diabetes is one of the most common chronic disorders of childhood. Unfortunately, it is increasing in incidence. The reason for this is unknown, although it is most likely related to the environment (see below). It is the most common form of diabetes to occur in people under age 40. Type 2 diabetes is the most common form after age 40. The list of famous people, sports stars, politicians, movie stars and artists who have type 1 or type 2 diabetes is long. Following diagnosis, children frequently discover classmates who also have diabetes. Their looks, personalities and activities are no different from those of anyone else.

It is important to differentiate type 1 diabetes from type 2 diabetes (discussed in Chapter 4). Type 2 diabetes is uncommon before puberty, but is increasing in frequency in overweight teenagers and adults. It does not have an autoimmune component as does type 1 diabetes (see below).

CAUSES

We know type 1 diabetes is not contagious, like a cold. We also know it isn't caused from eating too much sugar.

Three risk factors seem to be important in determining why a person develops type 1 diabetes:

1. inherited (or genetic) factors
2. self-allergy (autoimmunity)
3. environmental damage (e.g., from a virus, chemical or other cause)

> **TOPICS:**
> **Diabetes Disease Process**
>
> **TEACHING OBJECTIVES:**
> The teacher will:
> Design an educational knowledge foundation with the family that will ensure adequate knowledge on which to build.
>
> **LEARNING OBJECTIVES:**
> Learner (parents, child, relative or self) will be able to:
> 1. List two causes of type 1 diabetes.
> 2. Be aware of islet cell antibodies used to diagnose type 1 diabetes.

1. Inheritance (genetic)

The first important reason seems to be an inherited or genetic factor such as the way a person inherits the color of the eyes from a mother, father or other relative.

Facts about inheritance:

- People with type 1 diabetes are more likely to have inherited certain cell types (called **HLA types**). Those who don't have diabetes are less likely to have these HLA types.

- Nearly all people with type 1 diabetes have either a high-risk HLA type **DR3** or **DR4 gene**. There are also other genes that have been less frequently associated with an increased risk.

- Fifty-three percent of people with type 1 diabetes have one DR3 and one DR4, **with one of these coming from each parent.**

25

- Only three percent of people without diabetes have this DR3/DR4 combination. This combination makes a person more likely to develop diabetes. This is especially true if the person has a relative with diabetes.

- Over half of the families (up to 90 percent in one study) have no close relative with type 1 diabetes. Perhaps a family has either a DR3 or a DR4 gene, but no family member has ever married into a family with the other DR gene. If a family member with a DR3 gene then marries into another family carrying the DR4 gene, for example, the child may end up with the DR3/DR4 combination. They may then be at high risk for diabetes.

- It is now known there are also different genes that help to protect a person from developing diabetes.

- Children from a family who have a child with diabetes have a greater chance of developing it than do those without a family history. A brother or sister of a child with diabetes has about a 1 in 20 (five percent) chance of developing diabetes.

- The cause is not completely due to heredity. We know this from studies of identical twins. When one identical twin gets diabetes, only in half of the cases does the other twin also develop the disease. If it were entirely due to heredity, both twins would always develop it. We don't completely understand the inheritance factors. We do believe that **both** mother and father transmit the tendency to develop diabetes to their child.

2. Self-allergy (autoimmunity)

The second cause that seems to be important in type 1 diabetes is self-allergy (or autoimmunity). Normally, our immune systems protect our bodies from disease.

Facts about self-allergy (autoimmunity):

- In the case of type 1 diabetes and other autoimmune diseases such as lupus, arthritis and multiple sclerosis, the immune system turns against a body part. The immune system treats that body part like something it is allergic to and damages the body part.

- There can be evidence of this allergic reaction

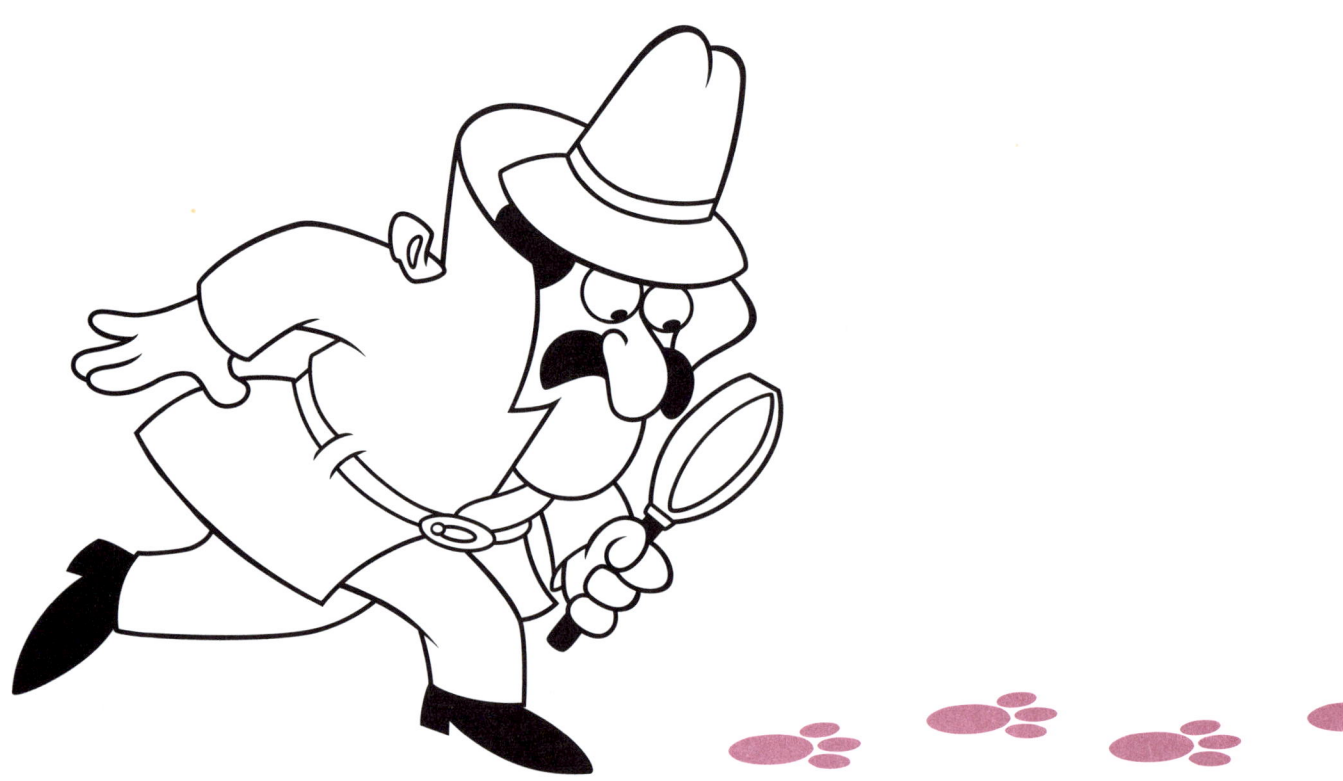

found in the blood. The allergic reaction in type 1 diabetes is against the cells in the pancreas (islet cells) that make insulin. The evidence in the blood is called an antibody or, more specifically, an **"islet cell antibody" (ICA)**. We now know that some people can have this antibody present in their blood for many years before they need insulin.

- Four specific diabetes-related antibodies can now be measured in the blood of people who are developing diabetes, including: "GAD" antibodies, insulin autoantibodies [IAA], ICA 512, and ZnT8 [zinc-transport] antibodies.

- Identifying these antibodies in the blood has made it possible to screen people who are at risk to develop diabetes. This screening has led to research trials (see Chapter 32) that are trying to prevent diabetes. We believe it is important for brothers, sisters and other relatives to have this screening.

- People with two positive antibodies are sometimes now classified as having Stage 1 diabetes. The risk for developing diabetes in the next three years is then 47 percent. The similar risk is 12 percent if only one antibody is positive.

- The antibodies may gradually disappear from the blood after the onset of type 1 diabetes.

- People who develop type 2 diabetes (previously called adult-onset) and those with MODY diabetes do not have these antibodies.

3. Environmental Damage (virus, chemical or other cause?)

A third factor is also believed to be important. This environmental factor may either be a virus or something in the food we eat or something we do not yet know about. This factor may be the bridge between the genetic (inherited) susceptibility and the allergic reaction.

THE DISEASE PROCESS

An example of the possible sequence of events is outlined below.

✓ A person inherits the tendency for diabetes.

✓ This tendency might allow a virus or other particle to injure the islet cells.

✓ Part of the damaged islet cell may then be released into the blood.

✓ The body would then make islet cell antibodies (an allergic or autoimmune reaction).

✓ The damage can attract white blood cells (WBCs) to the area of the islet cells. These now-active WBCs produce chemicals, which further injure the other islet cells (Figure 1).

✓ Anything that activates the WBCs in the future (viral infections, certain foods, stress, etc.) may result in more of the islet cells being destroyed.

We now know that most people who get diabetes don't just suddenly develop it. They have been in the process of developing it for many years. Most likely viral infections or other factors result in further damage and destruction of more islet cells. As more and more islet cells are destroyed, the person moves closer to having diabetes (see Figure 2, where onset of diabetes is represented by the broken line). The symptoms of diabetes have been discussed in Chapter 2.

TREATMENT

The treatment of type 1 diabetes is discussed throughout this book, and always involves insulin therapy (Chapter 8). Frequent blood/CGM sugar checking (Chapter 7) is important. Following a food plan (Chapter 12) and daily exercise (Chapter 13) are also important.

Often a **"honeymoon"** time begins a few weeks or months after a person with type 1 diabetes starts insulin shots. The insulin dose may go down and it may seem like the person does not have diabetes, but **THEY DO!** This period may last from a few weeks to a few years (see Chapter 2).

Checking **blood sugars** (Chapter 7) at least four times per day, or use of a continuous glucose monitor (CGM: see Chapter 29), is essential for people with type 1 diabetes. The use of an insulin pump (Chapter 28) or a CGM or an artificial pancreas (Chapter 30) may help make diabetes management easier.

The **MOST IMPORTANT RULE** for the patient with type 1 diabetes to remember is: **I MUST TAKE MY INSULIN EVERY DAY FROM NOW ON. IF I FORGET MY INSULIN, MY SUGAR LEVELS WILL BECOME VERY HIGH.** Even if I get sick, I still need insulin. I may need more or less insulin, but I must have it every day.

IMPORTANT: The only known difference about people who develop type 1 diabetes is that their bodies don't make enough insulin. THE PERSON AND EVERY OTHER PART OF THE BODY ARE OTHERWISE COMPLETELY NORMAL.

DEFINITIONS

Allergy: A special reaction of the body to some material. This is similar to what happens if you are allergic to something that makes you sneeze.

Antibody: The material we measure in the blood if someone has an allergy (example: milk antibodies might be present if someone has a milk allergy).

Autoimmunity (self-allergy): The process of forming an allergic reaction against one's own tissues. This happens in diseases such as lupus and arthritis. People with type 1 diabetes make an antibody against their islet cells (where the insulin is made).

Genetic (inherited): Features that are passed from both parents to children.

HLA type: The way to group cell types just as red blood cells are grouped into A, B, AB and O blood types. HLA stands for Human Leukocyte Antigen. A leukocyte is another name for a white blood cell. The white blood cell is the type of cell used in HLA typing.

Identical twins: Twins that come from the same egg. All their features (genetics) are exactly alike.

Islet cell (pronounced eye-let): The groups of cells within the pancreas that make insulin.

Islet cell antibody: The material measured in the person's blood to show they have had an allergy against the cells in the pancreas (the islet cells) that make insulin.

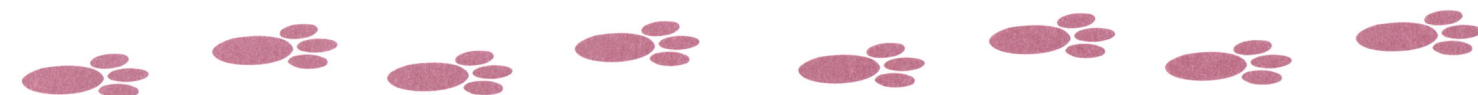

Questions and Answers from NewsNotes

Q: My daughter was in a car accident the week before the onset of her diabetes. Could that have caused the diabetes?

A: It is now accepted that diabetes comes on gradually over many months or many years. It is not just brought about by one event. After initial damage occurs to the islets in the pancreas (where insulin is made), islet cell antibodies may be positive, indicating some damage has occurred. We have followed many people with positive islet cell antibodies. Some have not needed to start insulin treatment for as long as ten years.

After the initial damage, many factors may cause activation of white blood cells (WBCs) in the islets. These factors may include some viral infections, content of the diet or even stress. When the WBCs in the islets are activated by these factors, they produce toxic chemicals that destroy a few more islets each time. Gradually, a person gets closer to having full-blown diabetes. Thus, the stress of the automobile accident may have been the final precipitating event, but it was most likely only one of several insults over many years.

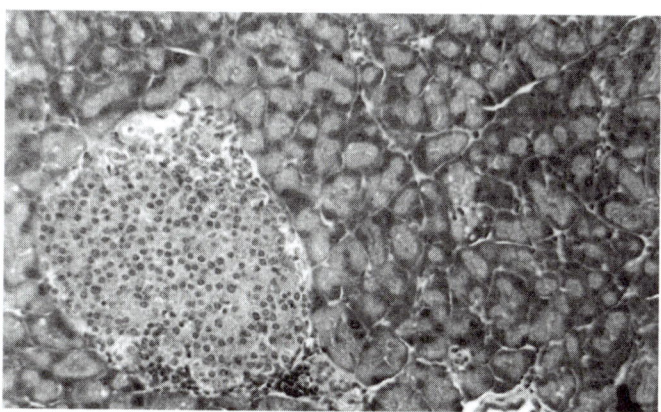 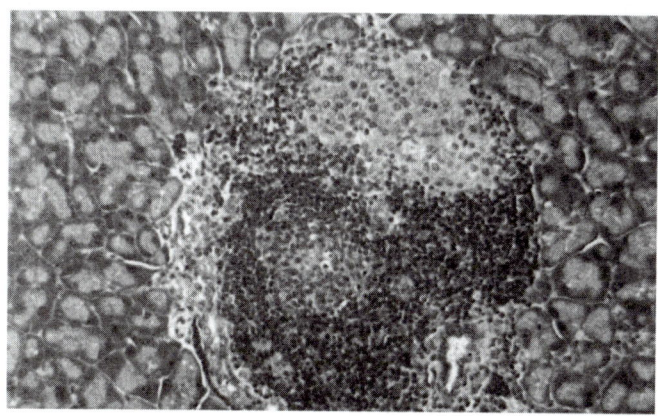

FIGURE 1

Microscopic Photograph of Pancreatic Islet
The photo on the left shows a normal islet (center) surrounded by other pancreatic tissue. This other tissue is responsible for making digestive enzymes. The photo on the right is from a diabetic animal. The white blood cells (WBCs) have invaded and destroyed most of the islet.

FIGURE 2
The Gradual Onset of Type 1 Diabetes

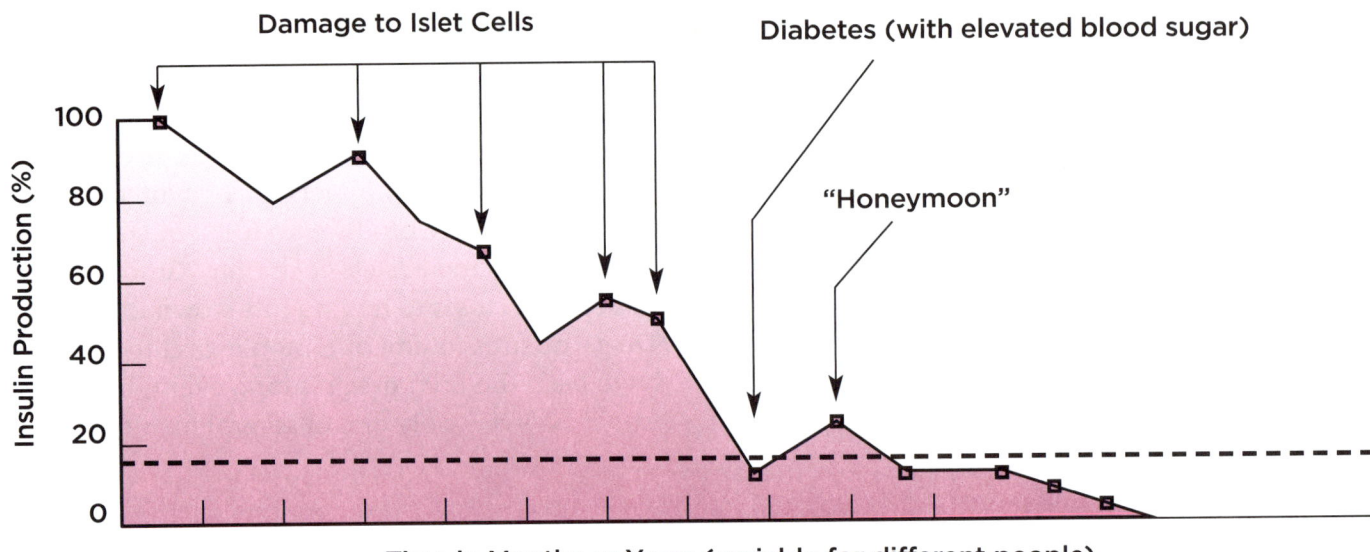

It is now believed that diabetes develops gradually, over many months or many years. It does not just come on suddenly in the week or two before the elevated blood sugars. Many insults (represented by the arrows in this Figure) likely result in further damage until the diagnosis of diabetes is made. The insults may include viral infections, stress, parts of the diet, or other agents. These agents may work by "activating" white blood cells in the islets to make toxic chemicals that cause injury to the insulin-producing cells (beta cells). However, a "genetic predisposition" (inherited factors) must be present for the process to start.

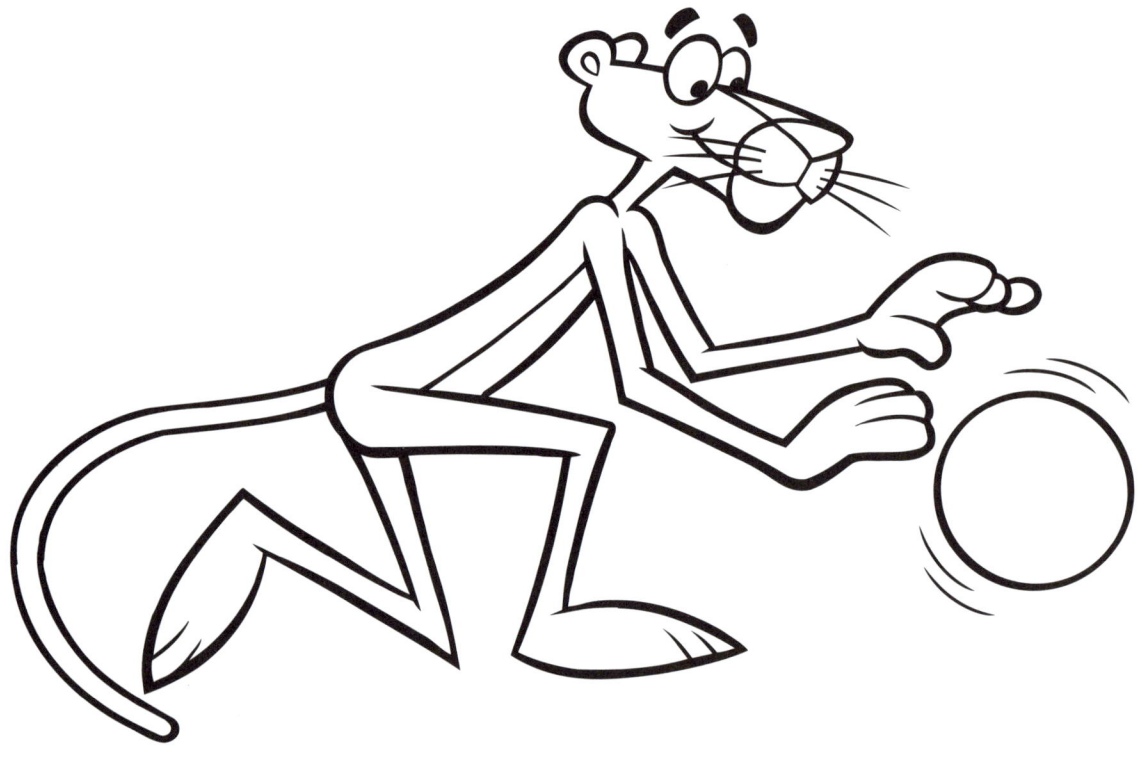

CHAPTER 4

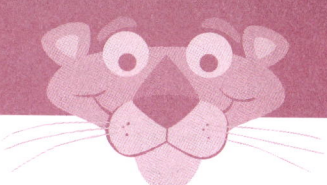

Type 2 Diabetes

INTRODUCTION

Type 2 diabetes (previously referred to as adult onset diabetes or non-insulin dependent diabetes) is the most common type of diabetes in adults over the age of 40. While it used to be uncommon in children and adolescents, type 2 is now appearing more often in overweight teenagers. It is rare in children before puberty or under 10 years of age, but in teenagers represents about 15 percent of all cases of diabetes in those who are white, 46 percent in Latinos, 58 percent in African-Americans, 70 percent in Asian-Pacific Islanders, and 86 percent in Native-Americans. Overall, it accounts for about 6 percent of all cases of diabetes in all youth under age 18 years.

Type 2 diabetes is often referred to as a **"disease of lifestyles."** For thousands of years in the past, people by necessity were very active. However, we now live in a world of automobile travel, television, cell phones, computers and video games. Physical activity is much less than in the past. In addition, high-calorie convenience foods, fast foods, and sugar-containing drinks have become a major part of our meals and snacks. The net result of these changes in diet and activity levels has been an increase in the incidence of being overweight and of type 2 diabetes in the U.S. and worldwide. Reducing the likelihood of type 2 diabetes in people at high risk is very important and is discussed in this chapter and in Chapters 12, 13 and 32. Education is a cornerstone both to the prevention and the self-management of type 2 diabetes.

TOPICS:
Type 2 Diabetes Disease Process
Medications (type 2 diabetes)
Nutritional Management
(also see Chapters 11 and 12)
Physical Activity
(also see Chapter 13)
Monitoring (checking blood sugars and ketones; also see Chapters 5 and 7)
Preventing, Detecting and Treating Acute and Chronic Complications
(also see Chapters 5, 15, and 23)

TEACHING OBJECTIVES:
The teacher will:
1. Present the basic concepts of type 2 diabetes and management.
2. Introduce the medications to be used, including dosing and side effects.
3. Assess current dietary habits and develop an individual nutritional management program.
4. Assess current activity level and develop an individualized exercise program.
5. Discuss monitoring blood sugars, ketones and laboratory tests.
6. Introduce acute and chronic complications.

LEARNING OBJECTIVES:
Learner (parents, child, relative or self) will be able to:
1. State the differences between type 1 and type 2 diabetes.
2. Identify the name, dose, schedule and side effects of medication(s) to be used.
3. Describe the planned nutritional management program.
4. Describe the planned exercise program.
5. Identify time frames for monitoring blood sugars, ketones and laboratory tests.
6. List one possible acute and two possible chronic complications.
7. State the goals for glycemic targets, exercise and management.

DIFFERENCES BETWEEN TYPE 2 AND TYPE 1 DIABETES

- In type 2 diabetes, the primary disorder is a problem with reduced action of insulin. This is called "insulin resistance" and is usually related to being overweight and inactive. Insulin resistance means that insulin cannot act normally to keep blood sugars in the desired range. If changes in lifestyle are not made, type 2 diabetes will be a progressive disease that may eventually require insulin injections.

- In response to insulin resistance, increased amounts of insulin are made initially. This is the opposite of type 1 diabetes, where the insulin levels are low or absent. Over time, individuals with type 2 diabetes produce decreasing amounts of insulin. This happens as the pancreas fails to keep up with the body's higher demands for insulin.

- In some cases, the increased insulin that the body makes to try to overcome the resistance causes darkening of the skin (called acanthosis nigricans). The most common areas for this darkening are the fingers, neck, armpits and elbows. By losing weight (eating fewer calories and exercising more), the sensitivity to insulin may return again, and the dark skin coloring may lessen or disappear.

- Laboratory measurements sometimes help in deciding whether someone has type 1 or type 2 diabetes. **ISLET CELL ANTIBODIES** (ICA: see Chapter 3) **ARE NOT PRESENT IN TYPE 2 DIABETES.** In type 1 diabetes, ICA antibodies are usually present. Measurements of C-peptide, a marker of how much insulin the body produces, may be normal or elevated in type 2 diabetes, but are generally low in type 1. However, sometimes the individual with diabetes must be monitored for a period to distinguish between the two types.

CAUSES

✓ **Inheritance (genetics)**

Type 2 diabetes has a stronger risk for inheritance than type 1 diabetes. In almost all cases, a parent and/or grandparent will also have the disease. In the case of identical twins, if one twin develops type 2 diabetes, the other twin has an 80 percent chance of also developing the disease. In type 1 diabetes, an identical twin has a 35-50 percent chance of developing the disease.

In type 2 diabetes, there are many different potentially-inherited (genetic) defects, which vary between families. There is not just one common defect in all families.

Children who are born to mothers with type 2 diabetes, or to mothers with gestational diabetes, have an increased risk of developing type 2 diabetes. Children born with a low birth weight for length ("small for dates") are also at an increased risk for developing type 2 diabetes, particularly if they have rapid weight gain during childhood.

✓ **Lifestyle**

Lifestyle Changes are IMPORTANT!

Most (but not all) people with type 2 diabetes are overweight or obese and do not lead active lives. Being overweight (BMI >85th percentile for age) or obese (BMI >95th percentile for age) are risk factors for developing type 2 diabetes. If the height and weight are known, the BMI can be easily determined using the graph in Chapter 12 (page 137). According to a study of a sample of U.S. children and teens, the obesity prevalence increased from 14.5 percent in 2000 to 17.3 percent (one in six) in 2012. Factors that can play a role in obesity include genetics, certain medications, eating on the run, recreational eating, eating foods higher in fat, increased portion size, increased TV and video time, and decreased physical activity. Dietary changes and increased exercise (see below) are essential in both the prevention and the treatment of type 2 diabetes.

DIAGNOSIS

Adults with type 2 diabetes can go several years with high blood sugar levels without other signs of diabetes. Then, with an illness or stress and decreasing function of the pancreas over time, symptoms begin, often gradually. In young people, this long period of time with high blood sugars before the appearance of symptoms may not occur. Instead, type 2 diabetes in young people is usually diagnosed around the time of mid to late puberty. This is because insulin resistance normally increases at this time. Type 2 diabetes before puberty is rare.

How it can be discovered

- Sometimes an elevated blood sugar is found during a routine check-up (Table 1). There may not be any other signs or symptoms.

- The increased urination and drinking of fluids may be absent or mild with type 2 diabetes

- Weight loss can occur (though variable)

- Increasing fatigue may be present

- During an illness, blood sugar levels (and/or ketones) may become very high. The illness may be a deep skin infection (abscess) or yeast infection.

- Trouble with vision (blurry/frequent change of glasses) may occur due to swelling of the lens of the eye from high blood sugars

Laboratory testing for diabetes can confirm the diagnosis.

✔ If the hemoglobin A1c (HbA1c) level is elevated (two values >6.5%, [>48 mmol/mol] Chapter 14), it is considered diagnostic.

✔ The 2-hour oral glucose tolerance test (OGTT) is a test done after fasting (no food for 10 hours). After a fasting blood sugar is drawn, the person then drinks all of a high sugar drink (e.g., Glucola) within five minutes. A second blood sample is drawn after two hours. See Table 1 for normal, borderline and diabetic blood sugar values.

✔ If a random blood sugar value is high (e.g., >200 mg/dL or 11.1 mmol/L) and there are symptoms, the glucose tolerance test (Table 1) may not be needed.

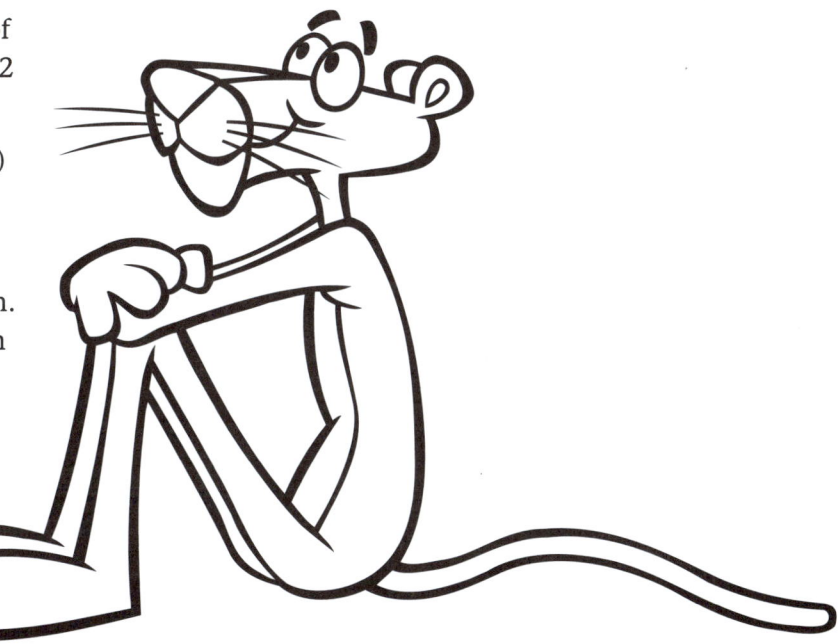

TABLE 1:
Oral Glucose Tolerance Test (OGTT) Blood Sugar Values (mg/dL and mmol/L)

	NORMAL		BORDERLINE		DIABETIC	
	mg/dL	mmol/L	mg/dL	mmol/L	mg/dL	mmol/L
FASTING	<100	<5.5	100-126	5.5-7.0	>126	>7.0
TWO HOURS AFTER DRINKING THE GLUCOLA	<140	<7.8	140-200	7.8-11.1	>200	>11.1

TREATMENT

The challenges of treating youth with type 2 diabetes have been described in the TODAY study (an acronym for The Treatment Options for Type 2 Diabetes in Adolescents and Youth [see reference 1 at end of this chapter]).

As in type 1 diabetes, the family must learn as much as they can, as diabetes is a family disease. In children with type 2 diabetes, there is typically a family member with this disease. However, the family member may have never received complete education regarding diabetes when diagnosed.

The family may initially need to learn how to give insulin shots (see Chapters 8 and 9) if:

✔ ketones are present (Chapter 5)
✔ symptoms of increased urination, thirst or severe weight loss are present
✔ there is uncertainty about the diabetes type
✔ if the HbA1c is >10% (>86 mmol/mol)

A) Nutrition

Medical nutrition therapy is now individualized for each person and family. Dietary changes are **very important** in type 2 diabetes, since weight loss and changes in the nutrients of the diet can reduce the insulin resistance. It is important to understand each family's attitude toward food, eating habits, and activities associated with eating (e.g., eating when stressed, snacking, rewarding behavior with food). For example, binge-eating is common in children/teens with type 2 diabetes. The individual in the family who does the grocery shopping and meal planning will be a key factor in dietary change. It will be important for this individual to know how to read food labels and to purchase and prepare healthy foods/meals.

Lowering calorie, fat, and carbohydrate intake through reduction of **portion sizes** and learning how to make **healthier food choices** are essential to losing weight and improving blood sugar levels (see Chapter 11). Usually, the most effective approach at the beginning is to keep dietary changes simple and achievable. Some simple, but important, changes include the elimination of sugary beverages and snacks, reducing portion sizes, and limiting the consumption of already prepared foods, fast food and restaurant food. Recent data suggests a low carbohydrate food plan (no grains, potatoes, foods with added sugar) may help some people. This is similar to the ketogenic diet (Chapter 12),

The plate method is a useful method for families to follow for meal planning (see Chapter 11). In this method, the plate is divided into 4 sections. One-fourth of the plate is devoted to grains, another fourth is devoted to protein (meat, fish, chicken, etc.), another quarter of the plate is devoted to vegetables (carrots, broccoli, green beans, etc.) and the final fourth represents fruits. A serving of milk and any free foods (e.g., lettuce) are on the side (see Figure in Chapter 11). For some families, carbohydrate counting may be useful, but takes practice.

The overweight individual may have trouble knowing what hunger feels like and/or what it feels like to be full. Reviewing these feelings can help with better food regulation. Behavioral habits such as putting the fork down between bites, chewing food slowly, using smaller plates/bowls, waiting 20 minutes before having seconds, and drinking a glass of water before eating can be simple and helpful tools in weight regulation. Food management is discussed in more detail in Chapters 11 and 12. Most important, the family **must** work with a knowledgeable dietitian. The dietitian will help to individualize the meal plan to fit personal preferences.

B) Exercise

Exercise is **equally important** for managing type 2 diabetes (Chapter 13). Some children with type 2 diabetes are not active and often do not enjoy being active. It is important to identify some activities that the child/adolescent might enjoy and to make physical activity fun, such as going on a family bike ride or playing basketball as a family. Then work on small achievable weekly exercise goals, such as "I will walk with my dog for 10 minutes, three days this week." The person will need to feel successful in order to stay active. Increase the physical activity and set new goals weekly. It is also helpful to establish rules to promote activity, such as restricting video games until after completion of the activity for the day. In order to motivate the child/adolescent to become more active, give them a choice between doing a household chore such as vacuuming, or going outside and riding a bike for 20 minutes. While most physical activity experts suggest **60 minutes of activity per day**, starting out slowly is more realistic and will reduce muscle soreness that will hinder daily exercise. In addition, it is important to reduce sedentary activity such as television, computer use and video game time. Finally, increasing general activity levels by walking (pacing) while talking on a phone or playing video games, taking the stairs instead of elevators and parking farther from the store can make surprising differences in weight and blood sugar levels.

It is important that the **entire family** make the same lifestyle changes. If family members are active along with the child/adolescent with diabetes, success will be more likely. Similarly, if foods with little nutritional value (e.g., sugary beverages, chips) are brought into the home by other family members, it will be more difficult for the person with diabetes to make healthy choices. It is important to praise all individuals in the family who have made healthy changes.

C) Blood Sugar (Glucose) Testing

Methods for blood sugar testing are covered in detail in Chapter 7. The blood sugar target range in an individual with type 2 diabetes is 70-140 mg/dL (3.9-7.8 mmol/L). In general, doing blood sugars for a person with type 2 diabetes who is on insulin is no different from a person with type 1 diabetes. Insulin may be started initially to lower the HbA1c (Chapter 14). If there is success in weight loss and returning the HbA1c level to normal, monitoring blood sugars is still important, but may be done less frequently. In people who are not taking insulin, the frequency of measuring blood sugars is often decreased to two times per day, approximately 3 days a week. This should be individualized and discussed with

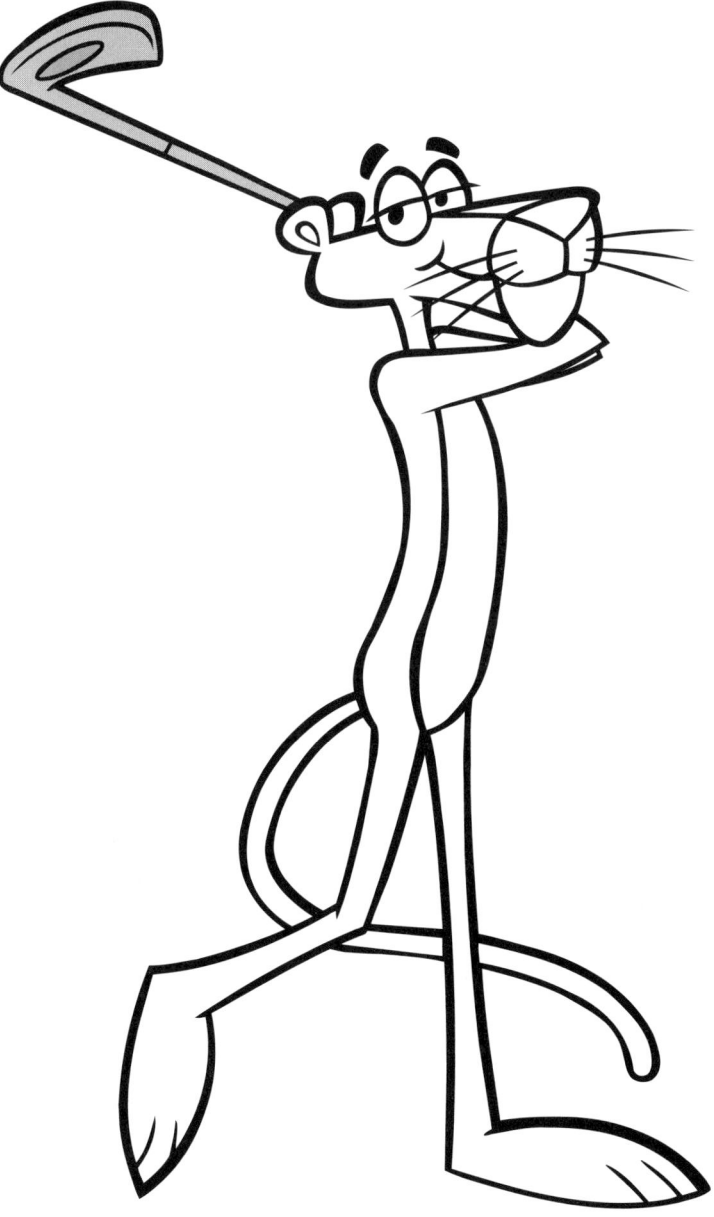

the diabetes care-provider. The aim would be to maintain the morning fasting or before meals sugar between 80 and 130 mg/dL (4.5-7.2 mmol/L). The values after any meal should be below 180 mg/dL (<10.0 mmol/L). However, it is essential to measure values more frequently during illness.

D. HbA1c (A1c)

The hemoglobin A1c (HbA1c) is discussed in Chapter 14. It reflects how high glucose levels have been in the past three months. The frequency of measurement will vary with the stage of treatment, but would ideally be every three months. A reasonable goal for most children and adolescents with type 2 diabetes would be <7% (<53 mmol/mol). More stringent A1c goals (such as <6.5% [<48 mmol/mol]) may be appropriate for selected individuals. Lower HbA1c values help to avoid chronic complications of diabetes (Chapter 23).

E. Support

Each person and family has different lifestyles and characteristics. The diabetes team should include a social worker or psychologist in addition to the nurse-educator, dietitian and physician. Ongoing evaluation of mental health, particularly related to depression, and disordered eating is important. Preconception counseling should be available for all girls starting at puberty (see Chapter 31).

F. Medications

Insulin (Chapters 8 and 9)

Some people with type 2 diabetes will always need to take insulin shots. Others will be able to take oral medications for several years. Eventually, those taking oral medications may need to take insulin shots. People with type 2 diabetes who have ketones or an HbA1c >10% (>86 mmol/mol) when their diabetes is diagnosed may need to be treated with insulin shots at the beginning. A once-a-day shot of Levemir/Lantus (Basaglar)/Tresiba insulin along with oral medicines is often very effective in improving blood sugars, even when they are very high. The basal U-100 insulin, Lantus, is also available as a more concentrated U-300 insulin (Toujeo) for youth, ages six years or older. Some people also need insulin with meals. People who are able to lose weight and become more active may be able to come off insulin shots and just take their oral medicine. However, they often need to return to insulin shots in later years due to the progressive nature of type 2 diabetes. The TODAY study found that after three years of type 2 diabetes, half of teenagers in the study needed insulin in order to control their blood sugar levels. An HbA1c level consistently above 6.5% (>48 mmol/mol) generally indicates a need to be on insulin therapy. It is important to remember that during times of illness, especially if ketones return, insulin shots may need to be given.

Other Medications

Oral tablets are NOT insulin. If taken orally, insulin would be destroyed by the stomach acid. Some of the tablets used for diabetes are medicines that make the person more sensitive to their own insulin. Some of the medicines also make the pancreas release extra amounts of insulin (Table 2 also lists some of these medications). Some new medicines work in entirely different ways. It should be noted that other than insulin, metformin, and Victoza (see section 4 below), none of the dozens of FDA-approved medications for adults with type 2 diabetes are approved for youth <18 years old.

1. **Metformin (Glucophage)** is the medication that is the most common first oral medicine for children/teens and adults with type 2 diabetes and the only oral medication that is FDA-approved for use in children. Metformin is usually very effective in bringing down the HbA1c in young people with type 2 diabetes. In addition to helping to control blood sugar levels, it may help with weight loss.

   - Main side effect: upset stomach, diarrhea, nausea, and bloating. These side effects can be reduced by always taking the medicine with food and increasing the dose slowly.

- Lactic acidosis is a very rare side effect that can occur if metformin is not stopped when a person has the stomach flu or severe illness. It can also happen during an x-ray procedure using dyes and during episodes of vomiting, diarrhea, pneumonia or with lung diseases.

♦ **Dosing**

- Start low with 500 mg (0.5 g) once a day with breakfast or dinner. Take metformin with some food, usually at breakfast or dinner.

- After one week, try this dose twice a day (with breakfast and dinner).

- After the third week, try one tablet (500 mg) in the morning with breakfast and two tablets (1000 mg) with dinner.

- The fourth week, if stomach upset is not a problem, try two tablets (1000 mg) with breakfast and with dinner.

- There is also a long-acting form of this medication. This can be taken at breakfast or dinner with the dosage gradually increased. Some people find that this has fewer stomach side effects. <u>Metformin needs to be stopped during times of severe illness or with vomiting or diarrhea</u>. If this continues for more than a day or two, it may be necessary to use insulin shots until the illness is over. This is why it is so important to be checking blood sugars during illness and contacting your healthcare-provider if the blood sugars are running high.

NOTE: We suggest not reading about the other oral medicines below unless there is a specific reason to do so.

2. **SGLT2 Inhibitors: Invokana® (canagliflozin), Farxiga™ (dapagliflozin), Jardiance® (empagliflozin), Zynquista (sotagliflozin) and others.**

These medications are scientifically referred to as "sodium-glucose-linked cotransporter 2" (SGLT2) inhibitors. They prevent sugar from being reabsorbed in the kidney, and it instead goes out in the urine. The HbA1c values may be lower and weight loss may occur. There is evidence in adults with type 2 diabetes that medications in this group reduce major adverse cardiac events (MACE), prevent or improve diabetic kidney disease, and also reduce all-cause mortality. Side effects are primarily genital yeast infections, urinary tract infections and episodes of diabetic ketoacidosis (Chapter 15). The Invokana is also available combined with metformin in a medicine called Invokamet™. None of these medications have been approved for use in individuals under age 18.

3. **Sulfonylureas**

The **sulfonylureas** (Table 2) have been around the longest and are commonly used in adults with type 2 diabetes. They act to make the person's own pancreas secrete more insulin and can lower the HbA1c, though not as well as metformin. Low blood sugar (Chapter 6) is a possible side effect, particularly in young patients. These medications are not commonly used in young people with type 2 diabetes because they can cause low blood sugars and weight gain. None have been approved by the FDA for use in children.

4. **Medications to Increase Levels of Glucagon-like peptide (GLP-1)**

GLP-1 is another hormone that is made in response to food. It works closely with insulin to regulate blood sugar. In recent years, the importance of GLP-1 in keeping the blood sugar normal has been recognized, and a number of new medications are related to this important hormone. Only Victoza has been approved by the FDA for use in children (ages 10 years and older). These medications have their effect by increasing insulin production, reducing the production of glucagon, a hormone that raises blood sugar, delaying stomach emptying and decreasing appetite.

There are two groups of GLP-1 medications:

i) **Medications that directly increase the amount of GLP-1, called GLP-1 receptor agonists (GLP-1 RA).** They include Victoza® (liraglutide), Byetta® (exenatide), Bydureon (exenatide once weekly), Lyxuma® (lixisenatide), and Trulicity (dulaglutide). These are proteins that react against the GLP-receptor to result in higher GLP-1 levels. All of these medications are taken by injection. Byetta is taken 60 minutes before breakfast and dinner. Victoza is taken once a day and Bydureon once a week. These medications cannot be taken in the same syringe as insulin. The most common side effects are nausea, diarrhea, vomiting, decreased appetite, and constipation. In addition to improving glucose control, they have been shown to reduce cardiovascular risk and mortality in adults with type 2 diabetes.

ii) **Medications that prevent the breakdown of GLP-1 so more remains in the body.** The second group are called DPP-4 inhibitors because they inhibit the enzyme that breaks down the body's own GLP-1. They include Januvia® (sitagliptian), Onglyza® (saxagliptin), Trajenta® (linaglitin), Galvus® (vidagliptin), and Nesina® (alogliptin) and other medications. None of these are currently approved by the FDA for use in children. These are oral medications taken once a day and have many of the same effects as the GLP-1 RAs in the first group, but do not cause weight loss and do not reduce cardiovascular risk. Some cases of pancreatitis have been reported with DPP-4 inhibitors.

MONITORING FOR COMPLICATIONS

Acute:

1. **Hypoglycemia:** Low blood sugars are less frequent with type 2 diabetes than with type 1 diabetes. However, they can occur. They are most frequently associated with use of insulin or sulfonylurea (Table 2). Treatment of low blood sugars is explained in Chapter 6.

2. **Acidosis/DKA:** Ketone production (Chapters 5 & 15) is less frequent with type 2 than with type 1 diabetes. However, diabetic ketoacidosis (DKA) can be present in some children at diagnosis, and ketones can occur during times of illness. Thus, it is wise to do a urine ketone check (Chapter 5) with any illness. A person who is receiving oral medications will usually need to use insulin shots when ketones are present. Youth who receive Victoza (or any GLP-1 medication) are at greater risk for DKA.

3. **Hyperglycemic hyperosmolar state** is a situation in which the blood sugars rise to dangerously high levels, leading to severe dehydration and changes in mental function. It can be caused by infections, medications, inconsistent use of diabetes therapies, substance abuse, undiagnosed diabetes, and other illnesses. This is a life-threatening emergency that is rare in children, but requires immediate treatment if it occurs.

Chronic (see also Chapter 23):

1. **High blood pressure (Hypertension):** High blood pressure is a common finding in children/adolescents with type 2 diabetes. In the TODAY study, more than one third of youth with type 2 diabetes had hypertension 4.5 years after diagnosis. Blood pressure should be assessed using the correct cuff size and using blood pressure standards that are based on gender, age, and height. The person should sit for five minutes prior to the measurement. The arm should be at the level

of the heart. A value of 130/80 or below the 90th percentile for age should be aimed for to help prevent long-term complications (Chapter 23). When hypertension is diagnosed in children, a type of blood pressure medicine called an ACE-inhibitor (Chapters 23 and 32) is commonly used. It may also have a positive effect on preventing diabetic kidney disease. Blood pressure should be monitored at each clinic visit.

2. **Abnormal blood lipids:**
Children/adolescents with type 2 diabetes may have decreased HDL (good cholesterol) and increased LDL (bad cholesterol) and triglycerides (blood fat). Recommended levels are provided in Chapter 11. Lifestyle changes with improved glycemic control will improve the lipids. Medications are used when lifestyle changes are not sufficient. Yearly screening is recommended.

3. **Obstructive sleep apnea:** This is most often found with overweight individuals. Symptoms include snoring with long breathing pauses when sleeping, frequent arousal during sleep, restless sleep, morning headaches, and daytime sleepiness. A sleep study should be performed if this condition is suspected.

4. **Polycystic ovarian syndrome (PCOS):** This condition is often associated with menstrual irregularity, increased hair on the face, and acne. Metformin may be effective in reversing these symptoms, although sometimes an oral contraceptive is added for a better effect. Metformin may improve irregular menses as well as fertility. The need for oral contraceptive pills to regulate menses is important to consider.

5. **Microalbuminuria:** This refers to increased protein in the urine, which can sometimes even be detected at diagnosis (see Chapter 23). This is an indication of early kidney damage from diabetes. The ratio of urine albumin to creatinine on a first morning void can also be used to screen for kidney damage. After 4.5 years of type 2 diabetes,

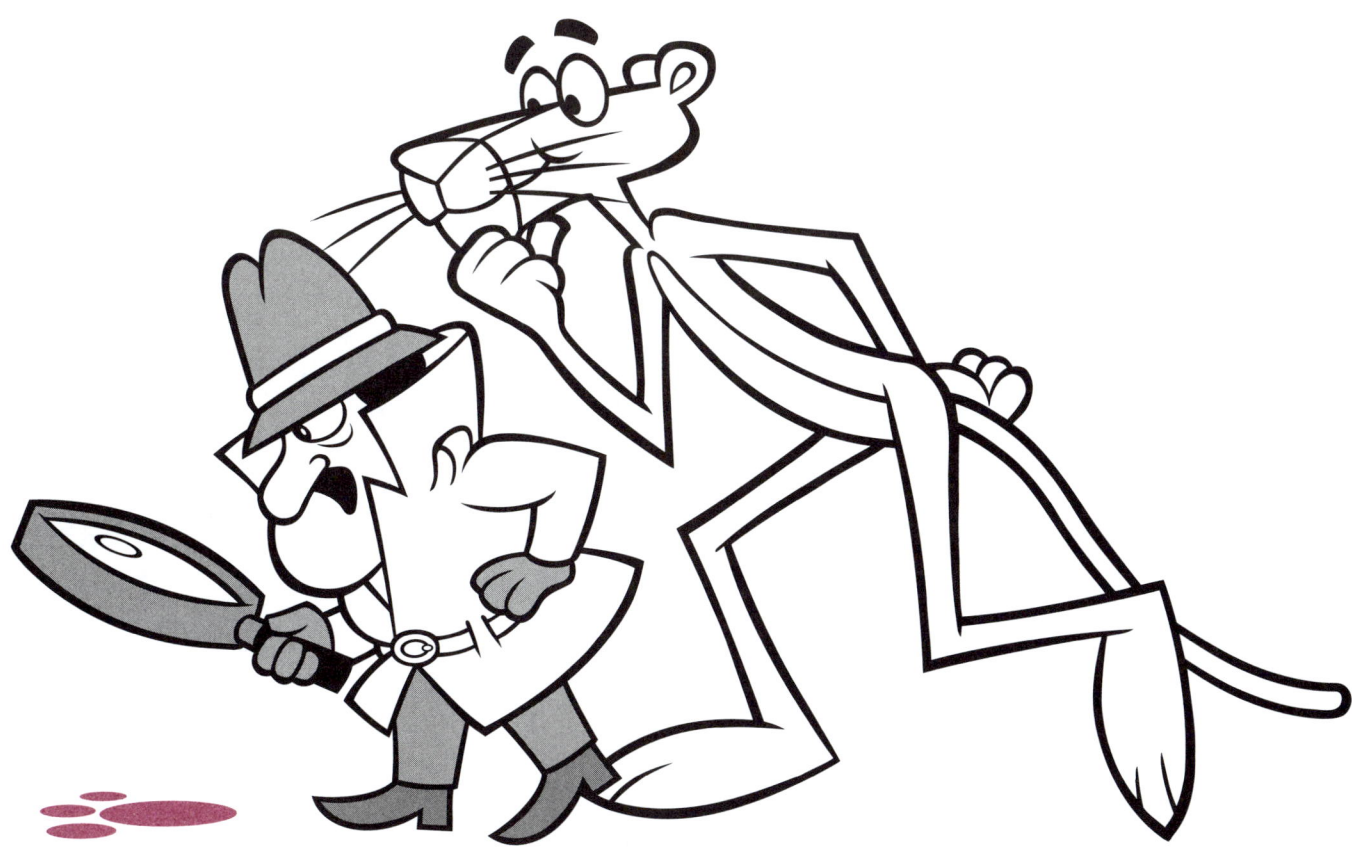

16.6 percent of the youth in the TODAY study had microalbuminuria. When found, ACE-inhibitors (see Hypertension above) are used because they may prevent worsening of kidney problems. Screening for microalbuminuria is recommended at onset and then yearly.

6. **Non-alcoholic fatty liver disease:** This consists of fatty deposits in the liver. It is diagnosed through laboratory testing, ultrasound, or CT scan. In this disease, the progression of chronic inflammation can lead to cirrhosis and liver failure. Weight loss, optimal glucose control and reduction in carbohydrates can help this condition in most individuals.

7. **Retinopathy:** A dilated eye exam is recommended at onset and yearly to identify early diabetic eye disease (see Chapter 23). In the TODAY study, 13.7 percent of youth with type 2 diabetes had retinopathy 4.5 years post-diagnosis.

8. **Social and psychological issues:** Overweight children are at risk for being teased about their weight by both their peers and family members. When children are teased about their weight, it can lead to unhealthy eating habits and binge eating behaviors. Overweight children/teens are also at risk for depression and low self-esteem.

Three references for those wanting more information specifically on type 2 diabetes in youth are:

1. Zeitler P, Hirst K, Pyle L, et. al. A clinical trial to maintain glycemic control in youth with type 2 diabetes. N Engl J Med. 366, 2247, 2012
2. American Diabetes Association. Diabetes Care 28 (Suppl 1) S4-S36, 2005
3. ISPAD Clinical Practice Consensus Guidelines 2014 Compendium. Type 2 Diabetes in the Child and Adolescent. Pediatr Diabetes. 15 Suppl 20:26-46.

DEFINITIONS

C-peptide: An insulin-related protein. It is split off from proinsulin when the active insulin is formed. It is easier to measure than insulin in the laboratory and is often used as a measure of insulin production.

FDA: Food and Drug Administration. The agency responsible for approving the use of new medicines in the U.S., and thus for our safety.

Glucagon-like peptide (GLP-1): An important hormone made by the body in response to food intake. It helps regulate blood sugar levels.

Lifestyle changes: In this chapter, exchanging sedentary (little exercise) habits for daily exercise, and decreasing high calorie and high fat food intake (particularly fast foods).

Oral glucose tolerance test (OGTT): Blood sugar levels are checked before and after drinking a highly sugared drink. It may be used to diagnose diabetes when the diagnosis is uncertain. Normal values are in Table 1 in this chapter.

Oral hypoglycemic agents: These are pills that help to make the body more sensitive to insulin or cause it to release more insulin. However, they are NOT insulin. Table 2 gives the names of a few of these agents. Many more are being developed that work in new ways.

Type 2 diabetes: The condition in which the body still makes insulin but is unable to use it effectively to metabolize sugar. This is the most common type of diabetes in adults over age 40. It is also becoming increasingly more common in overweight teenagers.

TABLE 2:
Examples of Type 2 Diabetes Medications

NAME	HOW TO TAKE	ACTION	MAIN SIDE EFFECTS
Biguinide			
metformin (Glucophage®, Glucophage XR® or metformin XR®)	Oral, 2-3 doses daily XR (long acting) once daily	Reduces liver secretion of glucose May help reduce weight	Stomach upset, diarrhea, nausea, bloating; acidosis with illness (rare)
Sulfonylureas			
Glyburide (DiaBeta, Micronase, Glynase)	Oral, 1-2 doses daily	Increases insulin production from the pancreas	Low blood sugar, weight gain, bloating, nausea, heartburn, anemia
glypizide (Glocotrol, Glucatrol XL)	Oral, 1-2 doses daily XL (long acting) 1-2 doses daily		
glimepiride (Amaryl)	Oral, once daily		
vildagliptin (Galvus)	Oral, 1-2 daily		
aloglipten (Nesina)	Oral, once daily		
GLP-1 Analogs (also called GLP-1 receptor agonists) [GLP-1 RA]			
exenatide (Byetta)	Injection, 1-2 doses daily	Increases glucose-dependent insulin secretion Decreases glucagon levels after meals Delays stomach emptying Decreases appetite	Nausea, hypoglycemia, diarrhea, dizziness, headache
exenatide extended release (Bydureon)	Injection, once weekly		
liraglutide (Victoza) lixisenatide (Lyxuma)	Injection, once daily		Headache, nausea, diarrhea, and anti-liraglutide antibody formation
DPP-4 Inhibitors			
sitagliptin (Januvia)	Oral, once daily	Prevents GLP-1 breakdown Increases glucose-dependent insulin secretion Decreases glucagon after meals Delays stomach emptying	Stuffy or runny nose, sore throat, headache, diarrhea, stomach or back pain, nausea, hypersensitivity, pancreatitis
saxagliptin (Onglyza)	Oral, once daily		
linagliptin (Trajenta)	Oral, once daily		
vildagliptin (Galvus)	Oral, 1-2 daily		
aloglipten (Nesina)	Oral, once daily		
Agents blocking sugar reabsorption in the kidney (SGLT-2 inhibitors)			
Invokana (canagliflozin)	Oral, once daily	Blocks sugar reabsorption in the kidney (± intestine)	Genital yeast infections Urinary tract infections Ketoacidosis (Chapter 15)
Farxiga (dapagliflozin)			
Jardiance (empagliflozin)			
Zynquista (sotagliflozin)			

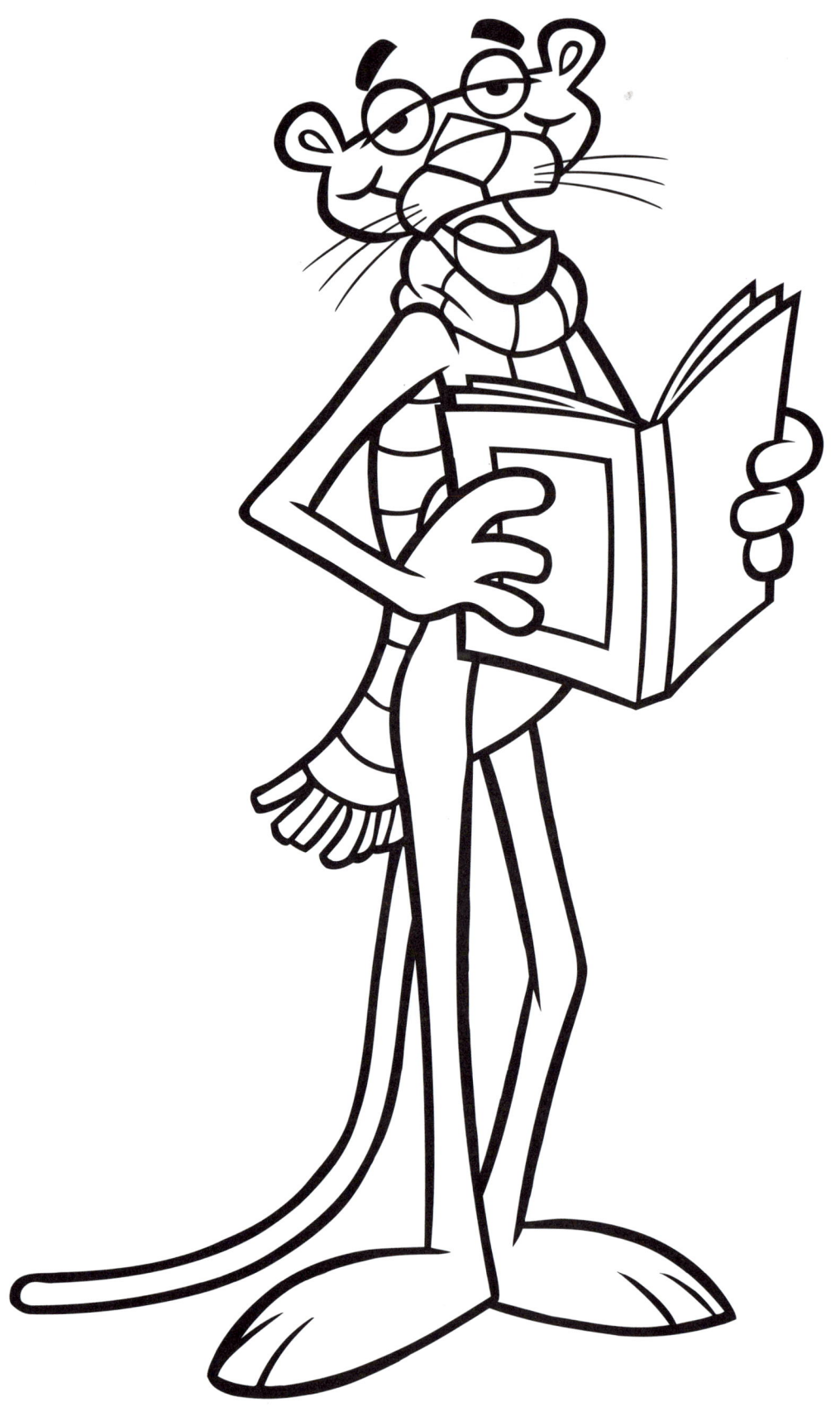

TYPE 2 DIABETES

Chapter 5

Checking Ketones

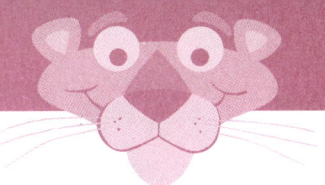

KETONES

Ketones are acidic molecules which appear in the urine and blood when body fat is used for energy. Ketones are a product of fat breakdown (see Chapter 15). It is best to treat ketones immediately.

Body fat is used for energy under the following circumstances:

- when there is not enough insulin to allow sugar to be burned for energy in the body (can build up to very large amounts).

- when not enough food has been eaten to provide energy (usually only trace or small amounts of ketones).

Ketone checking is **VERY** important. A method of testing for ketones must be kept in the home and taken on trips at all times.

We usually teach families how to do the urine ketone checks on the first day of diagnosis of diabetes. Frequent urine ketone tests are important following the diagnosis to determine if enough insulin is being given to turn off ketone production. **Turning off ketone production is one of the first goals in the treatment of newly diagnosed diabetes.** This often takes one or two days after starting insulin.

Another goal is to lower blood sugar levels (done primarily by giving insulin to turn off internal sugar production in the liver). This can take one or two weeks after starting insulin. Giving insulin helps to accomplish both goals.

> **TOPICS:**
> **Monitoring (ketones)**
> **Acute Complications (Prevention, Detection and Treatment)**
>
> **TEACHING OBJECTIVES:**
> The teacher will:
> 1. Discuss when ketone measurement should be done.
> 2. Introduce method to be used for measuring ketones.
> 3. Present the appropriate time to call the healthcare-provider.
>
> **LEARNING OBJECTIVES:**
> Learner (parents, child, relative or self) will be able to:
> 1. Define ketones and the importance of measuring ketones.
> 2. Identify and demonstrate when and how to measure for ketones.
> 3. State the appropriate time to call the healthcare-provider.

REASONS FOR MEASURING KETONES

It is important to check for urine or blood ketones because they can build up in the body. This can result in one of the two emergencies of diabetes, acidosis (also called diabetic ketoacidosis or DKA; see Chapter 15). In the past, it was only possible to test for urine ketones. The Precision Xtra™, the Nova Max Plus™ and the Keto-Mojo™ meters are available to do a home fingerstick test for blood ketones (see below). The diabetes care-provider should be notified when the urine ketone result shows moderate or large ketones or if the blood ketone test is above 1.0 mmol/L.

Usually, extra insulin is taken to help make the ketones go away. If the ketones are not detected and treated early, they will build up in the body and ketoacidosis (DKA) may result. This is particularly true during illnesses. Early detection of ketones and the treatment with rapid-acting insulin (Humalog/NovoLog/Apidra) can help avoid hospitalizations for DKA (see Chapter 15). Hospitalizations for ketoacidosis are still listed as the number one reason for hospitalizing children in the U.S. with known diabetes. **It is our belief that these hospitalizations are mostly avoidable. To accomplish this, the ketone checking must be done, the diabetes care-provider called when indicated, the fluid intake increased, and extra shots of insulin given.** As more youth use continuous glucose monitors (CGM), the alarms will alert people of the high glucose level and thus of a need to check ketones. Extra insulin can then be given to reduce the likelihood of DKA.

WHEN TO MEASURE KETONES

Ketones must always be checked if the blood/CGM glucose value is high (above 300 mg/dL [16.7 mmol/L]). They must also be checked ANY TIME THE PERSON FEELS SICK OR NAUSEATED (especially if he/she vomits, even once). If the person is sick, ketones can be present even when the glucose level is not high. Ketones should routinely be checked if a blocked insulin pump catheter is found.

A medicine called an SGLT-2 inhibitor causes sugar loss through the kidneys which may then result in low blood/CGM sugar levels in spite of elevated ketones.

Call your diabetes care-provider night or day if moderate or large urine ketones are present or for blood ketones ≥ 1.0 mmol/L. Tell the person answering the phone that the call is urgent.

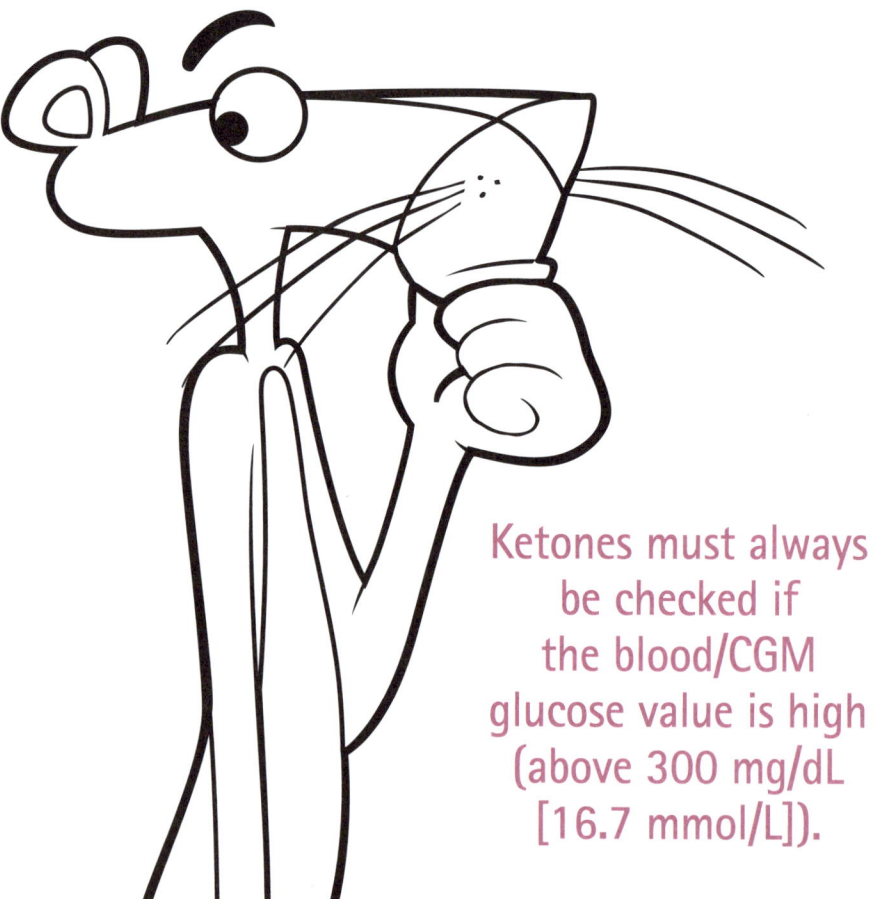

Ketones must always be checked if the blood/CGM glucose value is high (above 300 mg/dL [16.7 mmol/L]).

WHAT TEST MATERIALS ARE AVAILABLE?

Checking for Urine Ketones

The two strips that are most frequently used in checking for urine ketones are the Ketostix and the Chemstrip K®. If a child is not yet toilet trained, it is usually best to press a test strip (see section on Ketostix) firmly against the wet diaper. It is also possible to place cotton balls in the diaper where the diaper is most wet. Drops of urine can then be squeezed from the cotton ball.

Ketostix

Ketone strips are reliable for urine checking IF THEY ARE CAREFULLY TIMED WITH A SECOND HAND ON A CLOCK. The Ketostix are cheaper than the Ketodiastix (also measuring urine sugar) and it is not necessary to do the urine sugar, as a blood/CGM glucose level is more accurate. There is a place on the side of the bottle to write the date the bottle is opened. The strips can then last for six months.

The following procedure must be followed exactly:

1. Completely cover the colored square on the end of the strip by dipping into FRESH urine. Then immediately remove the strip from the urine. We suggest that the urine be collected in a cup and that the strip then be timed and read by two people. This helps to avoid errors due to color blindness or psychological factors. A supply of small paper cups might be kept in the bathroom medicine cabinet for this purpose.

2. Gently tap the edge of the strip against the side of the urine container to remove excess urine.

3. Compare the test area closely with the corresponding color chart. The timing is very important. READ KETONES AT **EXACTLY** 15 SECONDS AFTER DIPPING THE STRIP. HOLD THE STRIP CLOSE TO THE COLOR BLOCK AND MATCH THE COLORS CAREFULLY. These measurements must always be timed with the second hand of a clock. Counting is NOT accurate enough.

4. If the result is moderate (40), large (80) or extra large (160), extra insulin is needed every two hours and the person must drink extra fluids until the result is negative or small (see Chapter 15). If large or extra large, call the healthcare-provider and state the call is urgent.

Chemstrip K

The Chemstrip K (or Chemstrip uGK® with the urine glucose check) is the second method that can be used to check for urine ketones. The only difference from the instructions for the Ketostix is in the timing. Chemstrip K must be timed for one minute. Read as negative, small, moderate or large at exactly one minute.

Checking for Blood Ketones

The Precision Xtra (Abbott Labs), the Nova Max Plus (Nova Biomedical) and the Keto-Mojo meters are available for measuring blood ketones. The Precision Xtra test strips can be purchased in boxes of ten foil-wrapped beta ketone strips. Although the blood ketone strips are more expensive, they do not have to be replaced (like Ketostix) every six months. Thus, the cost is not all that different. When insurance will not cover the cost of the blood strips, some people screen with the urine strip and just do the blood test when the urine test is moderate or large. As discussed in Chapter 15, the blood ketone gives the ketone level at that minute. In contrast, the urine level may be hours behind (depending on how long urine has been in the bladder). An "approximate" comparison of results from urine versus blood ketone measurements is given in Table 1.

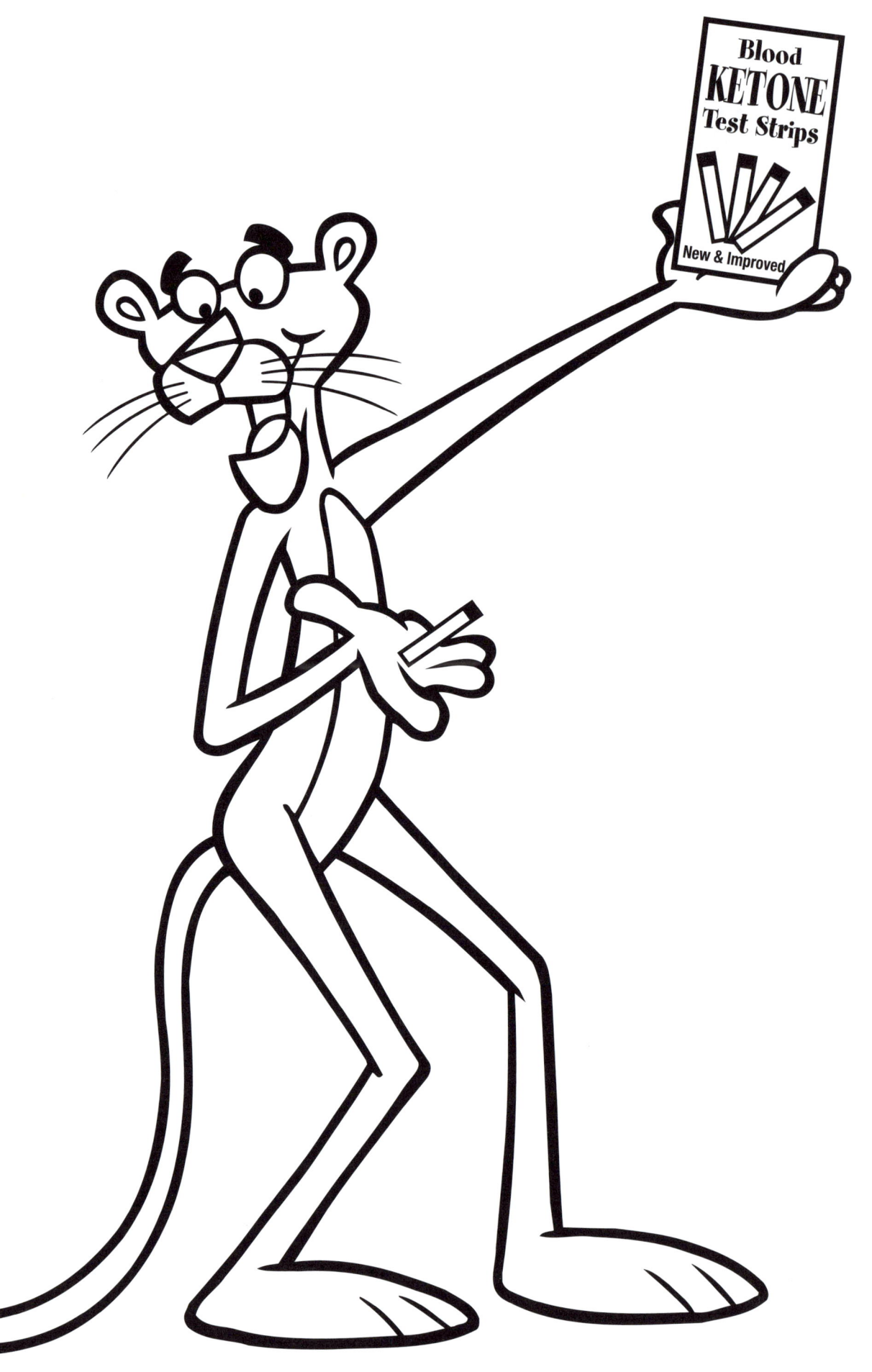

CHECKING KETONES

TABLE 1:
Comparison of Blood and Urine Ketone Readings

Blood Ketone (mmol/L)	Urine Ketone Strip color	Level	Action to take
<0.6	slight/no color change	negative	normal - no action needed
0.6 to 1.0	light purple	small to moderate	extra insulin & fluids**
1.1 to 3.0	dark purple	moderate to large*	call MD or RN**
>3.0	very dark purple	very large*	call MD or RN** <u>may need to go to the E.R.</u>

*It is usually advised to call a healthcare-provider for a blood ketone level greater than 1.0 or with urine ketone readings of moderate or large.

**If the blood glucose level is below 150 mg/dL (<8.3 mmol/L), a liquid with sugar (e.g., juice) should be taken so more insulin can be safely given.

Steps for use of the Precision Xtra Strips:

1. Open a strip and place it into the meter with the three black bars going first into the meter. Push the strip completely into the test port of the meter until it cannot go in any further.
2. After washing and drying the hand, lance the finger.
3. Place a drop of blood into the white target area at the end of the strip.
4. The result is then displayed on the meter in 10 seconds.

We suggest interpreting the readings as follows (in mmol/L):

    <0.6 = normal

0.6 – 1.0 = slightly elevated. Drink extra fluids.

1.0 – 3.0 = serious, call healthcare-provider and state the call is urgent. Take extra rapid-acting insulin every two hours (if ketones and blood/CGM glucose levels are still elevated) and drink extra fluids.

    >3.0 = **Call MD or RN. May need to go to the Emergency Room. Have someone take you!**

DEFINITIONS

Chemstrip K: Strips for measuring urine ketones (acetone). They are also available as Chemstrip uGK (for urine ketones and sugar).

Diabetic Ketoacidosis (Acidosis; DKA): What happens in the body when not enough insulin is available. Blood/CGM glucose levels are usually high at this time. Moderate or large urine ketones and blood ketones >3.0 mmol/L are usually present. This is the subject of Chapter 15.

Ketostix: Strips for measuring urine ketones (acetone). They are also available as Ketodiastix (for urine ketones and sugar).

Ketones (Acetone): The acidic molecules that appear when not enough insulin is present and fat is broken down. Ketostix or Chemstrip K strips measure urine ketones. The Precision Xtra, NovoMax Plus, and Keto-Mojo meters measure blood beta ketones.

mg/dL and mmol/L: The level in a measured amount (100 cc for dL or in 1,000 cc for L). Blood sugar (glucose) levels are expressed in mg/dL in the U.S., but they are usually expressed as mmol/L in Europe and other countries. It is possible to convert mg/dL to mmol/L by dividing by 18 (or multiplying by 0.0555). The opposite is done to go from mmol/L to mg/dL. A conversion table for glucose values is in the Appendix.

QUESTIONS AND ANSWERS FROM NEWSNOTES

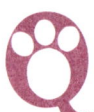**We recently obtained a meter that measures the blood ketones. How do the blood ketone measurements compare with the urine ketone measurements? When do we need to call our doctor or nurse?**

Like a blood sugar measured on a meter, the blood (serum) ketone value gives the ketone level at the time the measurement is done. The urine ketone measurement, like a urine sugar, can be hours behind. (The urine collected is since the last void.) The blood ketone value thus has the potential to be more representative of the current situation than the urine ketone measurement.

The measurement in blood is particularly helpful when a person cannot void frequently due to dehydration, or when a person has not voided for several hours, so that it is not possible to tell if the urine ketone measurement represents the current level.

Blood ketone measurements can be especially helpful for younger children. It would be wise to routinely call the diabetes care-provider when blood ketone values above 1.0 are obtained.

It has been shown that youth are more likely to check blood ketones with an illness (93 percent did) than to check urine ketones (only 53 percent did). Finding ketones earlier could save a hospitalization OR A LIFE!

Table 1 in this chapter gives an "approximate" comparison of urine and blood ketones.

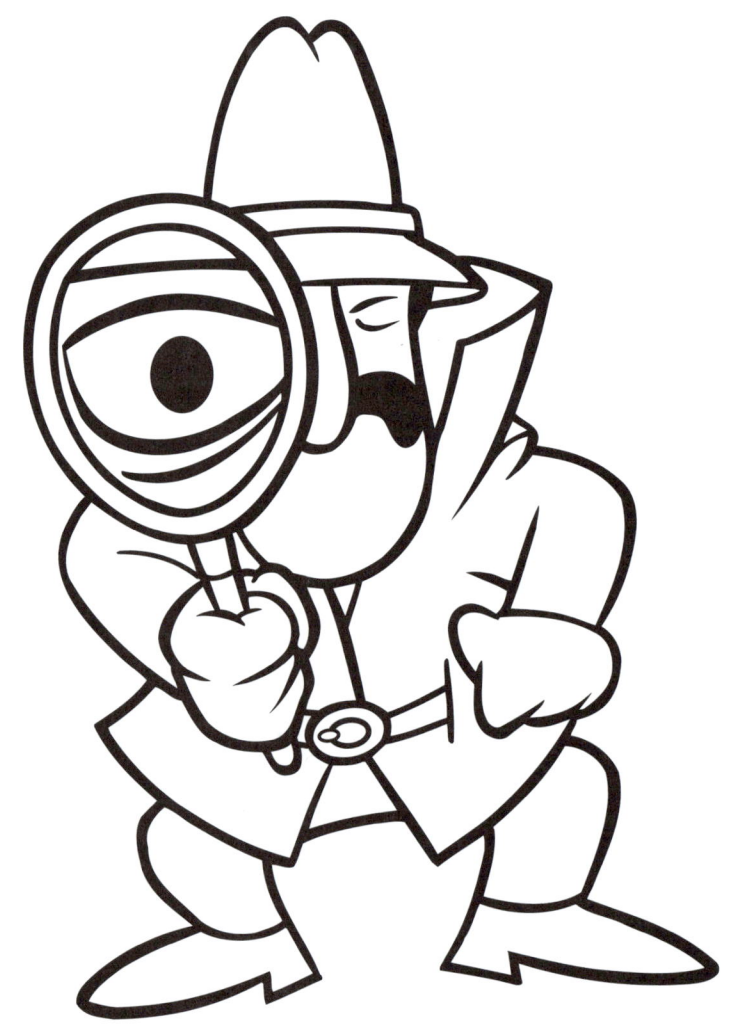

CHAPTER 6

Low Blood Sugar (Hypoglycemia or Insulin Reaction)

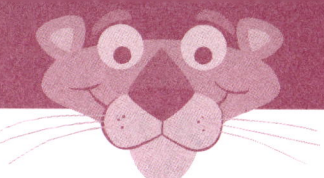

There are two emergencies relating to blood sugar levels in people with diabetes. The first, discussed in this chapter, is low blood sugar or hypoglycemia. The second is high blood sugar and ketoacidosis (Chapter 15). Low blood sugar can come on quickly and must be treated by the person, family or friends. Early treatment helps reduce the likelihood of a more severe reaction and possible hospitalization.

Any time a person has received a shot or bolus of insulin, or an oral diabetes medicine, there is a chance of a low blood sugar reaction. Education about low blood sugars is a key for avoiding lows in people of all ages. The family of a person with newly diagnosed diabetes must know the signs and symptoms of hypoglycemia before going home the first night.

A normal (non-diabetic) random blood/CGM glucose level is usually between 70-140 mg/dL (3.9-7.8 mmol/L). Normal fasting values are usually between 70 and 100 mg/dL (3.9-5.5 mmol/L). The American Diabetes Association (ADA) **defines a low blood sugar level as any level <70 mg/dL (<3.9 mmol/L).** This is the level at which the symptoms of hypoglycemia commonly occur. However, people who do **NOT** have diabetes can have occasional values between 60 and 70 mg/dL (3.3 to 3.9 mmol/L).

TOPICS:

Prevention, Detection and Treatment of Acute Complications (hypoglycemia, low blood sugar)

TEACHING OBJECTIVES:
The teacher will:
1. Present the symptoms, causes, and treatment of mild, moderate and severe hypoglycemia.
2. Identify the appropriate time to contact the healthcare-provider.

LEARNING OBJECTIVES:
Learner (parents, child, relative or self) will be able to:
1. Define mild, moderate and severe low sugar symptoms, causes and treatment.
2. State the appropriate time to contact a healthcare-provider.

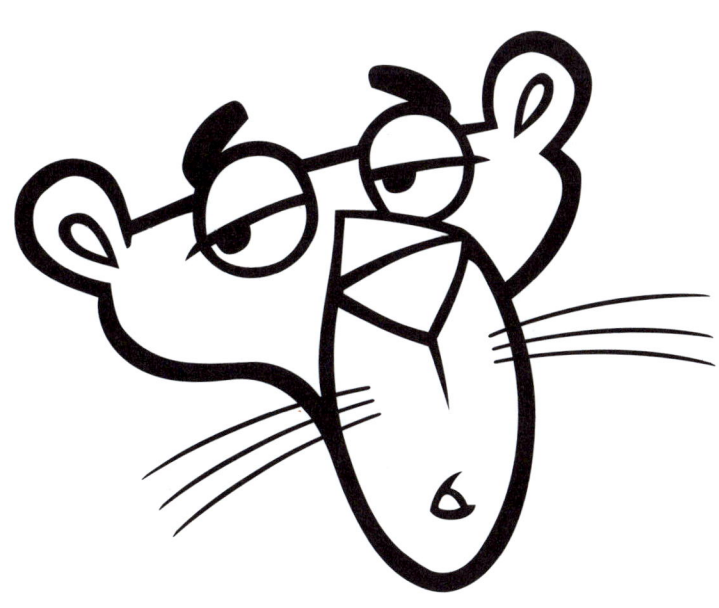

CAUSES OF LOW BLOOD SUGAR

Hypoglycemia (low blood sugar) occurs because of excess insulin activity. The level of sugar in the blood falls too low. Sometimes it is called an **insulin reaction**, a **reaction** or a **low**. Frequent causes are listed below:

- late or missed meals or snacks
- extra exercise (the low may be "delayed" until during the night)
- too much insulin/wrong dose
- taking a bath, shower or hot tub too soon after injection (dangerous)
- a previous low blood ("hypoglycemia can cause further hypoglycemia")
- illnesses, especially with vomiting
- alcohol intake

Avoiding low blood sugars (lows) is much wiser than having to treat the lows. One of the advantages of using a continuous glucose monitor (CGM) is that it has formulas to help predict low glucose levels and alarms to warn the person when a low sugar is about to happen or is happening (Chapter 29). If communicating with an insulin pump, the CGM may turn off insulin release from the pump to help avoid severe hypoglycemia (Chapter 30).

SYMPTOMS OF LOW BLOOD SUGAR

Usually the body gives a warning when low blood sugar or an insulin reaction is developing. DIFFERENT PEOPLE GET DIFFERENT WARNINGS.

These signs are the most common warnings of an insulin reaction:

- **Hunger:** the person may either feel hungry or have an upset stomach (nausea)
- **Shaky:** the person's hands or body may feel shaky
- **Sweaty:** the person may sweat more than usual (often a cold sweat)
- **Weak:** the person may feel weak and need to sit down
- **Color:** the face may become pale, gray or red
- **Headache:** sugar is the main "fuel" used by the brain
- **Confusion:** the person may feel or look spacey or may appear dazed
- **Sleepiness:** the person may yawn, feel sleepy (at unusual times) or may have trouble thinking clearly; preschoolers frequently get sleepy
- **Behavioral changes:** changes in behavior are quite common; often the person may cry, act intoxicated, or act angry; they also may feel weak or anxious or dizzy
- **Double or blurred vision:** the person may see double or the pupils of the eyes may get bigger; the eyes may appear glassy; the whites of the eyes may look blood shot
- **Loss of consciousness:** evidence suggests that at nighttime, in the absence of a bolus of insulin, the person usually has to have a low sugar for over two hours for this or a seizure to occur.
- **Seizure or convulsion:** both loss of consciousness and convulsion occur late in the reaction. They are usually the result of not treating a reaction quickly enough.

The first five initial symptoms (hunger, shakiness, sweatiness, weakness, and color) are due to the output of the "fight or flight" hormone, adrenaline (epinephrine is another name). The latter symptoms are more related to the lack of sugar to the brain. Sugar is the main source of fuel for the brain. If a severe low sugar continues too long, the brain can be harmed. It is particularly important to avoid low blood sugars in young children. The brain grows very rapidly in the first four years of life.

Children learn to tell if they have low blood sugar at different ages (see Chapter 18). It may be possible to train young children (or older people who have difficulty detecting low blood sugars) to recognize certain signs, and also to teach them words to express how they are feeling. For example, parents may frequently need to remind a young child:

"Remember how you felt shaky and you came and told me there was a 'tiger in your tummy?' You did a great job! Remember to tell a grown up if you feel that way again."

Ask the child how he/she feels when a low is found. This will reinforce their awareness of the symptoms. For very young children, the parent can often tell when the child has low blood sugar by the type of cry or fussiness he/she presents. Young children may be unaware of lows because they are busy playing. It is important for adults to be aware of the symptoms and of the need for snacks.

NIGHTTIME LOWS

People may wake up with symptoms (infants may just cry) when lows occur during the night. *The symptoms may be the same as during the daytime although there are sometimes special clues:*

- inability to sleep or waking up alert, hungry, restless, moaning, etc.
- waking up sweating
- waking up with a fast heart rate
- waking up with a headache
- sleep walking
- waking up feeling foggy-headed or with memory loss

DELAYED HYPOGLYCEMIA

Delayed hypoglycemia is also discussed in Chapter 13 on exercise. It often occurs from 4-24 hours after heavy exercise. For some people, blood/CGM glucose levels can be high during or after exercise. This may be due to the normal response of releasing adrenaline during exercise or from the extra snacks. Adrenaline causes sugar to come out of the liver and raise the blood sugar. At some point after the exercise, the adrenaline levels go back down (sometimes not until the time of sleep), and the sugar moves back into the muscle and liver. The result can be a low blood sugar or **"delayed hypoglycemia."** The symptoms are similar to those discussed above.

Avoiding hypoglycemia often involves lowering the insulin dose, particularly in relation to exercise (Chapter 13). This must be done after heavy exercise even though the blood sugar may be high. For people using an insulin pump, turning the pump off before and during extreme exercise, or use of a temporary basal rate, can be helpful. A 20 percent insulin reduction for six hours starting at bedtime has also been shown to be helpful in avoiding nighttime lows. For people receiving insulin injections and not using a CGM, a reduction in basal insulin and a blood sugar check during the night may be helpful. Exercise is essential for the heart and cardiovascular system. Therefore, it is important to always be thinking about ways to avoid post-exercise lows.

AVOIDING INSULIN REACTIONS (THINKING AHEAD)

A person's/parent's greatest fear is often of a severe hypoglycemic reaction. This fear is sometimes a factor in not achieving optimal sugar levels (and a low HbA1c level, Chapter 14). Unfortunately, the most common time for severe lows to occur is during the sleeping hours. This is because the adrenaline response to hypoglycemia is lower when sleeping and the person may not be awakened when the blood sugar falls. The good news is that the incidence of nighttime severe lows can now be greatly reduced with use of CGM and a partial artificial pancreas system (Chapters 29 and 30).

It is important to try to avoid lows. This may allow the stores of epinephrine and other "protective" hormones to build up so they are available when needed. Three important considerations in avoiding insulin reactions are outlined below:

Snacks – important when:

✔ heavy physical exercise or all day exercise is planned, such as hiking or skiing

✔ the bedtime blood/CGM glucose level is below 130 mg/dL (<7.2 mmol/L), especially after a day with much exercise

✔ a person has a low (but be careful not to eat in excess - see the "Rule of 15" below)

Insulin

✔ Use basal (Lantus [Basaglar], Levemir, or Tresiba) insulins rather than NPH (especially to cover nighttime hours).

✔ Reduce the dose of insulin which will be acting during and/or after the exercise period (see Chapter 13).

✔ Take the insulin injection AFTER a hot shower, bath or hot tub (not before).

✔ For days with heavy exercise, if doing insulin corrections for high blood sugars at bedtime or during the night, use half the usual dose and recheck the blood/CGM glucose level in 2 hours.

Blood/CGM glucose levels

✔ Check the blood/CGM glucose levels before, during (hourly) and after periods of exercise to help avoid lows and to plan for similar future activities.

✔ Knowing a blood/CGM glucose level can help decide the amount of treatment needed.

✔ Check the blood/CGM glucose level during the night if it was a heavy exercise day.

✔ **Always** do a recheck if the value was low (in approximately 15 minutes), especially if it was prior to the bedtime snack or during the night, to be certain it came back up.

✔ The CGM will give a warning alarm for a falling or low glucose level.

✔ The availability of the partial artificial pancreas system (Chapter 30) with the predicted and low glucose-suspend features can help to avoid severe lows.

TREATMENT FOR A LOW BLOOD SUGAR (see Tables 1 and 2)

The general rule is to **GIVE SUGAR IN SOME FORM AS FAST AS POSSIBLE.** If the reaction is not severe, do a blood sugar first. If unable to do a blood sugar, then just give juice or sugar pop (Table 1). A person with diabetes won't get sick from excess sugar in this situation. It will just cause high blood sugar and then be passed in the urine. Insulin reactions come quickly and should be treated at once by the person, parent, friend or teacher.

SOME PEOPLE USE THE "RULE OF 15": take 15g of carbohydrate and check again in 15 minutes. Then if the blood sugar is still below 70 mg/dL (<3.9 mmol/L), have another 15 g of carbohydrate and check again in 15 minutes. Use finger-stick blood sugar levels in follow-up, as CGM values are delayed and may result in overtreatment. Keep repeating until the blood sugar is back up. Then eat solid food or a meal. Following this rule may help to avoid secondary large rises in blood sugar levels. The grams of carbs may be less (e.g., 10g) for a small child, or higher (e.g., 30g) for a heavy adolescent or after excessive exercise. More carbs may also be needed if the blood sugar is very low (e.g., 50 mg/dL or 2.8 mmol/L) compared to when the value is higher. The best plan is to try a given amount of carbs and see if it works. If it doesn't, try a different dose the next time there is a low blood sugar. Some sources of quick-acting sugar with appropriate amounts for people of different ages are given in Table 1.

Different forms of sugar can be carried to treat low blood sugar. **PEOPLE WITH DIABETES SHOULD CARRY SUGAR PACKETS,**

TABLE 1:
Sources of Quick-Acting Sugar (Glucose) for Hypoglycemia

FOOD	AGE		
(Measured in grams of carbohydrate)	5 years or less (10g)	6-10 years (10-15g)	over 10 years (15-20g)
Glucose Tabs (4g each - check label; some = 5g)	2	3-4	4-5
Instant Glucose (1 tube = 31g)	1/3 tube	1/3-1/2 tube	1/2-2/3 tube
GLUCOSHOT/GLUCOGEL 1 tube (15g)	1/3 tube	1 tube	1 tube
Cake gel (1 small tube = 12g)	1 tube	1 tube	1-2 tubes
Apple juice (½ cup = 15g)	1/3 cup	1/3-1/2 cup	1/2-2/3 cup
Orange juice (½ cup = 15g)	1/4-1/2 cup	1/2-3/4 cup	3/4-1 cup
Sugar (1 tsp = 4g)	2 tsp	3-4 tsp	4-5 tsp
Honey (1 tsp = 5g; do not use if child is less than two years old)	2 tsp	2-3 tsp	3-4 tsp
Regular pop (soda) (1 oz = 3g)	3 oz	4-5 oz	5-6 oz
Milk (12g/cup)	3/4 cup	1 cup	1 1/2 cups
LIFE-SAVERS® (2.5g each)	4	4-6	6-8
Skittles® (1g each)	10 pieces	10-15 pieces	15-20 pieces
SweetTarts® (1.7g each)	6 pieces	6-8 pieces	8-12 pieces
Raisins (1 Tbsp = 7½g)	1-2 Tbsp	2 Tbsp	2 1/2 Tbsp
g = gram; tsp = teaspoon; Tbsp = Tablespoon			

LOW BLOOD SUGAR (HYPOGLYCEMIA OR INSULIN REACTION)

GLUCOSE TABLETS, OR ANOTHER SOURCE OF SUGAR IN THEIR POCKETS AT ALL TIMES FOR EMERGENCIES.** Glucose (dextrose) tablets have been shown to work just as fast as liquids with sugar. Candy is sometimes too tempting. It also may be taken by other children. A special pocket for sugar packets can be sewn inside of gym shorts. Some people carry them in a jogger wallet attached to a shoe. Others slip packets in high stockings. It is often best to wrap the packet in foil or a plastic bag in case of leaks. Insta-Glucose® comes in a tube and looks like toothpaste. It is available in most pharmacies. Walgreens has the GLUCO SHOT for about $3 U.S. A tube of clear cake gel from the grocery store will also work. **The initial sugar will be absorbed more quickly if the person waits before eating solid food.** After the blood sugar is back up, the person can eat some other longer-lasting solid food, like crackers or half of a sandwich. Gradually, each person will become familiar with the type of reactions that occur. The person will learn how severe the reactions tend to be, when they are most likely to occur and how best to treat them.

Eventually, as a person becomes more familiar with diabetes, it may be possible to treat the various reactions differently. Even though some CGM devices do not require fingerstick blood sugars, it is always wise to do a blood sugar if the reaction is not severe. (If severe, treat first and then do the blood sugar.) If the level is above 70 mg/dL (3.9 mmol/L), it is usually possible to treat the reaction with fresh fruit and solid food rather than juice or sugar pop.

Remember that it takes 10 to 20 minutes for the blood sugar level to rise, and it is wise to wait until the value is back up before returning to normal activity. It is important to repeat the blood sugar after the low to make sure it has returned to normal. This is particularly true when the low occurs late in the evening or during the night. **A PERSON WITH A LOW BLOOD SUGAR SHOULD NOT BE LEFT ALONE UNTIL THE BLOOD SUGAR HAS RETURNED TO NORMAL.**

Treatment by Severity of Reaction (see Summary, Table 2):

Mild Reaction (such as hunger at an unusual time, pale face, shakiness or irritability): If possible, do a blood sugar. If below 70 mg/dL (<3.9 mmol/L), give a small glass (4 oz) of juice or sugar pop (soda) or other quick acting sugar. Wait 10-20 minutes for absorption of the sugar and then recheck the blood sugar level. If the blood sugar is above 70 mg/dL (<3.9 mmol/L), give just solid food, without the juice or soda.

We are especially concerned about any blood sugar below 60 mg/dL (<3.3 mmol/L). When these are obtained frequently, the insulin dose or snacks should be changed so that further low values do not occur. In a child under five years old, we are concerned about values below 70 mg/dL (3.9 mmol/L). When values are below these levels at the time of an insulin injection, we usually recommend not giving the usual amount of rapid-acting insulin (or at least wait until after eating). If two or three values below 60 mg/dL (<3.3 mmol/L) are present at the same time of day in the same week, a decrease in insulin dose is probably needed. CALL THE DIABETES CARE-PROVIDER IF HELP IS NEEDED.

Moderate Reaction (very confused or spacey, very pale or very shaky): Give Insta-Glucose, Reactose™, Monojel™, cake decorating gel, or any source of simple sugar, such as sugar pop or juice if able to swallow. One-half tube of the Insta-Glucose can be placed between the cheeks and gums, and the person should be told to swallow. Always check for the risk of choking. Do a blood sugar as soon as possible. Repeat the blood sugar after 10-15 minutes to make sure it is above 70 mg/dL (>3.9 mmol/L). If not, repeat the initial treatment and wait another 10-15 minutes. Low-dose glucagon (see below) or intranasal glucagon can be used if not responding. Once the blood sugar has risen above 70 mg/dL (3.9 mmol/L), give solid food.

Severe Reaction: If the person is completely unconscious or has a seizure, it is risky to put the concentrated sugar around the gums. It

TABLE 2:
Hypoglycemia: Treatment of Low Blood Sugar (B.S.) When Possible, Always Check Blood Sugar Level!

LEVEL	MILD	MODERATE	SEVERE
Alertness	**ALERT**	**NOT ALERT** Unable to drink safely (choking risk) Needs help from another person	**UNRESPONSIVE** Loss of consciousness or seizure Needs constant adult help (position on side) *Give nothing by mouth* (extreme choking risk)
Symptoms	Mood changes, shaky, sweaty, hungry, fatigued, weak, pale	Lack of focus Headache, confused, disoriented *Can't* self-treat	Loss of consciousness or seizure
Actions to take	• Check B.S. • Give 2-8 oz sugary fluid (amount age dependent) • Recheck B.S. in 10-15 min. • B.S. *<70 mg/dL (<3.9 mmol/L), repeat sugary fluid and recheck in 10-20 min. • B.S. *>70 mg/dL (>3.9 mmol/L), give a solid snack • Slight risk for more lows in next 24 hours (after any low blood sugar)	• *Place in position of safety* • Check B.S. • If on insulin pump, may disconnect or suspend until fully recovered from low blood sugar **(awake and alert)** • Give Insta-Glucose or cake decorating gel - put between gums and cheek and rub in • Look for person to 'wake up' • Recheck B.S. in 10-20 min. • *Once alert* – follow "actions" under 'Mild' column • Moderate risk for more lows in next 24 hours • If not responding to oral treatment, may use low-dose glucagon (1 unit/year of age up to 15 units) or intra nasal glucagon (3 mg) if available	• *Place in position of safety* • Check B.S. • If on insulin pump, disconnect or suspend until fully recovered from low blood sugar • Glucagon: can be given with an insulin syringe like insulin: • Under 6 years: **30 units (3/10 cc)** • 6-12 years: **50 units (1/2 cc)** • Over 12 years: **100 units (all of dose or 1 cc)** • If giving 50 or 100 unit doses, may use syringe in box and inject through clothing if needed • **If intranasal glucagon (3 mg) is available, can use instead of injection** • Check B.S. every 10-15 min. until *>70 mg/dL (>3.9 mmol/L) • If no response, may need to call 911 • Check B.S. every hour for 4-5 hours • High risk for more lows for 24 hours (need to increase food intake and decrease insulin doses)
Recovery time	10-20 minutes	20-45 minutes	**Call RN/MD** Effects can last 2-12 hours.

* < sign means "less than"   > sign means "greater than"

LOW BLOOD SUGAR (HYPOGLYCEMIA OR INSULIN REACTION)

could get into the airway. It is better to just give glucagon as instructed in Table 3 in this chapter. If available, intranasal glucagon (3 mg) can be used instead of the injected glucagon. Remember to do the blood sugar level as soon as possible. Also, if using an insulin pump, remember to disconnect or suspend the insulin delivery. If the person does not improve after 10-20 minutes, it may be necessary to call 911 to get extra help. A second dose (same amount) of injected glucagon (from the same vial) can also be given. Approximately one of every 20 people with type 1 diabetes has a hypoglycemic seizure or coma each year. Every family must have glucagon available and know how to use it (see Table 3). Adjustments in the next insulin dose will be necessary. We recommend aiming for slightly higher blood sugars for several days after a severe reaction. Call your diabetes care-provider if you need help making this adjustment. Remember, it is always okay to call 911 for a severe reaction if you do not feel comfortable treating it yourself. Knowing how to administer glucagon, however, may help avoid emergency services.

One-sided Weakness (paralysis): It is not known why, but on rare occasions some people experience weakness (or paralysis) on one side of the body with a severe insulin reaction. This can last for one to 12 hours, but eventually clears. It is particularly worrisome to doctors in emergency rooms. They often insist on a very expensive evaluation to prove that a stroke has not occurred.

HYPOGLYCEMIC UNAWARENESS

Sometimes low blood/CGM sugars will be found during routine checking, and the person will not have had symptoms. This may be due to a very gradual fall in the blood sugar, or in young children, because they have not learned to recognize the symptoms. Some people with frequent lows fail to release adrenaline and may have the problem medically referred to as **"hypoglycemic unawareness."** In this case, they must not aim for such strict blood sugar management. Sometimes the insulin dose can be lowered. Use of a CGM to warn about low glucose values may help to reverse this condition. The use of the partial or complete artificial pancreas with predicted or low glucose suspend features (Chapter 30) can be VERY helpful. After blood/CGM glucose levels have been higher for two or three weeks, it may be possible to again recognize low blood sugars.

GLUCAGON

Glucagon is a hormone made in the pancreas, like insulin. It has the opposite effect of insulin and raises the blood sugar level. Glucagon injections are rarely needed, but all families must keep it on hand and to be prepared to use it if necessary. The expiration date on the box should be checked regularly and, if outdated, a new bottle should be

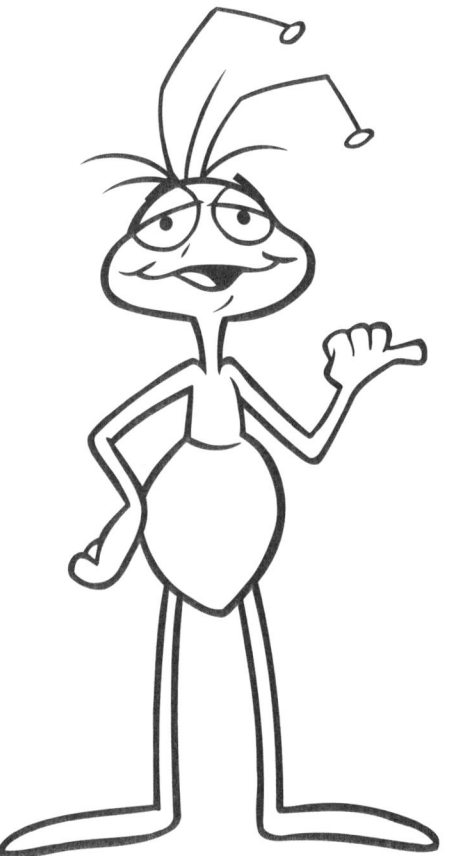

TABLE 3:
Glucagon Injections – When To and How To

- Use when a person is unconscious or having a seizure.
- Keep in a convenient and known place. Store in a refrigerator during hot weather. Protect from freezing.
- Keep a 3 cc syringe available or use the fluid-filled syringe in the emergency kit. An insulin syringe and needle can also be used (preferably a 1.0 cc syringe). Some people tape the syringe to the kit so they have this readily available.
- If you have the emergency kit, the fluid does not need to be withdrawn from bottle 1 (diagram at right) as it is already in the syringe. Put the liquid into the glucagon vial and swirl gently to mix. The large syringe that the liquid was in can also be used to give the glucagon injection. Draw up the dose indicated below. Clear the air pointing the needle upward.
- Withdraw from the mixed glucagon bottle:
  If using an insulin syringe, put needle into center of stopper.

  (Estimate dose if using the emergency kit syringe.)

  0.3 cc (30 units) for a child less than six years old
  0.5 cc (50 units) for a child 6-12 years of age
  1.0 cc (100 units) for a person over 12 years of age
- If using the syringe that comes in the emergency kit, inject into deep muscle (in front of leg or upper, outer arm) though it is OK to inject into the subcutaneous fat. Inject through clothing if needed. If the glucagon is drawn into an insulin syringe then give it just as you would an insulin shot. If a blood sugar has not yet been done, it can be done now.
- Wait 10-20 minutes. Check blood sugar. If still unconscious and blood sugar is still below 60 mg/dL (3.3 mmol/L), inject second dose of glucagon (same amount as first dose).
- If there is no response to the glucagon, or if there is any difficulty breathing, call paramedics (or 911).
- As soon as he/she awakens, give sips of juice, sugar pop or sugar in water initially. Honey may help to raise the blood sugar for children over the age of 1 year. After 10 minutes, encourage solid food (crackers and peanut butter or cheese, sandwich, etc.).
- Notify diabetes care team of severe reaction prior to next insulin injection (so dose can be changed if needed). Complete recovery may take 1-6 hours.

Please copy this page as often as you wish. Tape a copy to the box of glucagon.

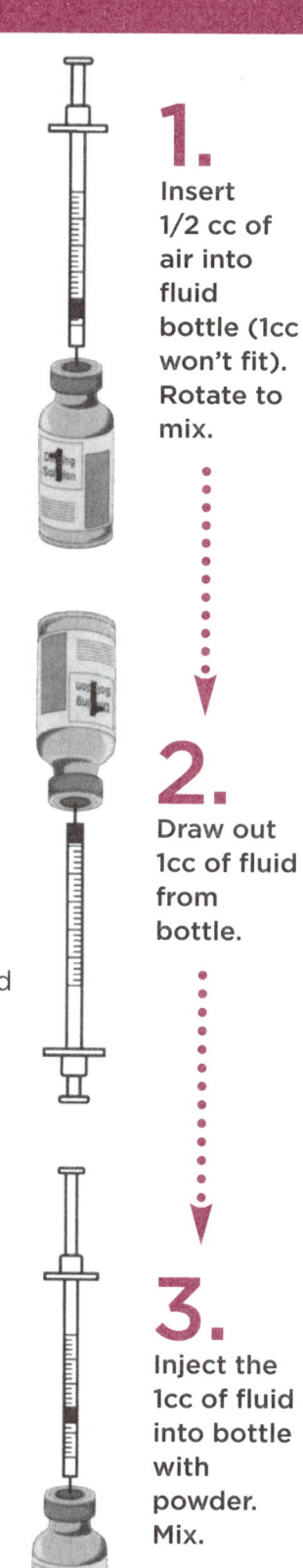

1. Insert 1/2 cc of air into fluid bottle (1cc won't fit). Rotate to mix.

2. Draw out 1cc of fluid from bottle.

3. Inject the 1cc of fluid into bottle with powder. Mix.

LOW BLOOD SUGAR (HYPOGLYCEMIA OR INSULIN REACTION)

obtained. If a very severe reaction occurs and the person loses consciousness or has a seizure, glucagon should be given promptly. It can be stored at room temperature. It should not reach a temperature above 90° or below freezing. It can be taken in a cooler with the insulin and blood sugar strips for trips away from home. If available, intranasal glucagon (3 mg) can be used instead of injected glucagon (see below).

Use of Glucagon

1. Severe Low Blood Sugar

Glucagon comes in a bottle containing 1 mg as a tablet or powder. There is a syringe containing diluting solution in the emergency kit. The method for giving glucagon is shown in Table 3. **This table may be copied and attached to the glucagon kit.** A video from Eli Lilly and Co giving instructions for glucagon use is also available as a link on our website, www.barbaradaviscenter.org. Novo Nordisk also provides a "Hypokit"™ to instruct people on glucagon usage.

At the time of this writing, a new pre-filled syringe (PFS) for glucagon injection (Gvoke™ PFS) had just been approved by the FDA. It is stable at room temperature, does not have to be mixed, and is available in two doses – one for children ages two and up (0.5 mg), and one for adults (1.0 mg). In addition, Fresenius Kabi has introduced a glucagon emergency kit that makes the mixing of the liquid and glucagon powder easier.

Sometimes vomiting will occur after a severe reaction. This may be from the glucagon that was injected. It usually does not last very long, and if the blood sugar is above 150 mg/dL (8.3 mmol/L), it is usually not a big problem. If the person is lying down, the head should be turned to the side to avoid choking. Urine or blood ketones should be checked (see Chapter 5) as they can sometimes also form. If the family is concerned about the ketones, or if the blood sugar did not rise, or if the vomiting continues, the diabetes care-provider should be called.

Do not be concerned that the instructions are simplified in the school setting (Chapter 25) to just give 0.5 cc glucagon if below age 16 years or 1.0 cc if age 16 or older. It is important to just get some in.

2. Low Dose Glucagon

Sometimes the blood sugar can be low (<70 mg/dL [<3.9 mmol/L]) and the person cannot keep any food down (such as with vomiting or diarrhea). In this case, a very low dose of Glucagon can be given just like insulin – using an insulin syringe (Table 3). The dose is one unit per year of age up to age 15 years. Older people can just use the 15 units.

For example: a five-year-old would get five units or a 10-year-old would get 10 units.

If the blood sugar is not higher in 20-30 minutes, the same dose can be repeated. This treatment has saved many ER visits. If available, intranasal glucagon (3 mg) can be used instead.

3. Intranasal Glucagon (Baqsimi™ nasal powder [pronounced, "Back see-me"]):

The availability of intranasal-glucagon makes the treatment of moderate to severe hypoglycemia much easier. This is particularly true for the school or work setting, where a nurse or trained family member may not be available. Severe lows can occur rapidly during the day, with altered eating, exercise or insulin boluses. In contrast, they usually occur at night only if the glucose level has been below 60 mg/dL (3.3 mmol/L) for over two hours.

Baqsimi comes in a compact, portable and ready-to-use dispenser as a single 3 mg dose. The device should be kept wrapped (don't pull red opener) until it is to be used. It is approved for children age four years and above, so insurance may not cover it for younger children (approximate price = $286 U.S.). The plastic device for administration of the intranasal-glucagon requires only one step for administration, the depression of the plunger.

It raises the blood sugar to above 70 mg/dL (3.9 mmol/L) in an average of 16 minutes (compared to 13 minutes for intramuscular-glucagon). This difference is inconsequential. If there is no response in 15 minutes, a second dose can be given. The intranasal-glucagon has been shown to still be effective with nasal congestion. It may be easier to carry outside of the home than the injectable glucagon. Storage is the same as for injectable glucagon (i.e., below 86 degrees, can carry in pocket, but not left in car or hot sun).

Record All Insulin Reactions

Record low sugar readings in your record book or download from your glucose meter or CGM. If from CGM, note if the person had symptoms when the readings were low. Many families circle all values <60 mg/dL (<3.3 mmol/L). Try to identify and record the cause of any low or high blood/CGM sugars (Table 4). If more than two mild insulin reactions occur in a short time period, adjust the amount of insulin or call the diabetes care-provider. It is usually possible to call during office hours, but if a severe reaction occurs during other than office hours, call the on-call care-provider prior to giving the next regularly scheduled insulin shot.

Medical Identification

In case of a severe insulin reaction, EVERYONE needs to know that the person has diabetes. This includes teachers, strangers, police, co-workers, friends and medical personnel. The person with diabetes should wear a bracelet or necklace with this information. A card in the wallet is not enough; this may not be found by paramedics. A diabetes ID card can also be stapled to the registration of the car in the glove compartment. Bracelets, necklaces, or ID tags can be found at most pharmacies or medical supply houses. Listed below is contact information for various products. Product and services vary:

The MedicAlert tag includes a number that can be called 24 hours a day for information concerning both the person and the doctor.

The MedicAlert Foundation
(provides MedicAlert tags)
2323 Colorado Avenue
Turlock, California 95382
888-633-4298
www.medicalert.org

A bracelet, necklace or medallion with your personal medical information (name, condition and medications) can be engraved and ordered through American Medical Identifications, Inc.

American Medical Identifications, Inc.
P.O. Box 925617
Houston, Texas 77292
800-363-5985
www.americanmedical-id.com

Colorful sports bracelets are sometimes preferred and can be ordered from FIFTY 50 PHARMACY.

FIFTY 50
1420 Valwood Parkway, Suite 120
Carrollton, Texas 75006
Phone: 800-746-7505
www.fifty50.com

Other possible sources include:

www.tah-handcrafted-jewelry.com,

and www.laurenshope.com (800-360-8680).

For people who will not wear a necklace or bracelet, a watch or shoe tag may be the next best choice. There are medallions that stick to the front of a wallet, cell phone, insulin pump, etc. These can be purchased from LIFETAG, Inc. (888-LIFETAG or www.lifetag.com).

Toddlers should not wear a neck chain (too risky), but they often do well with ankle bracelets, charms or a medallion laced in the shoe. The sports bracelet described above works quite well around the ankle.

Rubber bracelets can be purchased at http://coolmedid.com.

DEFINITIONS

Adrenaline (used collectively to include epinephrine and non-epinephrine): The excitatory hormone. This is released with a low blood sugar or a rapid fall in blood sugar, which then causes the symptoms of low blood sugar.

Glucagon: A hormone also made in the pancreas (like insulin) that causes the blood sugar to rise. It is available to give to people who are unconscious from a severe insulin reaction.

Hypoglycemia: The term used for a low blood sugar (insulin reaction).

Hypoglycemic unawareness: The term used to describe low blood sugars without having any warning signs or symptoms.

Insta-Glucose, Monojel, or Reactose: Sources of concentrated sugar that can be purchased. These can be given to a person experiencing low blood sugar.

Ketoacidosis (Acidosis, DKA): What happens in the body when not enough insulin is available. The blood sugar is usually high at this time. Moderate or large ketones (acetone) are in the urine (see Chapter 15).

Seizure (Convulsion): Loss of consciousness with jerking of muscles. This can occur with a very severe low blood sugar (insulin reaction).

TABLE 4:
Some Factors That Change the Blood Sugar

Lowers:

✔ Insulin

✔ Hot bath, showers or hot tubs may increase insulin absorption and cause a low blood sugar

✔ Exercise, although for some people, the values may be higher immediately following exercise

✔ Less food or eating late

Raises:

✔ Sugar intake

✔ Missed insulin

✔ Hormones such as glucagon, adrenaline, growth hormone and cortisol (steroids, prednisone); their action is opposite to that of insulin

✔ Illness (which may cause ketones)

✔ Rapid growth; teenagers usually require more insulin with increased growth Menstrual periods (may cause ketones)

✔ Emotions such as anger and excitement; some younger children can have lower blood sugars with extra excitement

✔ Inhalers given for asthma which have epinephrine derivatives in them

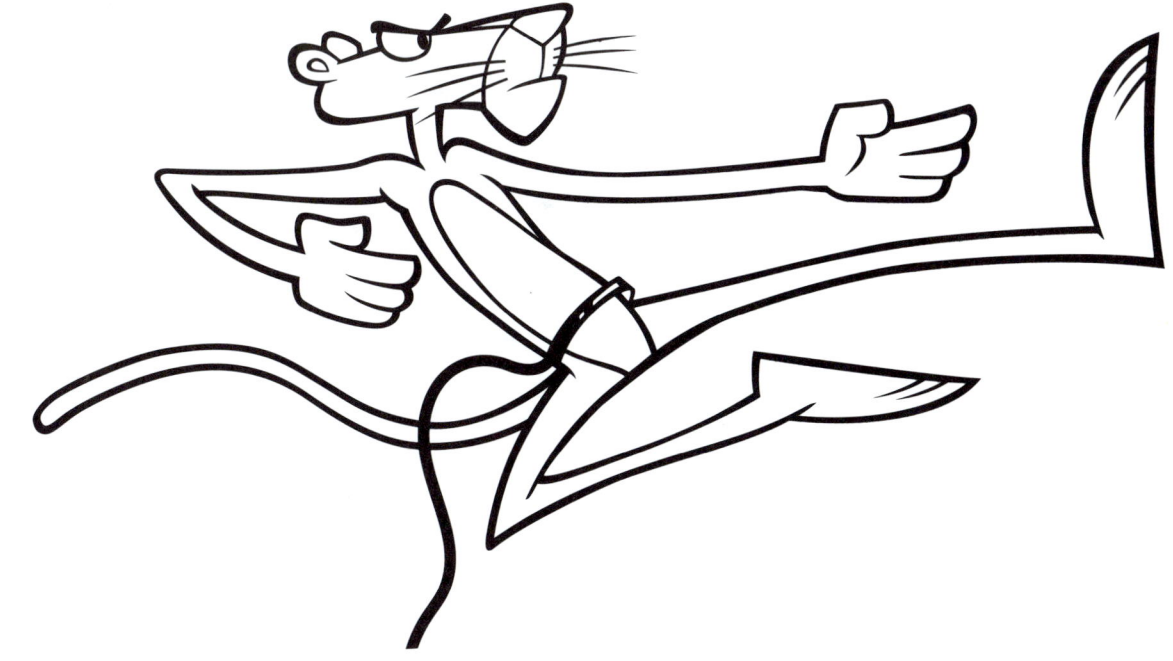

QUESTIONS AND ANSWERS FROM NEWSNOTES

Q: Do we still need to keep glucagon?

A: YES! The current statistic (from three studies) is that four to 13 percent of standard insulin-treated patients have one or more severe episodes of hypoglycemia each year. Glucagon should be given anytime there is loss of consciousness without being able to arouse the person. If paramedics are to be called, it is still wise to give the glucagon before they arrive.

Two studies have shown it will work just as fast when given subcutaneously (the same place as insulin) as when given into muscle. People used to think it always had to be given into muscle.

Some people have rebounding, a high blood sugar and even ketones after glucagon. Vomiting can also occur, but these side effects can be handled.

If intranasal glucagon is available, it can be used instead of injectable glucagon (see text).

Q: Since I have lowered my hemoglobin A1c (HbA1c), I don't seem to feel low blood sugar reactions. Is this common?

A: Unfortunately, this is not unusual. It is called hypoglycemic unawareness. People with diabetes often do not make the counter-regulatory hormones as effectively as they did previously. Adrenaline (epinephrine) output is also sometimes reduced in people with frequent low sugars. This is probably the most important hormone involved, which normally increases with low blood sugar and then causes the symptoms (shakiness, sweatiness, rapid heartbeat, etc.). Sometimes it is possible to reduce the insulin dose to let the blood sugars run a bit higher for two or three weeks in order to regain the ability to feel low blood sugars.

Q: We were recently told at a clinic visit that our child should not be given insulin just prior to a hot bath, shower or hot tub. Would you please explain the reason for this?

A: The hot bath, shower or hot tub increases blood flow to the skin. As more blood flows to this area, more insulin is rapidly taken up by the blood (probably primarily Humalog, NovoLog, Apidra or Regular insulins). This can then result in a severe low blood sugar. The answer is to always take the insulin after the hot shower or bath. The shower or bath should not be taken in the 10-15 minutes after Humalog/NovoLog/Apidra or in the first hour after taking Regular insulin.

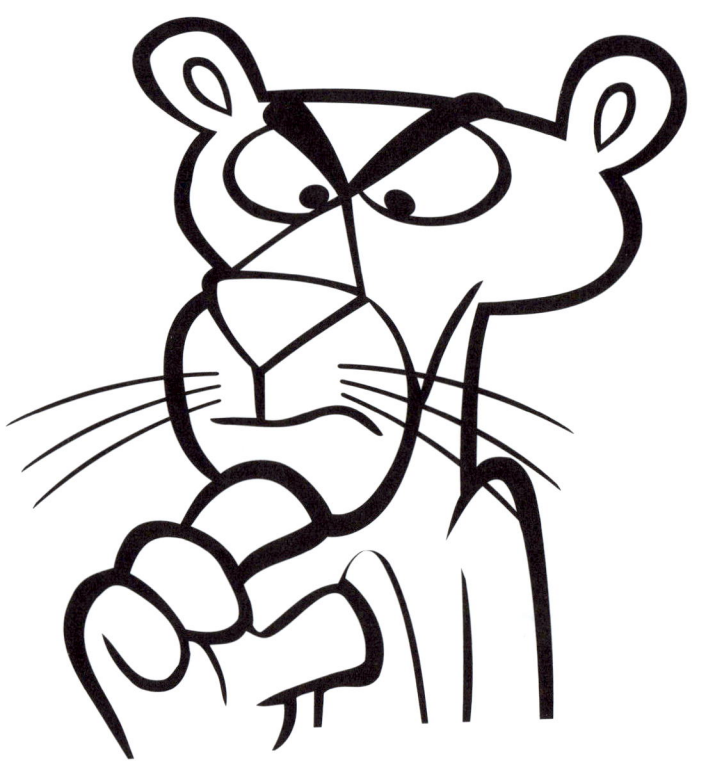

CHAPTER 7

Blood/CGM Sugar Monitoring*

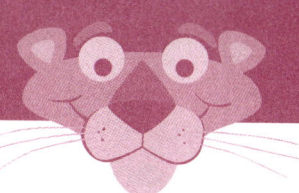

MEASURING BLOOD SUGARS

The ability of people (or families) with diabetes to check blood sugar levels quickly and accurately changed diabetes management greatly. Prior to this, diabetes was primarily managed by measuring urine sugars, which were very unreliable. The people in the intensive treatment group of the Diabetes Control and Complications Trial (DCCT) did at least four blood sugars every day (see Chapter 14). They were able to achieve improved glucose levels as a result of frequent blood glucose (BG) monitoring, more frequent dosages of insulin and following a dietary plan. The improved diabetes management was shown to significantly reduce the risk for the eye, kidney, nerve and cardiovascular complications of diabetes. Clearly, for people who are able to check blood sugars more frequently, or to consistently use a continuous glucose monitor (**CGM**), improved diabetes management is now possible. Use of a CGM is discussed in Chapter 29.

For people with type 1 diabetes, we recommend a minimum of checking blood/CGM sugar levels before meals (and snacks) and at bedtime. Additional blood/CGM sugar checks may be needed with exercise, driving, on sick days, and with hypoglycemic episodes (and in follow-up). An ADA Position Statement on type 1 diabetes stated that **checking blood sugars 6-10 times daily** may be needed to safely achieve HbA1c goals. Although every person/family must learn to check blood sugars at the time of diagnosis, the eventual use of a CGM may reduce the number of blood sugar checks needed.

> **TOPICS:**
> **Monitoring Diabetes (checking blood sugar levels)**
>
> **TEACHING OBJECTIVES:**
> The teacher will:
> 1. Present blood sugar (glucose) concepts: rationale, times, frequency and desired ranges for the individual.
> 2. Provide instruction for the glucose meter.
> 3. Discuss how to troubleshoot problems with the meter.
> 4. Introduce the concept of following blood/CGM sugars and observing trends.
>
> **LEARNING OBJECTIVES:**
> Learner (parents, child, relative or self) will be able to:
> 1. Describe rationale for checking blood sugars and list times, frequency and desired ranges.
> 2. Demonstrate use of meter, including setting time and code when necessary.
> 3. Locate and state the 1-800 number listed on the meter to call for problems.
> 4. Choose and apply a method for following blood/CGM sugar results and recognizing trends.

The terms "sugar" and glucose are used interchangeably in this book. The use of blood/CGM indicates that the measurement may be by either method of checking.

FIGURE 1
Blood Sugar (or CGM) Values

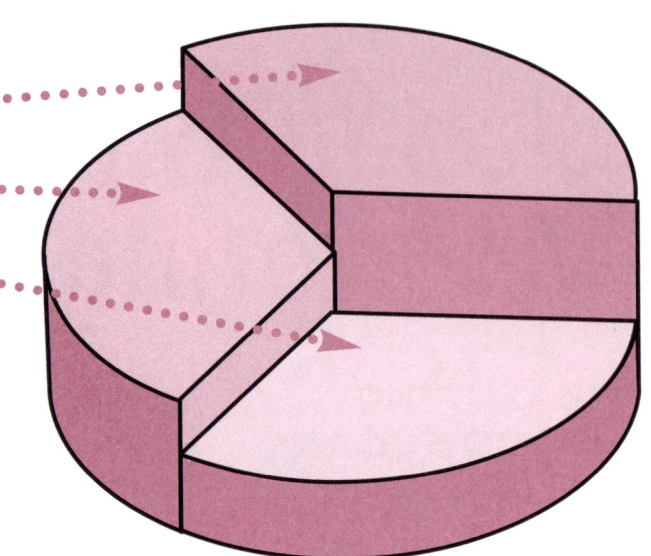

High = 35%
OK = 36%
Low = 29%

Graphs can be obtained from some of the blood sugar meters when they are brought to the clinic. This young man had a HbA1c (see Chapter 14) of 7.1 percent (54 mmol/mol), but was having too many high and low values. At least 70 percent of values should be in the target range (see suggested ranges for different ages in Table 4).

WHY DO BLOOD/CGM GLUCOSE MONITORING?

There are many reasons why checking blood/CGM sugars at home has become a "cornerstone" of diabetes care. Blood sugar measurements are usually used initially in diabetes management. Then, when the person/family is ready, CGM use can be initiated. CGM measures subcutaneous rather than blood sugar levels. Although Chapter 29 is devoted to CGM, reference to CGM is also included in this chapter.

Some of the reasons why measuring sugar levels is important are outlined below and in Table 1:

- **For safety:** A big reason for the use of blood/CGM sugar checking relates to safety. Almost no one feels all the low blood sugars that occur, and very young children may not report feeling any lows. Checking the blood/CGM sugar level before bedtime may help in choosing ways to reduce the occurrence of low blood sugars during the night. Doing a blood/CGM sugar check prior to driving is an absolute necessity.

- **To reduce the risk of hypoglycemia (Chapter 6) or diabetic ketoacidosis (DKA: Chapter 15):** Some people do not feel all of their low or high blood sugars. Checking blood/CGM sugar values (or hearing a CGM alarm) may reduce the likelihood of an acute episode of hypoglycemia or DKA.

- **To improve diabetes management:** Studies have clearly shown that doing a minimum of four blood sugars daily (or consistently using a CGM) and using the results wisely can result in overall improved sugar management. This results in a reduced risk for diabetic complications. Children and teenagers who reduce the number of blood sugar checks per day (if not wearing a CGM) usually have a rise in the HbA1c level.

- **To adjust the insulin dosage:** If blood/CGM sugar values are checked regularly, and the results are analyzed to look for patterns of lows or highs, the insulin dosage can be adjusted as needed. Chapter 22 provides examples of insulin adjustments based on blood/CGM glucose levels. People who take a rapid-acting insulin (Humalog or NovoLog) before meals can use the blood/CGM sugar value, along with the amount of food to be eaten and planned exercise, to decide how much insulin to take.

TABLE 1: Reasons for Blood/CGM Glucose Levels

- ✔ For safety (especially before driving a car)
- ✔ To reduce the risk of hypoglycemia and DKA
- ✔ To improve diabetes management
- ✔ To adjust the insulin dosage
- ✔ To manage illness/surgery
- ✔ To understand the effects of various foods, insulin doses, exercise or stress
- ✔ To discriminate a true low from a false low sugar episode
- ✔ To know the blood/CGM sugar level immediately
- ✔ To give people a sense of security
- ✔ As an indicator to check the urine or blood ketone level
- ✔ To know the time spent in range (CGM) and the time below or above range

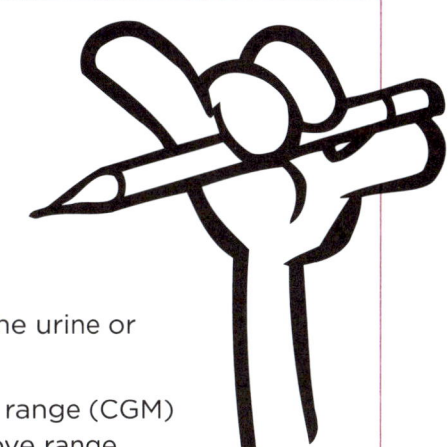

- **To manage illness/surgery:** Being able to check blood/CGM sugar values at home when a person is sick or before or after surgery allows for safe management at home. People who do not check their sugar levels frequently during an illness are more likely to become seriously ill and to be admitted to the hospital.

- **To understand the effects of various foods, insulin doses, exercise or stress:** By checking blood/CGM sugar values two hours after eating a certain food or doing a certain amount of exercise, one can better plan the insulin dose the next time. Pizza, for example, tends to raise blood sugars higher and longer than other foods for some people. If this is found to be true, extra rapid-acting insulin can be considered for the next time it is to be eaten. Similarly, some people lower or raise their blood sugar with a certain exercise, whereas others do not. Knowing the blood sugar value after doing the exercise a few times will help in future planning.

- **To discriminate a true low from a false low sugar episode:** Some people report symptoms of an insulin reaction when the blood sugar is still above 70 mg/dL (3.9 mmol/L). This may occur when the blood sugar falls rapidly (for example, from 300 to 150 mg/dL [16.7 to 8.3 mmol/L]) or for other unknown reasons. Checking a blood/CGM sugar level will help determine whether the symptoms are due to a true low sugar. If the level is above 70 mg/dL (3.9 mmol/L), it is helpful to eat food that is not high in sugar.

- **To know the blood sugar level immediately:** A blood/CGM sugar value will give helpful immediate results. For example, a child may be irritable and the cause unknown. The blood/CGM sugar value will help the parent decide whether the irritability is due to a low blood sugar level or to another cause. Another person may have an important event and just want to know the blood/CGM sugar value prior to starting the event.

- **To give people a sense of security:** Many people feel better knowing how their blood/CGM glucose values are running. However, it is important to remember that there may not always be an exact relationship between the blood sugar level and what one expects it to be. There are always unknown factors that result in occasional high or low levels. This can be upsetting for the person who expects blood/CGM sugar values to always be in the target range. It is important not to become

BLOOD/CGM SUGAR MONITORING

discouraged when results do not match the expected values. We emphasize that sugars are "in target" or "high" or "low," but not "good" or "bad." Questions or concerns about the blood/CGM sugar values should be discussed with the diabetes team.

- **As an indicator to check the urine or blood ketone level:** Blood/CGM sugar values above 300 mg/dL (16.7 mmol/L) indicate a need to check the blood or urine ketone level. (Some meters now even flash this advice.) Checking for blood or urine ketones when the sugar level is high may help to avoid an episode of ketoacidosis (see Chapter 15).

- If using a CGM, **knowing the time in range and the time below or above range** can be very helpful (see Chapter 29).

HOW TO DO SELF-BLOOD SUGAR LEVELS

• Finger-poking

A finger-poking (lancing) device is used to get the drop of blood. Families tend to choose their favorite device. Most lancing devices now have various intensity settings for different depths. For example, the ACCU-CHEK® FastClix has intensity settings from 0.5 to 5.5 and six lancets built-in for ease of changing. The adjustable pokers are particularly helpful for young children who have tender skin and may not need much lancing depth.

The hands should be washed with warm water (to increase blood flow and to make sure they are clean). **Any trace of sugar on the finger may give a false elevated reading.** We do not recommend routinely wiping with alcohol, because any trace of alcohol left on the skin will interfere with the chemical reaction for the blood sugar determination (Table 2). Alcohol also dries and toughens the skin. Occasionally, when away from home (e.g., camping, picnics), it is necessary to use alcohol-free travel wipes to cleanse the finger. Air dry the finger before doing the blood sugar check.

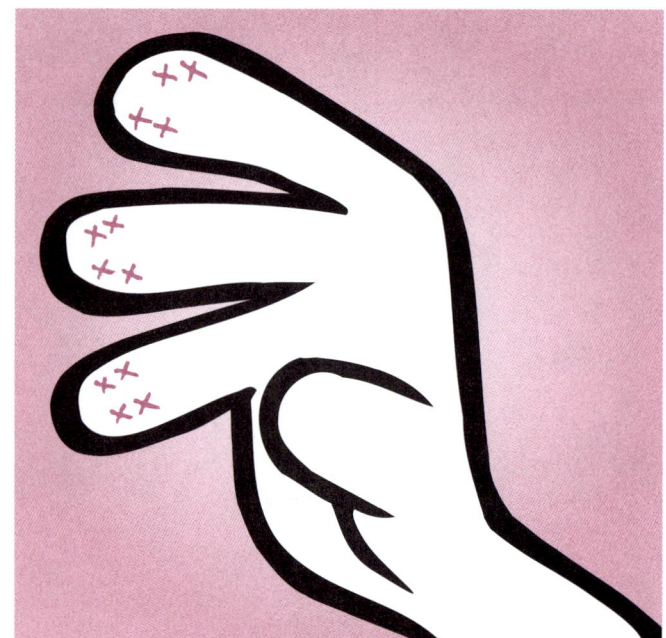

It is often helpful to place the finger to be used on a tabletop. This avoids the natural reflex of withdrawing the finger and not getting an adequate poke. The side of the finger should be used rather than the fleshy pad on the fingertip, which is more painful. If the drop is not coming easily, hold the hand down to the side of the body to increase the blood in the finger. IT IS IMPORTANT TO ROTATE FINGERS SO THAT ONE FINGER DOES NOT BECOME TOO "ABUSED." If the fingers become sore, the toes or the ball at the base of the thumb may be used.

• Alternate Sites for Blood Sugars

Some people use poking sites other than the fingers or toes. These sites are used because they may not hurt as much. The poker may need to be "dialed" to the maximum depth to get enough blood. The most common site is the forearm. The main problem has been that the blood flow through the arm is slower than through the fingertips. The slower blood flow means the blood sugar value from the arm may be 10 minutes or more **behind** the fingertip. It is important to rub the site to be used on the arm prior to doing the stick. The rubbing will increase the blood flow in the area. (The person may feel low or have a low value from a fingerstick, but the arm level will not be low.)

We advise **use of the fingertip if the person is feeling low.** Also, people who do not feel their lows (hypoglycemic unawareness, Chapter 6) should always use their fingertips for blood sugars. **Remember** to change the lancet every day. A sharp lancet will lessen injury to the site and help avoid an infection.

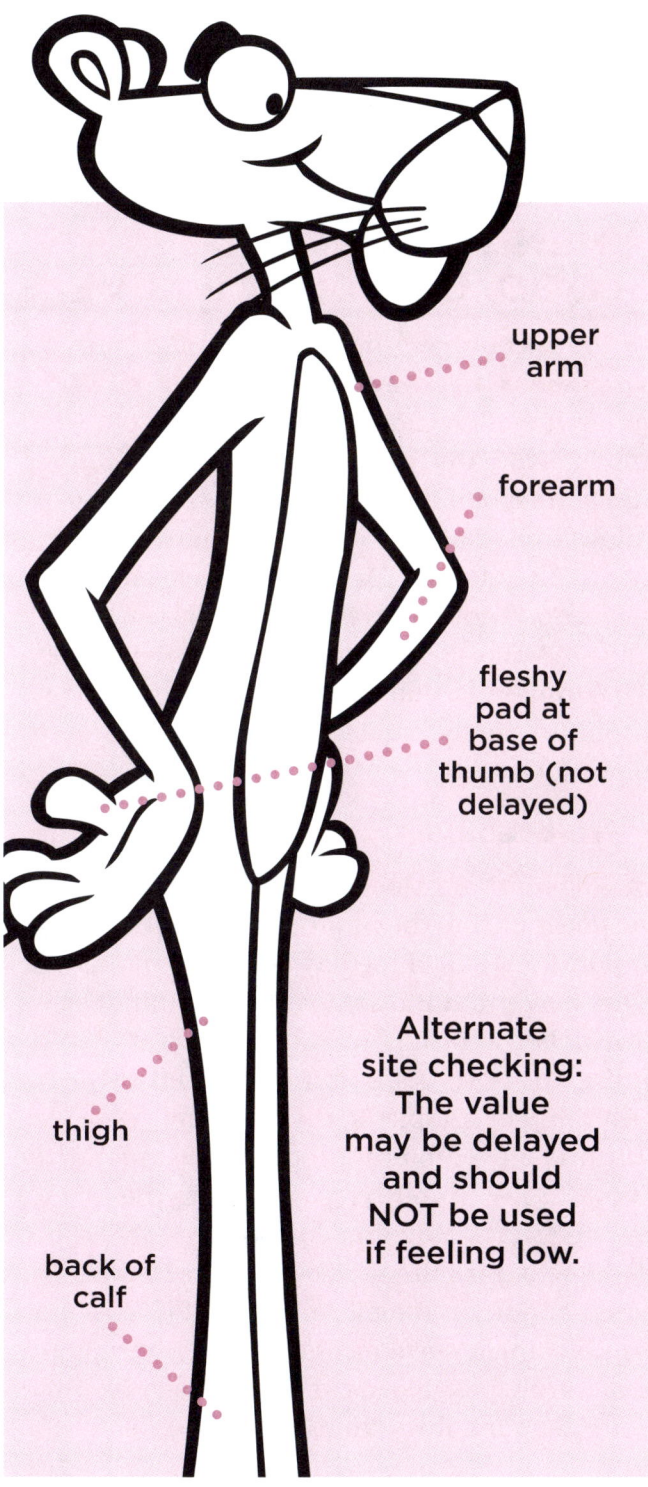

upper arm

forearm

fleshy pad at base of thumb (not delayed)

thigh

back of calf

Alternate site checking: The value may be delayed and should NOT be used if feeling low.

• Blood Sugar (Glucose) Meters

Some of the features in selecting a meter are listed in Table 3. The meter chosen should meet the person's needs. Some people leave a meter at school or at work. If using more than one meter, try to use the same brand. This will help with downloads. Families tend to prefer small meters that are easy to slip into a pocket. They also prefer meters that take a short time for the glucose determination. Particularly for younger children, the need for only a small amount of blood is helpful. Most of the strips now have a capillary action to pull the blood into the strip. This may be helpful for a small child who has difficulty holding still. For some people, accuracy in cold, heat, high humidity or high altitude is important. If a strip has been in a cooler or refrigerator (most strips spoil above 90° or if they freeze), they should always be brought to room temperature before using.

Often the main reason one meter is selected over another in the U.S. is that the family's health insurance will pay for that meter and its strips. The glucose strips usually add up to a cost of four or more U.S. dollars per day, so insurance coverage is important. The cost of strips is usually a more important factor than the cost of the meter. Some common problems causing inaccurate blood sugar results are shown in Table 2.

We do request that families choose a meter with a memory for at least the last 100 glucose values. **The meter(s) must always be brought to the clinic visit** so that it can be downloaded. The values as well as graphs, such as the pie-chart (Figure 1), can be printed. Some families like to download their blood sugar results in their homes. During the "honeymoon" phase (Chapter 2), or when the body still makes much of its own insulin, most of the blood/CGM sugar values will be in the desired range for age. For other people with diabetes, the goal should be to get 70 percent of the values at any time of day within range for that person's age. In contrast to our suggestion of different blood sugar targets

TABLE 2:
Common Problems Causing Inaccurate Blood Sugar Results

- Finger is not clean and dry (sugar on finger will raise result; alcohol or water will interfere)
- Strips have expired
- Strips have been exposed to heat (>90º, e.g., left in hot car) or frozen (e.g., left in cold car)
- Inaccurate meter

for different aged children (Table 4), the ADA recommended in 2015 that all children aim for levels of 90-130 mg/dL (5.0-7.2 mmol/L) before meals and levels of 90-150 mg/dL (5.0-8.3 mmol/L) at bedtime or overnight.

There are many different blood glucose meters available. Some inexpensive meters purchased in chain stores are not as accurate as meters obtained through reputable health insurance plans. Some meters offer more complex features, such as alarms, wireless connectivity, insulin dosing instructions, or transmission of data directly to a specific insulin pump or CGM. Our Center does not recommend one meter over another. However, four commonly used meters are the ONETOUCH® Verio Flex, the Contour® next ONE, the ACCU-CHEK® Guide, and any of the four FreeStyle meters. Features of the latest meters are readily available online.

WHEN TO CHECK BLOOD/CGM SUGAR LEVELS

We encourage people to do at least four blood sugar checks every day or to use a CGM. Values are often checked before breakfast, before lunch, before the afternoon snack before dinner, at bedtime, and during the night. Occasional values should also be done two hours after meals. The blood/CGM sugar goals for before meals and bedtime/overnight are shown in Table 4. Values should not exceed 180 mg/dL (10.0 mmol/L) at any time after meals. Some important times for checking (and the reasons) are as follows:

1. Pre-breakfast

The morning blood/CGM sugar value reflects the levels during the night and is the most important value of the day related to diabetes management. It is also used to determine the dose of basal insulin, no matter when it's given during the day. As shown in the figure at the beginning of Chapter 2, this value reflects the "turning off" of internal sugar production by the liver. It is not usually elevated due to the bedtime snack or eating during the night. The rapid-acting insulin dose at breakfast is also based in part on the morning blood/CGM sugar result. Using a basal insulin or an insulin pump, it is usually possible to get the majority of fasting sugar values "in range" (see Table 4).

TABLE 3:
Desired Features of Blood Glucose Meters

- Accurate (in environment where it is to be used)
- Strips are paid for by the family's insurance
- Storage of at least the last 100 values
- Able to be downloaded at clinic and/or at home
- Small in size
- Short determination time
- Small drop of blood (capillary action of strip)
- Wireless connectivity
- Insulin dosing assistance
- A control solution or strip can be used to check for accuracy

TABLE 4:
Blood/CGM Glucose Levels in mg/dL (mmol/L)

NON-DIABETIC NORMAL VALUES*

Normal (fasting)**	70-100 (3.9-5.5)
Normal (random)	70-140 (3.9-7.8)

GOALS FOR PEOPLE WITH DIABETES*

Diabetes management recommendations always need to be tailored to the individual. Higher targets may be considered if: history of hypoglycemic unawareness/severe hypoglycemia, use of NPH at bedtime, poor access to blood sugar strips or CGM, very low insulin requirements, athletes, and infants or toddlers. In young children, use of a CGM and/or an insulin pump may be necessary to reach goals safely.

	Before Meals/Fasting	Bedtime/Overnight
0-5 years	70-150 (3.9-8.3)	100-180*** (5.5-10.0)
6-17 years	70-130 (3.9-7.2)	90-150*** (5.0-8.3)
18 years and up	70-130 (3.9-7.2)	90-150*** (5.0-8.3)

Low Values*		Possible Symptoms
Low	Below 70 (Below 3.9)	Sweating Hunger Shakiness
"True low"	Below 60 (Below 3.3)	Confusion. If not treated, can lead to seizure or unconsciousness episode

Desired Range	70-180 (3.9-10.0)	

High Values*		Possible Symptoms
High	180-400 (10.2-22.2)	Low energy Frequent urination
Very high	400-800 (22.2-44.4)	Stomachache Rapid breathing If not treated, can lead to DKA

Remember to check ketones if >300 mg/dL (16.7 mmol/L)

*Blood/CGM glucose levels in mg/dL (mmol/L)
**Most values for non-diabetic children are in this range. However, occasional values down to 60 mg/dL (3.3 mmol/L) are still normal.
***If a very heavy exercise day, 130 mg/dL (7.2 mmol/L) might be a better lower level.

BLOOD/CGM SUGAR MONITORING

TABLE 5: Daily Record Sheet

To Nurse Educator: _____ Physician: _____

Patient _____ Date of Birth _____ Parents: _____

Phone: _____ Best time (8 a.m. - 5 p.m.) to reach you: _____

Date		Breakfast		Other (optional)		Lunch		Other (optional)		Dinner		Bedtime		Comments (Activity, illness, snacks, etc. …)
		Results	Insulin Dose	Results	Insulin Dose	Results	Insulin Dose	Results	Insulin Dose	Results	Insulin Dose	Results	Insulin Dose	
	Time:													
	BG/Ket:													
	Time:													
	BG/Ket:													
	Time:													
	BG/Ket:													
	Time:													
	BG/Ket:													
	Time:													
	BG/Ket:													
	Time:													
	BG/Ket:													
	Time:													
	BG/Ket:													

Ket = Ketones

Problem Area(s) Noted: _____ Suggested Solution(s): _____

Please note: Make sure insulin doses are included under "Insulin Dose" heading.

BLOOD/CGM SUGAR MONITORING

2. Pre-lunch

A blood/CGM sugar value before lunch helps to decide if the morning rapid-acting insulin (or Regular insulin) dosage is correct. For people using morning NPH insulin, it may also be having an effect at this time. Families of school children should routinely request that a value be done prior to eating lunch. The value, along with expected carbs to be eaten, is used to determine the lunch insulin dose. For most children (and schools), doing a blood sugar is not a problem and can be done without interfering with the child's normal school life.

3. Pre-dinner

The blood/CGM sugar value before dinner reflects the dose of morning NPH insulin (if taken) and/or the dose of rapid-acting insulin given at lunch. It may also reflect afternoon sports activities and the food eaten for an afternoon snack. **Youth who eat a large afternoon snack (or at other times) should use Humalog or NovoLog to cover the food to be eaten.** The pre-dinner value will then tell if the dose given was correct. The value also is used along with the expected carbs to be eaten in determining the dinner insulin dose.

4. Bedtime

The blood/CGM sugar value prior to bedtime is important for all people with diabetes. It is particularly important for:

- people who tend to have low sugars during the night
- people who play or exercise after dinner or who have had heavy exercise that day
- anyone who did not eat well at dinner
- knowing if the rapid-acting insulin dose given at dinner is correct

As can be seen in Table 4, suggested bedtime blood/CGM sugar values are given for the different ages. **If the values are below the lower level (three stars), doing a follow-up blood sugar check during the night is wise.** These values may be different for each person.

5. After meals

In recent years, more emphasis has been placed on checking blood/CGM sugar values two hours after eating a meal. The highest blood sugars of the day occur after meals, and these values add to the HbA1c value (Chapter 14). More people are now using carbohydrate counting. They may inject insulin 20 minutes prior to meals based on their expected carbohydrate intake (Chapter 12) and the pre-meal glucose. The blood/CGM sugar values two hours after the meal confirm if the **I**nsulin to **C**arbohydrate ratio (**I/C** ratio – Chapter 12) and the estimated carbohydrates were correct. **The blood/CGM glucose values listed in Table 4 by age can also be the goals for two hours after meals.** The American Diabetes Association recommends that all post-meal values be below 180 mg/dL (10.0 mmol/L). The use of CGM has been very helpful in monitoring post-meal values. We would recommend that families check blood/CGM glucose values two hours after each meal a few times each week. If a log is kept, values obtained two hours after meals can be flagged by a symbol such as a star.

6. Nighttime

It may be necessary to occasionally check blood/CGM glucose values in the middle of the night (see Chapter 6 on Low Blood Sugar) to make sure the value is not getting too low. This is particularly true after a heavy exercise day. The diabetes care-provider may suggest this if very erratic results are noted for the morning blood sugars. The use of CGM can be very helpful in evaluating nighttime values.

A nighttime blood/CGM glucose value is particularly important for people who tend to have reactions (low blood sugars) during the night. More than half of the severe low sugars occur during the nighttime hours. Many families will routinely do a level during the night. Others choose to do a value once or twice weekly. **IT IS IMPORTANT TO CHECK THE LEVELS ON NIGHTS WHEN THERE HAS BEEN**

EXTRA DAYTIME PHYSICAL ACTIVITY. For a younger child, it might be playing hard outside during the day or on a nice summer evening. The best time to do a check varies with each person. For some, between midnight and 2 a.m. is the best. For others, the early morning hours are the most valuable – perhaps when a parent is getting ready for work. Table 4 gives suggested values for during the night. The use of a CGM in combination with an insulin pump may allow suspension of insulin with a low or predicted low glucose level (Chapters 28 and 29). This has been very helpful in reducing the frequency of severe nighttime lows.

7. With low blood sugar

As noted above, doing a blood sugar when feeling low helps to separate a "false low" from a "true low" (<70 mg/dL [or <3.9 mmol/L]). A food with sugar must be given for a "true low," whereas other food may be given (e.g., cheese, peanut butter) for values above 70 mg/dL (>3.9 mmol/L).

RECORD KEEPING

An example of a daily record sheet is included in this chapter (Table 5). Many families will fax or email the page or download data from their meter or CGM to their diabetes care-provider if they have concerns. If this is done, make sure the insulin dosages and instructions for return fax or phone contact are included. These sheets may be copied and stored in a notebook to bring along to clinic visits. Evaluating records to look for patterns in blood sugar fluctuations is essential. **Patterns of high or low blood/CGM glucose levels will be missed if results are not analyzed at regular intervals.** It is important to note all reactions and possible causes. Some people also circle or highlight all values below 60 mg/dL (<3.3 mmol/L) or put a star on days of reactions so that these can be easily noted by the diabetes care-providers. If times of heavy exercise are recorded, it may be possible to see the effects of exercise on blood/CGM glucose values. Illnesses,

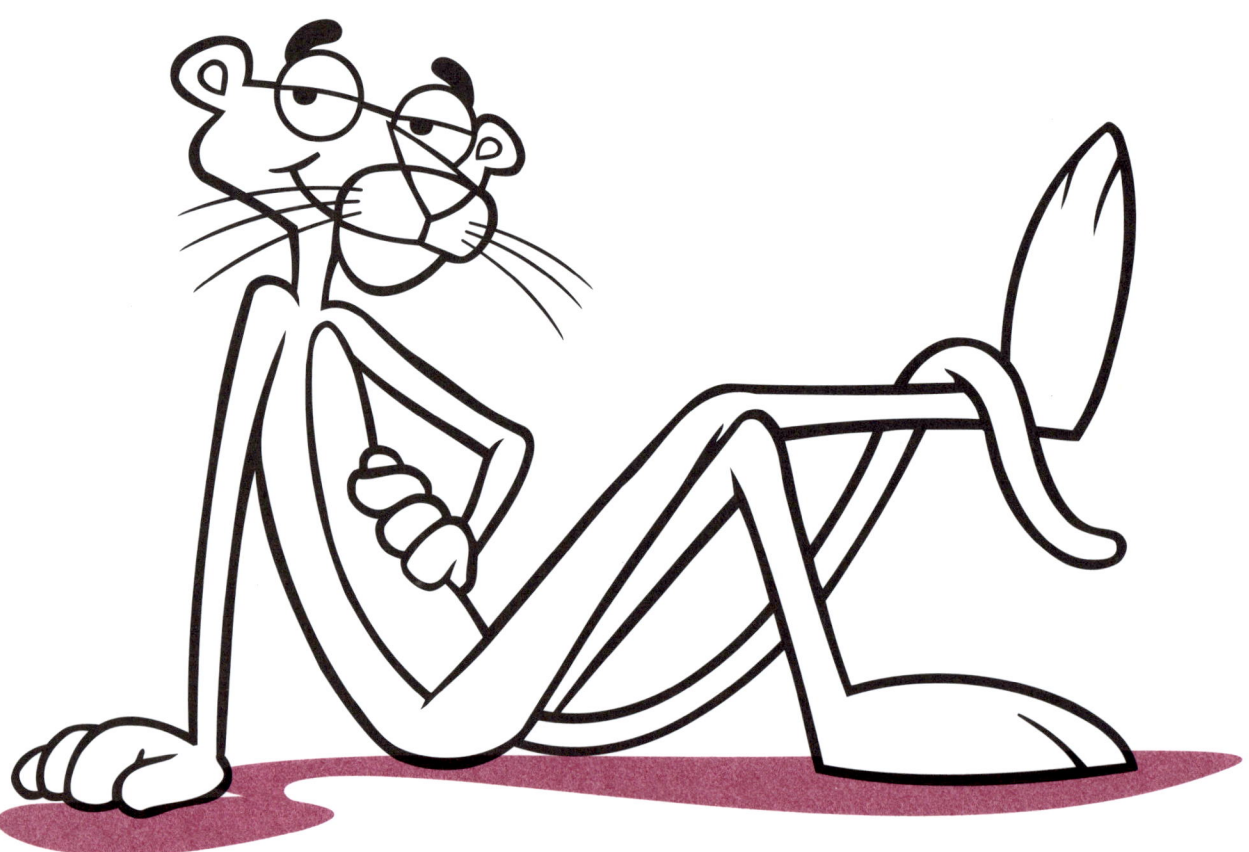

stress and menstrual periods may increase the blood sugar and should be noted. It may be helpful to record what was eaten for the bedtime snack and if there was heavy exercise to see if these are related to morning blood/CGM glucose values. Also included is a place to record urine or blood ketone checks, as newly-diagnosed people must check their ketones frequently. Ketone checks (Chapter 5) are essential with any symptoms of illness or anytime the blood/CGM glucose level is above 300 mg/dL (>16.7 mmol/L).

The insulin dose can be recorded with the units of rapid-acting insulin on top (e.g., 5H or 5NL) and the units of intermediate-acting insulin on the bottom (e.g., 15N).

Fastidious record keeping (or regular viewing of computer downloads) and bringing the results to clinic visits allow the family and diabetes team to work together most effectively to achieve optimal diabetes management. Complacency and not following values often results in missing patterns of high blood/CGM glucose values and a resultant high HbA1c value. We also encourage families who send blood/CGM sugar results and who have questions to suggest solutions, which can be discussed with the doctor or nurse.

DEFINITIONS

Artificial Pancreas: The combination of a CGM, insulin pump and algorithms (mathematical formulas) to automatically change (or temporarily discontinue) insulin dosages.

Continuous Glucose Monitor (CGM): Medical devices that measure a person's glucose levels every five minutes. They use a small sensor that is placed under the skin (see Chapter 29).

DCCT: Diabetes Control and Complications Trial. This trial was completed in June 1993 and clearly showed that eye, nerve and heart complications of diabetes were related to glucose management (see Chapter 14).

Glucose: The scientific name for the sugar in the blood or urine. It is used interchangeably with the word sugar.

Insulin reaction (hypoglycemia): A term for a blood/CGM sugar level that is too low (see Chapter 6).

mg/dL and mmol/L: Milligrams of material in 100 cc of fluid or millimoles of material in one liter of fluid. Blood sugar (glucose) levels are expressed in mg/dL in the U.S., but they are usually expressed as mmol/L in Europe. It is possible to convert mg/dL to mmol/L by dividing by 18 (or multiplying by 0.0555). The opposite is done to go from mmol/L to mg/dL. A conversion table for glucose values is in the Appendix.

Monitoring: As used in this chapter, keeping track of and following blood sugar levels at home and analyzing them in a record book or with a computer download.

Subcutaneous: Under the skin (but not in a blood vessel).

QUESTIONS AND ANSWERS FROM NEWSNOTES

Q: What is the best range for my morning blood/CGM glucose values?

A: There is not one answer for all people. It depends on the individual person and family as well as the age of the person with diabetes. Textbooks list a normal fasting level (or when no food is taken for two or more hours) as 70-100 mg/dL (3.9-5.5 mmol/L). It is unrealistic for most people with diabetes to aim for normal non-diabetic fasting sugar levels. Suggested values by age for people with diabetes are given in Table 4. However, these are "generally suggested ranges" for fasting or if there is no food intake for at least two hours, and each individual or family must adapt these to their situation. In contrast, the 2015 ADA recommendations for glucose levels for all pediatric age groups are 90-150 mg/dL (5.0-8.3 mmol/L) at bedtime and overnight, and 90-130 mg/dL (5.0-7.2 mmol/L) before meals (no age differences).

A person who has had severe episodes of unrecognized hypoglycemia might be wise to choose a higher range. This might help to reduce the severe insulin reactions.

It is wise to discuss the levels of blood/CGM glucose values to aim for with your care-provider at each clinic visit.

Q: Do I need to check my child's blood/CGM glucose value every morning at 2:00 a.m.?

A: For most children, this is NOT necessary. However, occasional checks during the night are helpful. Special circumstances that make nighttime checks more important include any illness, a low blood/CGM glucose value before bedtime, or previous frequent lows during the night.

Q: With most glucose meters and CGMs having memories of glucose values which can be printed out in the clinic, do I still need to write down every blood sugar value?

A: Most meters and CGMs can be downloaded using the family's home computer. FAMILIES MUST DEVELOP A SYSTEM TO LOOK AT VALUES TOGETHER AT REGULAR INTERVALS. They are otherwise not making optimal use of their data. We often ask for weekly faxes or emails if diabetes management is suboptimal and we think the family needs extra help.

Q: Our family does everything by email now. Is there a way I can get the blood glucose fax sheets from Chapter 7 of the Pink Panther book on my computer?

A: Yes, this can now be easily done. Table 5 in this chapter can also be scanned and emailed. Families wanting to use these electronic forms to email to their doctor or nurse can get them from the Barbara Davis Center home page at: www.barbaradaviscenter.org. Next, go to Books Online, to *Understanding Diabetes*. You can then select pages and email them to your doctor and nurse at your Center. The email address at my clinic is:

_____

It is <u>essential</u> for you to give phone numbers and the time to get back to you, as it is often best to actively discuss the blood sugar/CGM results and insulin doses.

CHAPTER 8

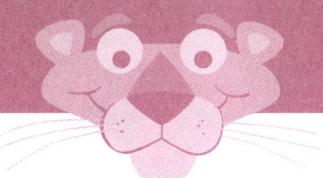

Insulin: Types and Activity

INSULIN

Before insulin was discovered in 1921, there was no successful treatment for people who had type 1 diabetes. Since then, millions of people all over the world have been helped by insulin.

Insulin is a hormone made in the pancreas, an organ inside the abdomen (see picture in Chapter 2). Special cells called "beta cells" make the insulin. These cells are located in a part of the pancreas called the "islets" (pronounced eye-lets). When a person has type 1 diabetes, there is a loss of the cells which make insulin. Most people with diabetes now use human insulin or insulin analogs. The human insulin does not come from humans, but has the same make-up as human insulin. There are no known advantages of one brand of insulin over another brand. The analog insulins have slight changes that make their activity more closely resemble normal insulin activity.

Insulin must be stored so that it does not freeze or get over 90° F (32° C), because it will spoil. Otherwise, the insulin vial being used can be kept at room temperature for 30 days.

WHAT DOES INSULIN DO?

Food (carbohydrate) is converted to sugar for the body's energy needs. The insulin allows the sugar to pass from the blood into the cells. There it is burned for energy. The body cannot turn sugar into energy without insulin (see diagram in Chapter 2). If insulin is not available, sugar cannot pass into cells, so it builds up in the blood and spills into the urine. Insulin also turns off the production of sugar from the liver (see Chapter 2). The goal of insulin treatment is to use insulin shots to replace what the body's pancreas normally does.

People who have type 1 diabetes can't make enough insulin. These people have to get their needed insulin through injections. Insulin cannot be taken as a pill, because the stomach acid destroys it. There are no known vitamins, herbs or other medications that can take the place of insulin injections. People who have type 2 diabetes still make insulin (although not enough to keep their sugars in a normal range; see Chapter 4). They can take pills to help them

---

TOPICS:
Medications (Insulin)

TEACHING OBJECTIVES:
The teacher will:
1. Describe insulin and what it does in the body.
2. Present the types of insulins to be used and their actions.
3. Discuss the schedule for insulin injections.
4. Identify who and when to call for insulin doses.

LEARNING OBJECTIVES:
Learner (parents, child, relative or self) will be able to:
1. State why the body needs insulin.
2. List the specific types of insulins to be used and their actions (onset, peak and duration).
3. State the schedule for insulin injections (including before or after meals).
4. Identify who and when to call for insulin doses.

Two of the most common methods of using Lantus (Basaglar), Levemir or Tresiba insulin:

FIGURE 1-A

Use of Lantus (Basaglar), Levemir or Tresiba Insulin

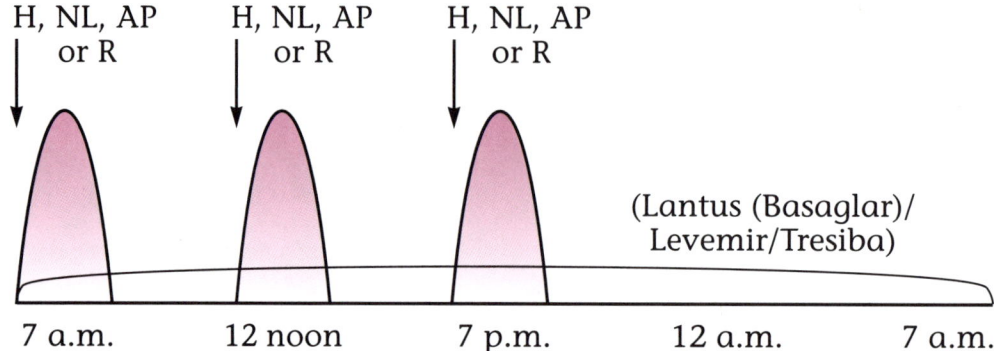

In the first example, Lantus (Basaglar), Levemir or Tresiba is used as the basal insulin (given in the a.m., or at dinner or at bedtime) and a rapid-acting insulin is taken 20 minutes prior to meals and snacks. This is often referred to as basal-bolus insulin therapy.

FIGURE 1-B

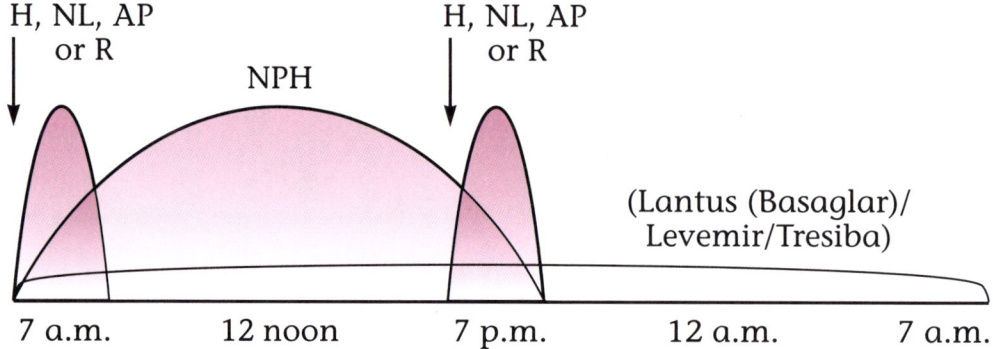

In this second example, NPH and a rapid-acting insulin are taken in one syringe in the a.m. A rapid-acting insulin is taken alone at dinner. Lantus (Basaglar), Levemir, or Tresiba is taken consistently either in the a.m., at dinner, or at bedtime.

make even more insulin or to be more sensitive to their own insulin. However, these pills <u>are not</u> insulin, nor are they effective for type 1 diabetes.

Insulin can be given using a syringe (and a vial of insulin) or by an insulin pen (Chapter 9). Although using a pen is more convenient, it is sometimes more expensive (depending on the insurance company). It is not possible to mix two insulins in a pen.

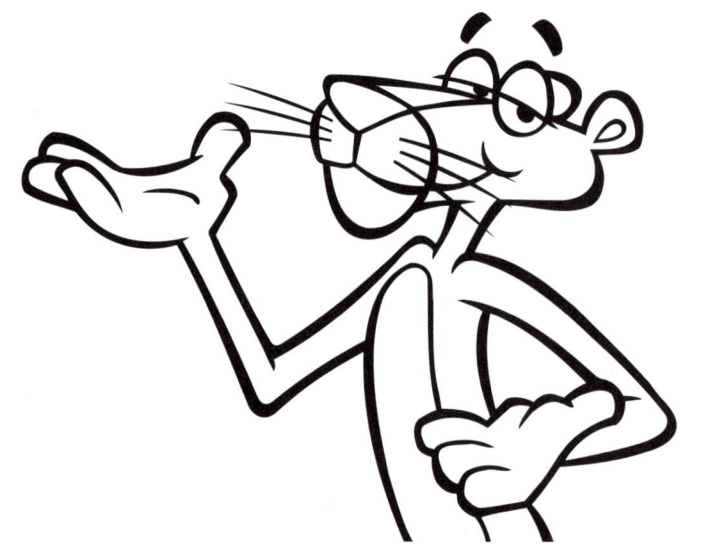

INSULIN: TYPES AND ACTIVITY

TABLE 1: Insulin Activities

Type of Insulin	Begins Working	Main Effect	All Gone
Normal (RAPID-ACTING/SHORT-LASTING			
Humalog (Admelog)/NovoLog/Apidra	15 minutes	90 minutes	3-4 hours
Regular	30-60 minutes	2-4 hours	6-9 hours
INTERMEDIATE-LASTING			
NPH	1-2 hours	4-8 hours	12-15 hours
LONG-LASTING/BASAL			
Lantus (Basaglar)	1-2 hours	2-22 hours	24 hours
Levemir	1-2 hours	2-20 hours	20-24 hours
ULTRA-LONG-LASTING			
Tresiba (insulin Degludec)	1-2 hours	24 hours	72 hours
PRE-MIXED INSULINS			
70/30 NPH/Regular	30-60 minutes	3-8 hours	12-15 hours
75/25 NPH/Humalog	20 minutes	90 minutes - 8 hours	12-15 hours

TYPES OF INSULIN

Several companies make many different types of insulins.

The four broad classes of insulin are:
1. "rapid-acting/short-lasting" (such as Humalog [H], NovoLog [NL] and Apidra [AP]) and, to a lesser extent, Regular (R) insulin
2. "intermediate-lasting" (such as NPH [N])
3. "long-lasting" such as Lantus® (Basaglar) and Levemir®
4. "ultra-long-lasting" such as Tresiba (Degludec)

Insulin action (when it begins working, when it peaks in activity and how long it lasts) may vary slightly from person to person. The action may also vary from one day to the next in the same person. The site of the shot and exercise may influence the insulin action. Increased temperature (bath, shower, hot tub, sauna) may increase blood supply to the skin and cause the insulin to be absorbed more rapidly. Physical activity, or lack of it, can also have an effect. Average times of action for different insulins are shown in Table 1. Commonly used insulins are listed in Table 2.

1. Rapid-Acting/Short-Lasting Insulin (lasts 3-4 hours) and Regular Insulin (lasts 6-9 hours)

Humalog (Admelog), NovoLog or Apidra (H, NL or AP) insulins are rapid in **onset** of activity (10-20 minutes) and are short-lasting. They have a **peak** activity in approximately 90 minutes and effectively last three to four hours. They are usually given to allow the sugar in meals to be used by the body. Figure 1 shows the activities of the rapid-acting insulins given prior to all meals (1-A) or prior to breakfast and

FIGURE 2
Blood Glucose Levels Before or After a Meal

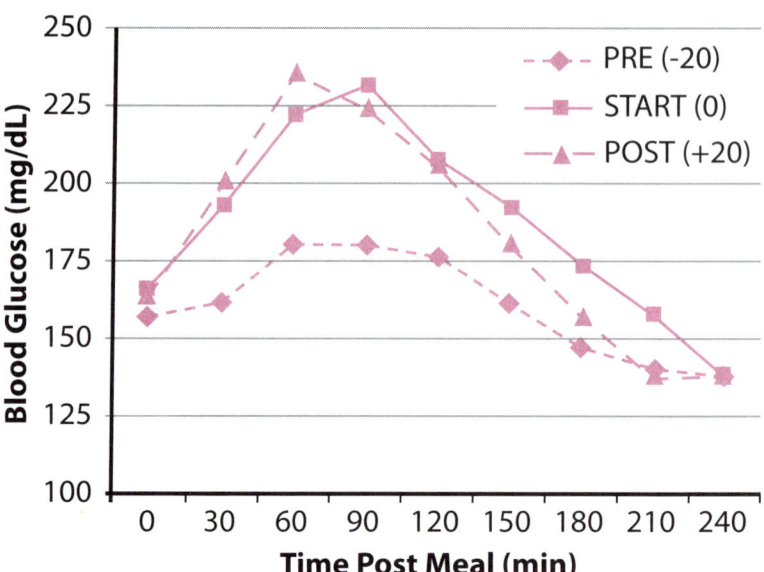

Blood glucose levels when a rapid-acting insulin was given 20 minutes prior to a meal ("PRE"), at the beginning of the meal ("START"), or after the meal ("POST"). The ADA goal for blood sugars at any time after a meal is to not exceed 180 mg/dL (10.0 mmol/L).

(Reproduced with permission of Diabetes Technology and Therapeutics 12:173, 2010)

---

dinner (1-B). After the honeymoon period, the rapid-acting insulins are usually also given to cover snacks and high blood sugars. All three rapid-acting insulins are similar in activity. We use the term "rapid-acting insulin" to indicate that the insulin used may be any one of the three (H, NL or AP). Although these rapid-acting insulins have been an advance over Regular insulin in terms of onset of action, they still do NOT start working or reach a peak in activity as quickly as desired. This is because the blood (or continuous glucose monitor [CGM]) glucose level usually peaks in 60 minutes after food is eaten, whereas H, NL, and AP do not peak in activity until 90 minutes after being given. By taking the H, NL or AP 20 minutes prior to eating, the insulin peak and blood/CGM glucose peak are more closely matched. As a result, the blood/CGM glucose values are not as high after meals (Figure 2).

Fiasp® (fast-acting insulin aspart) is a faster-acting form of NovoLog. It is available in a Fiasp® FlexTouch® Pen or Penfill® cartridge.

Lyumjer® (fast-acting Humalog) was approved by the FDA in June, 2020. This new *Insulin lispro aabc* is available as a U-100 or U-200 insulin.

Regular insulin begins to act approximately 30-60 minutes after being injected. It is thus best taken 30 to 60 minutes prior to a meal. It has its peak effect two to four hours after the injection and lasts six to nine hours. There is variability in these times from person to person.

Humalog/NovoLog/Apidra (H/NL/AP) insulins have several advantages over Regular insulin:

- They start working in 10-20 minutes, rather than in 30-60 minutes as does Regular insulin. They also reach peak activity more rapidly (approximately 90 minutes) than does Regular insulin (approximately 2 to 4 hours). Finally, they do not last as long (3-4 hours) as Regular insulin (6-9 hours).

- Because the rapid-acting insulin does not last as long as Regular insulin, there is less danger of lows several hours after meals or during the night.

- Use of rapid-acting insulin after meals in toddlers who eat varying amounts can help to avoid hypoglycemia as well as food struggles (Chapters 18 and 19). In this case, the higher blood/CGM sugar values are a compromise for safety.

FIGURE 3

Example of Two Injections/Day Using a Rapid-Acting Insulin (or Regular) and NPH (H=Humalog, NL=NovoLog, AP= Apidra, R=Regular insulin)

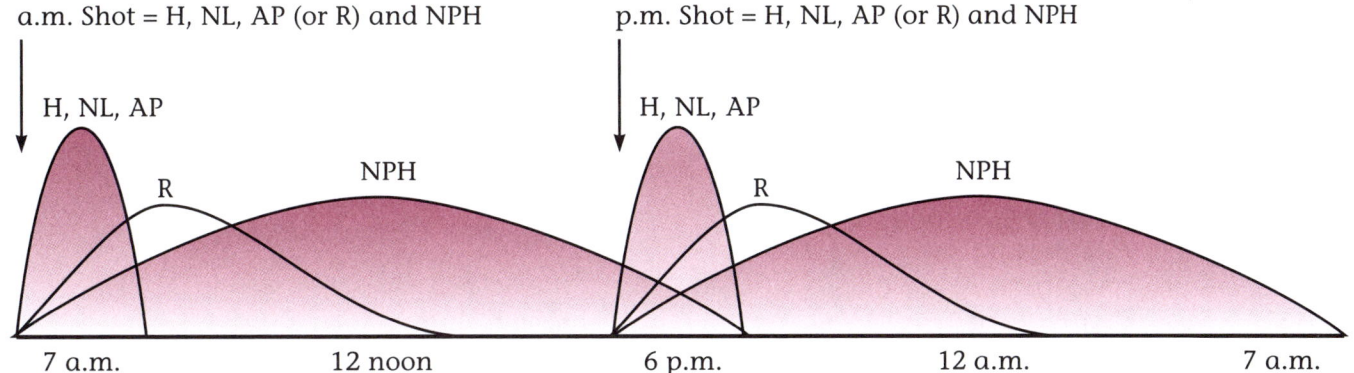

Many people receive two injections per day. NPH and a rapid-acting insulin (or Regular) are given prior to breakfast and dinner. When possible, the insulin should be given 20 minutes prior to the meal.

It is important to remember to avoid taking a warm shower or bath, or getting into a hot tub for one to two hours after taking a rapid-acting or Regular insulin. The warm water increases the blood flow to the skin and causes the insulin to be absorbed faster. This faster rate of absorption could cause a low blood sugar.

2. Intermediate-Lasting Insulin (lasts 10-13 hours)

✓ **NPH (N) insulin**, also referred to as "cloudy" insulin, is made with a protein that allows it to be absorbed in the body more slowly. The letters NPH stand for **N**eutral **P**rotamine **H**agedorn. Protamine is the protein added to the insulin to make it longer-acting. Hagedorn is the name of the man who developed it. Human NPH has its peak activity four to eight hours after the injection in most people. It is often taken twice daily (Figure 3) in countries in which a basal insulin is not available. If it is taken in the morning, the peak action usually comes in the midday to afternoon. NPH insulin can be used in the morning for children who are unable to receive a noon injection of H, NL or AP (Figure 1-B). Human NPH insulin lasts an average of 13 hours. The peak in NPH insulin activity and the duration of activity may vary in the same person from day to day. NPH insulin may be pre-mixed with Regular or H, NL or AP insulin without changing the activities of either insulin. NPH is often called "N" on the bottles.

✓ **Pre-mixed Insulins:** The pre-mixed insulins are used primarily by people who do not have access to basal or rapid-acting insulins or do not wish to draw the insulins from separate vials prior to injecting. They have the disadvantage that the percentage of each insulin is fixed and the individual insulins cannot be varied (for blood sugar, exercise, food, illness, etc.). There are many mixtures available and only a few examples will be given.

• **70/30® and Mixtard®:** Different combinations of pre-mixed NPH and Regular insulin are available. The most frequently used are 70/30 and Mixtard, both of which have 70 percent NPH and 30 percent Regular insulins. (In Europe and

INSULIN: TYPES AND ACTIVITY

many countries, the order of the insulin mixture is reversed, i.e., 30/70 meaning 30 percent Regular and 70 percent NPH.) The usual times of activity are shown in Table 1.

- **Humalog mix 75/25** (Lilly) is also a combination of a rapid (25 percent) and an intermediate-acting (75 percent) insulin.

- **NovoLog Mix 70/30** (Novo-Nordisk) is a mixture of 70 percent NPH and 30 percent NovoLog (or 30/70 in Europe and many countries).

3. Long-Lasting (basal) Insulins (last 20-24 hours)

✓ **Lantus (or Basaglar)** is a clear insulin that lasts 24 hours with almost no peak (a basal insulin). Its profile is similar to the basal insulin put out by a normal pancreas. It is often compared with the basal insulin of an insulin pump (Chapter 28).

✓ **Levemir (Insulin detemir)** is made by Novo-Nordisk and is also a basal insulin. Its duration is 20 to 24 hours. It may need to be taken twice daily by some people. It is a clear insulin. There is also some evidence it may help with weight loss.

4. Ultra-Long-Lasting Insulin

✓ **Tresiba (Degludec)** lasts up to 72 hours and is also a clear insulin. Although it has some activity over 36 hours, its main activity is over 24 hours. Levels are very consistent, which may help to reduce nighttime lows.

USE OF BASAL INSULINS (Lantus [Basaglar], Levemir or Tresiba insulin):

- The basal insulin can be taken once daily (either consistently in the morning, at dinner or in the evening). A rapid-acting insulin (H/NL/AP) is then taken 20 minutes before each meal (see Figure 1-A). The pre-meal insulin is often taken with an insulin pen. An advantage of taking the Lantus (Basaglar) or Levemir in the morning is that if some of the injection is accidentally given into muscle, there may be a peak in early activity (after two to four hours). If this occurs, it is better to have it happen during the daytime. As discussed in Chapter 9, intramuscular injections are least apt to occur when using the buttocks. There may also be an increase in peak insulin activity when taking large doses of Lantus or Levemir insulin. The best time to take the basal insulin should be considered jointly between the family and care-providers.

- If the activity does diminish at 22-24 hours, it may be best to have this happen in the early morning hours, **especially for very young children or those in the honeymoon phase.**

- For infants or those who have trouble with shots, the basal insulin can be given (often in the buttocks) while they are sleeping. Lantus tends to last the full 24 hours more readily than Levemir, which sometimes has to be given twice daily. However, Lantus (initially) may sting more than Levemir. Tresiba has consistent activity over 24 hours.

- In addition to the morning basal insulin, a mixture of NPH and H/NL/AP is sometimes taken 20 minutes prior to breakfast (see Figure 1-B). For children who are unable to take a noon shot at school, this is an option. However, NPH at breakfast to cover lunch and afternoon snacks does not match up as well as multiple doses of rapid-acting insulin. Some people who take a noon shot still do better with a small amount of NPH insulin in the morning.

Lantus (Basaglar), Levemir or Tresiba Dose: The starting dose is often half the total units of intermediate-acting insulin (e.g., NPH) taken per day (a.m. and p.m.).

For example:

If 40 units of NPH insulin was taken in the morning and 20 units at dinner, a total of 60 units was taken per day. We would then start the person on 30 units of basal insulin.

This dose can then be increased or decreased depending on morning blood/CGM glucose levels. The basal insulin dose is adjusted based on morning glucose values, no matter when the dose is given.

The goal for the morning and pre-meal blood/CGM glucose values (Chapter 7) is:

Under 6 years of age: 70-150 mg/dL (3.9-8.3 mmol/L)

6-17 years of age: 70-130 mg/dL (3.9-7.2 mmol/L)

>18 years: 70-130 mg/dL (3.9-7.2 mmol/L)

It is important to bring morning fasting blood/CGM glucose levels in range. If the day starts with high values, subsequent values are also often high from continued liver production of sugar (Chapter 2).

Basal-Bolus Insulin Therapy/Intensive Diabetes Management

Intensive Diabetes Management involves:

- Four or more shots of insulin per day (or use of an insulin pump)
- Checking blood sugar levels four or more times per day (or use of a CGM)
- Paying attention to food intake
- Frequent communication with the healthcare-provider
- Daily exercise

The Diabetes Control and Complications Trial (DCCT) used Intensive Diabetes Management to show that sugar levels "closer to normal" helped to reduce the likelihood of the chronic complications of type 1 diabetes (Chapter 14). Similar studies have shown this to also be true for type 2 diabetes. Most diabetes doctors now recommend intensive diabetes management for all people with type 1 diabetes (after the honeymoon period). The goal of intensive management is to keep the blood/CGM glucose levels as close to normal as possible without hypoglycemia. For intensive therapy to be safe, frequent blood/CGM glucose values are needed. An ADA Position Statement on type 1 diabetes advised six to 10 blood glucose checks daily (or use of a CGM) to safely achieve HbA1c goals. Intensive diabetes management can be accomplished using Lantus (Basaglar), Levemir, or Tresiba insulin (once daily) and a rapid-acting insulin 20 minutes prior to food intake. Insulin pumps (Chapter 28) provide an alternative and have become safer and more popular in recent years.

Comparison of Lantus (Basaglar)/Levemir or Tresiba Insulin with NPH Insulin:

- The differences in activity can be seen in Figure 1-B.

- The basal insulins are more consistent in absorption and activity than the NPH insulin. NPH varies in its peak activity even in the same person from one day to the next. The basal insulins do not have as great a peak as NPH insulin (unless accidentally injected into the muscle).

- Because they are clear insulins, they do not need to be turned up and down to mix (as with NPH). There is no settling in the vial and insulin concentrations do not vary from one shot to the next.

- Studies have shown a decrease in low blood/CGM glucose values, particularly during the night, when compared with using NPH insulin twice daily. This is due to less of a peak in activity (particularly at night, see Figure 3), as well as to more consistent absorption.

- When using a basal insulin, three or more shots per day of rapid-acting insulin will be needed to cover food intake. Because they are clear, care must be taken not to confuse them with the rapid-acting insulins, which are also clear.

HOW OFTEN IS INSULIN GIVEN?

One Injection Per Day

A few people have optimal blood/CGM glucose values by taking insulin once a day. This is particularly true during the "honeymoon" period that occurs shortly after diagnosis. A basal insulin, Lantus (Basaglar), Levemir or Tresiba, is usually taken in the morning or, less commonly, at dinner. It has very little "peak" (unless accidentally given into muscle) and lasts about 24 hours (see Table 1). Some people with type 2 diabetes who need insulin may do well with one injection of a basal insulin each day.

People who take one insulin injection per day may do better on two or multiple injections per day if they:

- do not have an optimal HbA1c level or 70 percent of glucose values "in range"
- have frequent low blood/CGM glucose values
- have to take a very large dose in one injection
- have many changes in their daily lives
- come out of the honeymoon phase

Multiple Injections Per Day (see Basal-bolus insulin therapy above)

Most people attain better diabetes management using multiple injections of insulin per day. Most doctors now believe it is best to treat all patients with type 1 diabetes with multiple daily injections (MDI) or pump therapy (Chapter 28). When a person receives multiple injections per day, there are multiple small peaks of insulin activity. Each of the small peaks in insulin activity can be adjusted to fit the person's schedule. In countries in which a basal insulin is not available, it may be necessary to use two injections per day of NPH insulin combined with a rapid-acting insulin (see Figure 3). There is then a greater risk of low blood/CGM glucose values during the night. The risk for night-time lows has been shown to be slightly reduced if the second shot of NPH is taken at bedtime rather than at dinner, which will mean a third daily shot.

Figure 1-B shows three injections of insulin per day using a rapid-acting insulin and NPH in the a.m. and Lantus (Basaglar), Levemir or Tresiba insulin (at breakfast, dinner or bedtime) and a rapid-acting insulin at dinner.

During adolescence, diabetes managment may become more difficult for a variety of reasons. Teens usually need more insulin due to pubertal hormones causing insulin resistance. The growth and sex hormones make it more difficult for insulin to work. Blood sugar goals can often be achieved more easily with three or more injections of insulin per day or use of an insulin pump.

AMOUNT OF INSULIN

Insulin is measured in "units" per cc (ml). Most insulins normally used contain 100 units per cc (ml). They are called U-100 insulin. Some insulins are also available with 200 units/ml (e.g., Tresiba) so it is important to always check. Standard insulin syringes hold either 3/10 cc (30 units), 1/2 cc (50 units) or 1 cc (100 units). The 3/10 cc syringes have larger distances between the unit lines and are easier to use if it is necessary to measure small doses. They also have lines for 0.5 unit markings.

Insulin dosage is based on body weight, blood/CGM glucose results, planned exercise and food intake (especially carbohydrate). After the initial diagnosis and treatment, people are usually started on approximately ¼ to ½ unit of insulin per pound (½ to 1 unit per kilogram [kg]) of body weight per day. The dose is then gradually increased as needed up to ½ to ¾ units per pound body weight (1.1 to 1.65 units per kg body weight). After a few weeks to months, many people go into a "honeymoon" or "grace" period when much less insulin is required (see Chapter 2). Frequent telephone contact with the diabetes team is important when the honeymoon starts. The insulin dosage must then be reduced to help avoid low blood sugars. We generally recommend continuing the injections during this period. After the honeymoon, most people gradually increase to an average insulin dosage of ½ unit per pound (1.1 units per kg) body weight. During the teenage growth spurt, the growth hormone level is high and blocks insulin activity. The insulin dosage may increase to 3/4 units per pound (1.5 units per kg) body weight. The dosage then goes back down after the period of growth is over. Insulin dosages can and should be adjusted to fit the person's lifestyle and needs. *For example, seasonal changes are common.*

In the winter, when it is cold outside, children may not go out to play after dinner. They may need more H/NL/AP insulin before the evening meal.

In the summer, when they go outside to play after dinner, the evening H/NL/AP insulin dose often can be decreased. Chapter 22 deals with how to adjust insulin dosages.

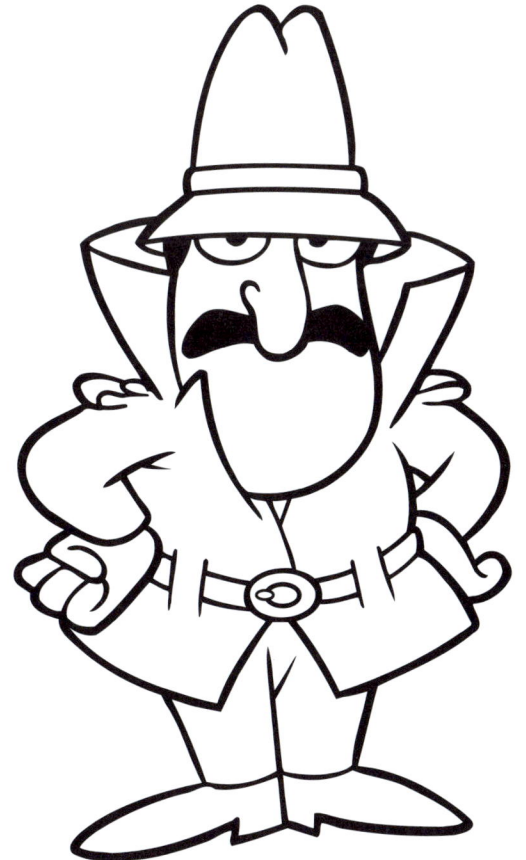

DEFINITIONS

Admelog: A generic form of Humalog insulin.

Analog: A form of insulin with a slightly different make-up that results in different times of onset and duration of activity. Humalog (Admelog), NovoLog and Apidra are examples of insulin analogs modified to have a rapid onset of activity.

Basaglar: A generic form of Lantus insulin.

Basal-bolus insulin therapy: Use of a basal insulin (Lantus [Basaglar], Levemir or Tresiba) with injection of a rapid-acting insulin prior to meals, or use of an insulin pump.

Beta cells: The cells in the islets of the pancreas which produce insulin.

cc (cubic centimeter; same as ml or milliliter): A unit of measurement. Five cubic centimeters (cc) equals one teaspoon; 15 cc equals one tablespoon; 30 cc equals one ounce; 240 cc equals one cup.

Fiasp: A faster-acting form of Novolog insulin.

Hormone: A chemical made in certain glands and secreted into the blood for action elsewhere. An example is insulin that is produced by the pancreas and carried by the blood for activity throughout the body.

Lantus (Basaglar) insulin (insulin glargine): A basal insulin that is flat in activity and lasts 24 hours. It has an acid pH in contrast to other insulins, which all have a neutral pH.

Levemir (insulin detemir): A basal insulin that is flat in activity and lasts up to 24 hours. It has a fatty acid attached that binds to plasma albumin, resulting in slow release.

Insulin pump: A pager-sized device designed to give a preset steady (basal) injection of insulin throughout the day, as well as pre-meal supplements (boluses) of insulin which are regulated by the user. See Chapter 28 for more details.

Tresiba (Deglude c): An ultra-long-lasting insulin (72 hours) that has its main effect in the first 24 hours.

QUESTIONS AND ANSWERS FROM NEWSNOTES

Q I sometimes have low sugars in the middle of the night. I take NPH and Regular Insulins.

A You may be helped by changing to "basal-bolus" insulin therapy. This is usually considered one injection per day of Lantus (Basaglar), Levimir or Tresiba (Degludec) and at least 3 injections per day of Humalog, NovoLog or Apidra insulins (pre-meal plus as needed for snacks or high blood sugar levels). There are two main reasons why this might help your number of lows decrease. The first is that the rapid-acting insulins do not last as long as the Regular insulin (for example, if taken to cover a bedtime snack or high blood sugar). The second is that basal insulins do not peak during the night (especially when given in the morning) as does dinner or evening NPH insulin.

Q What are the main advantages of the insulin analogs, Lantus (Basaglar), Levemir or Tresiba (Degludec)?

A By far the main advantage is in reducing the likelihood of low blood/CGM glucose levels during the night. This is because, when given in the morning, there is no peak in activity during the night as occurs with dinner or bedtime NPH insulin. In addition, the use of a true basal insulin helps to avoid the large "swings" in blood sugars often seen with NPH insulin.

Q Our son is about to go hiking in a very hot part of the U.S. Is there any way to keep his insulin, blood sugar strips and glucagon cool so they don't spoil?

A You can order the FRIO Cool Pouch at www.medicool.com. Hopefully all will fit in their larger pack.

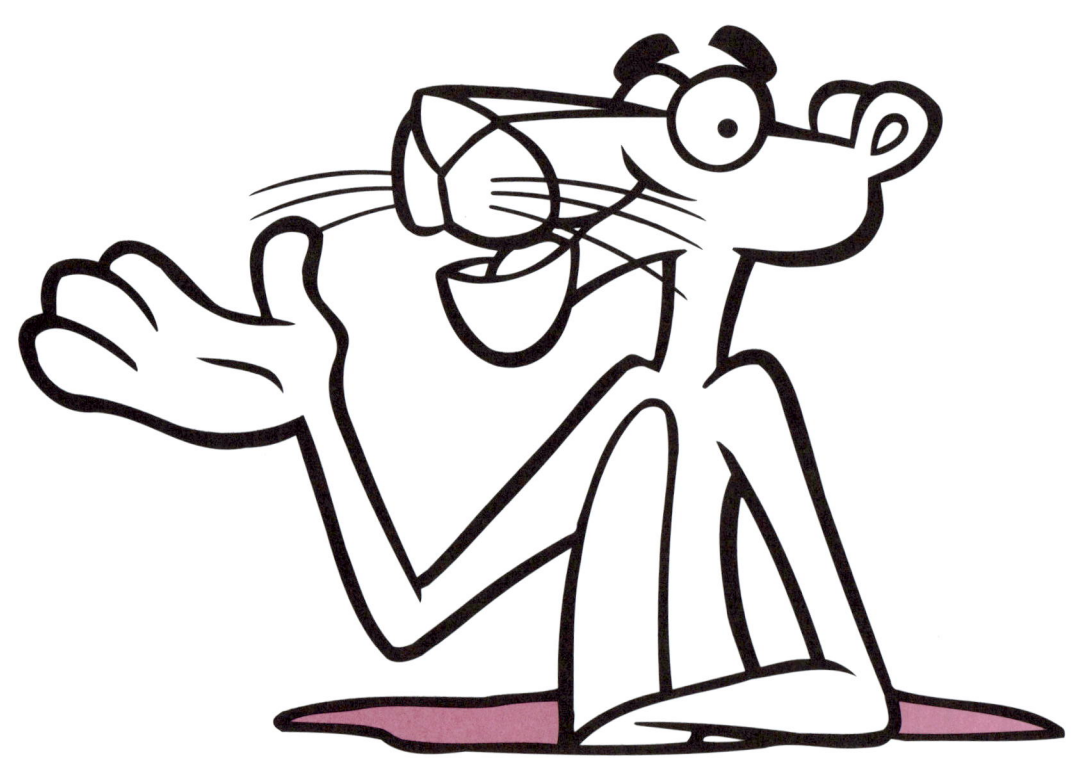

CHAPTER 9

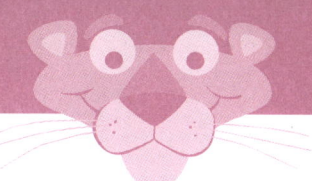

Drawing Up and Giving Insulin

WHERE TO INJECT THE INSULIN

Insulin is injected into the fat layer beneath the skin. Proper techniques must be learned so that the insulin is not injected too shallow into the outer skin (which may cause a lump, pain or a red spot) or too deep into the muscle (which may cause pain and insulin to be absorbed too quickly). If the injections are given in the recommended areas (Figure 1), it is very unlikely that a large artery or vein will be entered. The only problem if this were ever to happen would be that the insulin would last only a matter of minutes rather than hours. Also, it is not true that injecting a bubble of air into someone (even into an artery or vein) would harm them. These are common, but unnecessary worries. Most people are pleasantly surprised to know that they can learn how to give shots just as well as medical providers. Possible places to give insulin are the following (see Figure 1):

- buttocks (seat): slowest absorbing
- abdomen (holding pinch of fat): fastest absorbing
- arms (holding a pinch of fat) – intermediate absorbing
- thighs (holding a pinch of fat) – intermediate absorbing

These are the sites with the most subcutaneous fat (listed in order). Select at least two or three of the usual four areas for injections and skip areas that are not well tolerated. Injections should be moved around within the sites that are used (example: six to nine areas in each buttock site). If there are swollen or lumpy areas, injections should not be given into these sites, as the insulin may be absorbed at a different rate, causing high or low blood or continuous glucose monitor (CGM) glucose values.

Insulin is absorbed more rapidly from the abdomen than from the arm, and more rapidly from the arm than from the thigh or buttock. However, the differences are not great for most people. The buttock should generally be used for injections of Lantus (Basaglar)/Levemir/Tresiba

> **TOPICS:**
> **Medications: Insulin Mixing and Administration**
>
> **TEACHING OBJECTIVES:**
> The teacher will:
> 1. Demonstrate technique for mixing (if applicable) and drawing up insulin.
> 2. Identify age-appropriate injection sites.
> 3. Instruct on injection technique.
> 4. Observe family members/self giving insulin injection.
>
> **LEARNING OBJECTIVES:**
> Learner (parents, child, relative or self) will be able to:
> 1. Complete accurate demonstration for mixing (if applicable) and drawing up insulin.
> 2. Choose two age-appropriate sites for injections.
> 3. Demonstrate correct injection technique using saline.
> 4. Demonstrate correct injection technique using insulin.

insulin to make certain it is given into the fatty tissue. You may also use an area where a large pinch of fat can be held.

Based on studies done in Sweden, it is best to take a pinch of the skin when using most needles. The exceptions may be the buttock area or the central abdomen if there is a sufficient amount of fat tissue and either the BD Ultra-Fine Mini ™ or the BD Ultra- Fine™ Nano needles are being used.

Rapid-acting insulin may be absorbed even more quickly when the shot is given in an area that is then exercised. Injecting into an arm or leg which will be used in an activity may increase the likelihood of low blood sugars during exercise, due to the increased blood flow to the area being exercised. For example, if you are to play tennis, don't inject into the arm that will be used to swing the racquet. A low blood sugar could be more likely.

Insulin should also not be injected just prior to a bath, shower or hot tub. The warm water will draw more blood to the skin, causing a rapid absorption of the insulin and resulting in a serious low blood sugar. If the water is warm enough to turn your skin pink, then the insulin will be absorbed more quickly. Wait at least 90 minutes after giving rapid-acting insulin to get into hot water.

INSULIN SYRINGES/NEEDLES

(See picture diagram of insulin syringes and Table 1)

There are several brands of disposable insulin syringes with varying needle widths (measured in gauges, with a larger number for a thinner needle) and varying lengths. The needles are thin and are sharp for easy

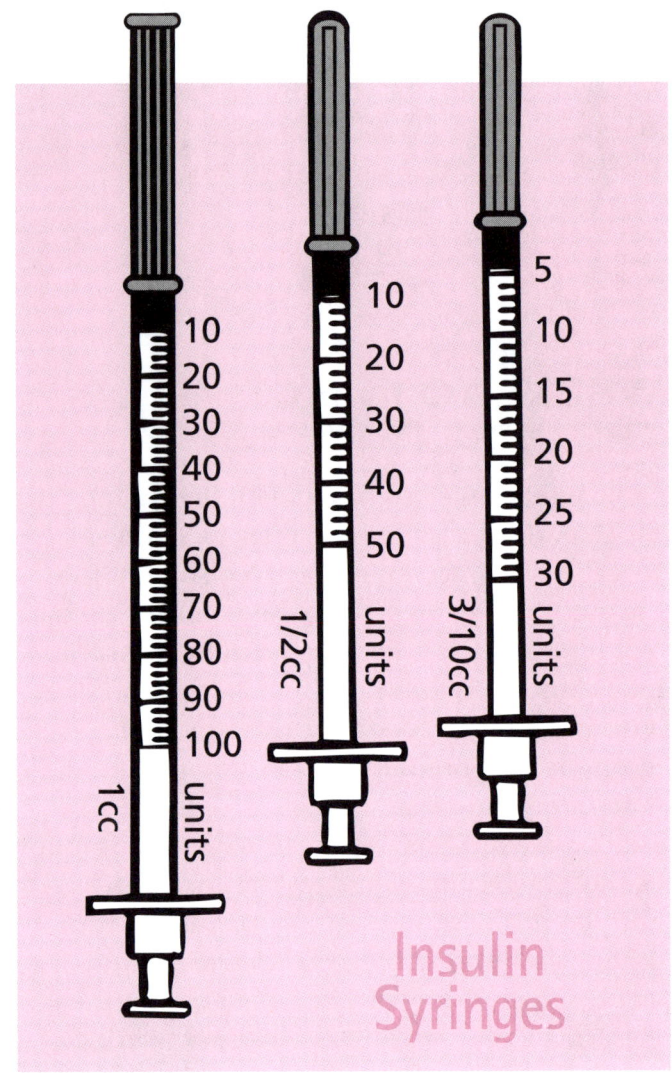

Insulin Syringes

insertion. The amount of insulin the syringe will hold varies. There are 3/10 cc and 1/2 cc syringes for people using less than 30 or 50 units of insulin per injection, or 1 cc syringes for those using more than 50 units per injection (see drawings). There are also 3/10 cc syringes with ½ unit markings allowing for smaller doses of insulin to be measured. This syringe can be helpful for young children.

The BD Ultra-Fine II short needles are just 5/16 inch (8mm) in length (compared with the usual ½ inch [12.7mm] length) and at 30 gauge are very thin. These are particularly helpful for young children.

FIGURE 1
Insulin Rotation Chart

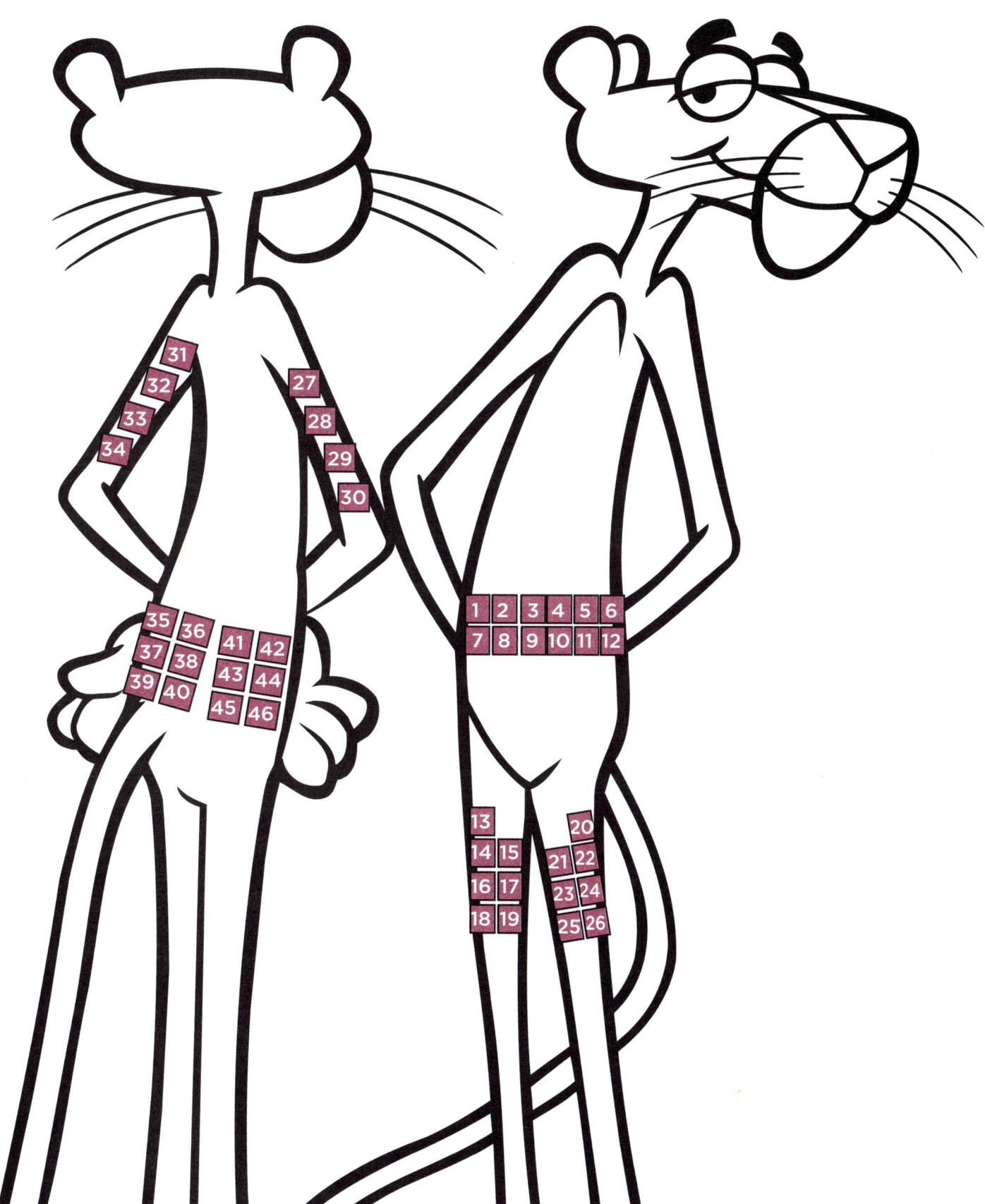

DRAWING UP AND GIVING INSULIN

DRAWING UP THE INSULIN

Although the use of insulin pens is easier and more convenient then drawing insulin from a vial, we have included pen use later in this chapter. This is because everyone must know how to draw insulin from a vial in case a pen is not available.

You will be shown how to draw the insulin into the syringe. YOU SHOULD LEARN BY PRACTICE AND FORM CORRECT HABITS FROM THE START. When possible, wash your hands first. Figure 2 shows how to draw up insulin and give an injection. Our families often start by doing "air" shots into a doll or mannequin. The next practice step is drawing up sterile salt water (saline) and doing the injection into each other. This helps family members to realize how little pain is caused from the shots. In addition, Table 1 gives a checklist to follow. The nurse will go over the checklist with you at regular intervals.

These are the steps:

- Get everything together: alcohol, insulin and a syringe.

- Wash your hands.

- Push the plunger of the disposable syringe up and down before drawing in the insulin. This will help soften the rubber at the end of the plunger and smooth the plunger action.

- Wipe the top of the insulin bottle(s) with alcohol and allow to air dry (don't blow on it).

- Insert the needle through the rubber top of the bottle of rapid-acting (Humalog/NovoLog/Apidra) or Regular insulin with the bottle sitting upright on the table. Turn the bottle (with the needle inserted) upside down. To remove any air bubbles, draw out about five more units of insulin than needed and push quickly back into the bottle. This can be repeated several times as needed until air bubbles are cleared. "Flicking" the syringe barrel with the finger is not recommended as it can cause the needle to bend. After the air bubbles are gone, adjust the top edge of the rubber plunger to be in line with the exact number of units needed. The needle can then be removed from the vial and held or the cap put on the needle.

- If also drawing NPH insulin into the syringe, some families leave the needle in the rapid-acting insulin bottle until the NPH insulin is mixed. Others hold the syringe in one hand while mixing the NPH insulin (turning up and down 20 times) with the other hand. NEVER lay the syringe down on the table with the needle touching anything, as this may lead to bacteria collecting on the needle and causing an infection. Insert the needle into the bottle of the NPH insulin while the bottle is upside down. This helps avoid air from the vial getting into the syringe. With the bottle turned upside down, slowly draw the number of units of the NPH insulin needed. The total number of units in the syringe will be the sum of the rapid-acting units plus the NPH units.

  After mixing the two types of insulin, never re-inject insulin from the syringe back into the intermediate insulin bottle. This will give you an incorrect dose of insulin. If you draw up too much insulin you will need to throw your syringe away and draw up your doses again.

- The NPH insulin needs to be mixed gently. Do not vigorously shake the NPH insulin, as this may break it down and cause the insulin to absorb differently. Some people roll the bottle between the palms of their hands. **The NPH bottle should be turned or rolled gently 20 times to mix thoroughly**. Avoid touching the rubber stopper of the vial if it has already been wiped with alcohol. Clear insulins do not need to be mixed.

- **Venting the insulin bottles**

  In the past, we instructed families to inject air into the insulin bottles with each dose. This was to help keep a vacuum from developing, which would pull the insulin drawn out back into the bottle.

TABLE 1: Drawing Up Two Insulins Into a Syringe

A. Gather supplies: Insulin, syringe, alcohol wipe for tops of bottles, log book with insulin dosage. **Do not confuse the rapid-acting insulin vial with the Lantus (Basaglar)/Levemir/Tresiba vial (all three are also clear).**

B. Technique:

- Know correct insulin dosage
- Wipe tops of insulin bottles with alcohol swab
- Either "vent"* the bottles weekly (smaller doses) or put air into the long-acting (cloudy) insulin with the bottle upright and remove the needle. Put air in the clear insulin and leave the needle in.
- Draw up clear (rapid-acting) insulin, get rid of air bubbles and remove the needle
- Mix the cloudy NPH insulin vial by gently turning the bottle up and down 20 times; this ensures that the insulin gets well mixed
- Slowly draw up the NPH (or long-acting) insulin into the syringe, making sure not to push any insulin already in the syringe back into the vial. For people mixing Lantus insulin with a rapid-acting insulin, the clear Lantus insulin will become cloudy as it is pulled into the syringe holding the rapid-acting insulin. This does not usually cause problems with needle-plugging.
- If insulin vials have been in the refrigerator, you can warm up the insulin once it is mixed in the syringe by holding the syringe in the closed palm of your hand for 1-2 minutes; it will be less likely to sting if brought to room temperature
- Give insulin injection

An option now used by some people is to not put air into the bottles, but to just "vent" the bottles to remove any vacuum once weekly (see text).

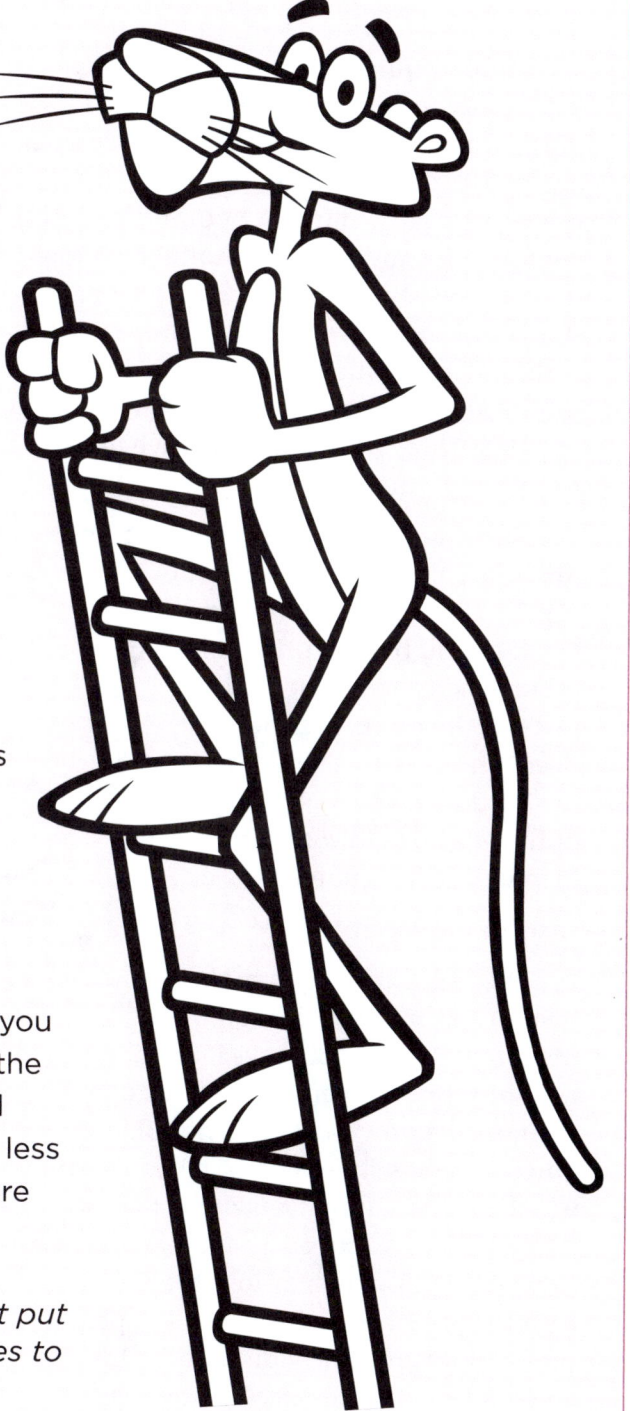

DRAWING UP AND GIVING INSULIN

Most families now prefer to "vent" their insulin bottles once a week. This is done by using a new syringe and removing the plunger from the syringe barrel. With the insulin vial sitting upright on the table, insert the needle into the rubber stopper and allow air to equalize in the insulin bottle. This will remove any vacuum that may be inside the bottle. This will only take a moment. Pick one consistent day of the week to vent the bottles.

Some families may prefer to inject the air when drawing up the insulin. This is particularly true when large doses are being given. The amount of air injected into a bottle equals the number of units of insulin being withdrawn. The air should be added to the NPH insulin bottle first. The rubber stopper of the bottle should first be cleaned with alcohol. With the bottle sitting upright, insert the needle into the bottle and push in the air within the syringe. Remove the needle from the bottle.

Draw air into the syringe again, the amount equal to the dose of the rapid-acting insulin. With the rapid-acting bottle upright on a table, insert the needle and push in the air. Leave the needle in the bottle and turn upside down. Follow the steps outlined above to withdraw the insulin doses required.

- **Insulin Longevity**

The companies who make insulin recommend changing insulin vials every 30 days if the bottle is kept at room temperature. This is due to the possible growth of bacteria. Blood/CGM glucose values should be watched carefully when the insulin bottle is almost empty or if the 30 days are exceeded. If the values start to be unusually high or low, the last bit of insulin should be discarded. Some people prefer to just routinely discard the insulin when it only fills the neck of the turned bottle. The expiration date on the bottle should always be checked and the insulin discarded if that date is reached. Unopened refrigerated insulin is useable until the manufacturer's expiration date on the top of the box.

Insulin used in an insulin pump usually retains activity for three days (with no differences between the three brands of rapid-acting insulin). An exception is when traveling to a very warm climate (e.g., summer in Mexico). It might then be easier to temporarily switch to an injected basal insulin.

In summary, BE PRECISE ABOUT THE DOSAGE. An overdose can cause an insulin reaction (low blood sugar). If you ever take an incorrect dose, be sure to notify your diabetes care-provider. It is wise to have the dosages posted on the refrigerator or some obvious place to avoid confusion. Children below age 10 do not usually have the fine motor abilities and concern for accuracy to draw up insulin by themselves. Parents should assist them with these tasks (see Chapter 18).

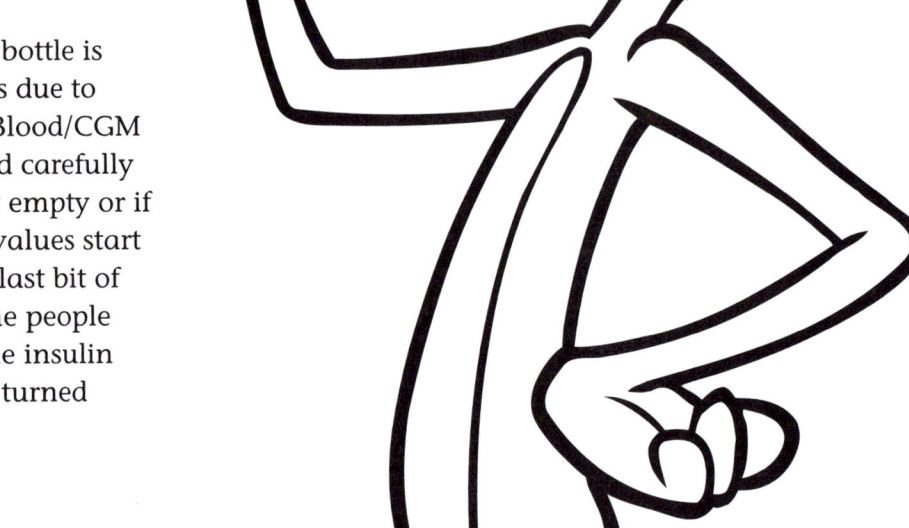

TABLE 2:
Giving the Insulin (see Figure 2)

- Choose the area of the body where you are going to give the shot. Use four or more areas and use different sites within the area (see Figure 1).
- Make sure the area where you will be giving the shot is clean.
- Relax the chosen area (see "Different Age Children" section for techniques).
- Pull up the skin with the finger and thumb (even with short needles).
- Touch the needle to the skin and "punch" it through the skin.

If Short Needle:
a 90° angle for the 5/16-inch (short) or the BD Ultra-Fine Nano needle. These hurt less and are not as likely to go into muscle.

If Longer Needle:
use a 45° angle for the 5/8-inch needle (only).

A 90° angle looks like this ↓

A 45° angle looks like this ↘

- Push in the insulin slowly and steadily; wait three seconds to let the insulin spread out.
- Let go of the skin pulled up.
- Put a finger or dry cotton over the needle as it is pulled out; gently rub a few times to close the hole where the needle was inserted; press your finger or the cotton down on the area where you gave the shot if bruising or bleeding happens.
- <u>Look to see if a drop of insulin comes back through the hole the needle made ("leak-back"); make a note in your log book if this happens.</u>

The nurse will teach the right way to give shots so that a drop of insulin does not leak back. A drop can contain as much as five units of insulin.

HOW TO INJECT THE INSULIN

(See Table 2 and Figure 2)

- Clean the site of injection with soap and water (or an alcohol swab or hand sanitizer if camping or in a hospital). Alcohol dries and toughens the skin and is not routinely recommended.

- Lift the skin and fat tissue between the thumb and the first finger. **If you are using the BD Ultra-Fine Nano needle and the fat in the area of injection is adequate, the needle can be inserted at a 90° angle without pinching (usually only the buttock [seat area] on younger children).**

In other areas, where there is not as much fat, a "gentle pinch" should still be used during the injection. Touch the needle to the skin, holding the syringe at a 90° angle (or less). It is generally best to push the needle all the way into the skin. If the needle is not in far enough, the insulin may not be injected into the fatty layer. If it goes into the layer directly under the skin rather than into the lower fatty layer, it will sting and may cause a bump or redness and itching. To ensure injection into fat, the "gentle pinch" can continue to be held during the injection of the insulin.

- Inject the insulin by pushing the plunger down with a SLOW and steady push as far as it will go. Some people like to wait a few seconds to let the insulin "spread out" after each five units of insulin is injected. A smooth injection is important. AFTER THE INSULIN IS IN, **WAIT THREE SECONDS BEFORE REMOVING THE NEEDLE.** THIS WILL HELP AVOID INSULIN LEAKAGE FROM THE INJECTION SITE. A loss of one drop of insulin may be equal to two to five units. Loss of insulin is a common reason for variations in the blood/CGM glucose levels. If "leak-back" continues to be a problem, move to a new site. A strategy to avoid "leak-back" is to draw two units of air into the syringe after removing the needle from the insulin bottle. Then flick the side of the syringe with a finger to make the air rise up under the plunger. The air will then be injected after the insulin and will help to avoid "leak-back."

- After the injection, place a finger or dry cotton ball over the site. Press firmly for a few seconds to suppress any bleeding. Gently rub the site to close the needle track. Some bleeding may occur after the needle is pulled out; this is not harmful, although some insulin may be carried out with the blood. Some people put a finger on the site where the needle came out and rub gently. The finger should be clean. (If you are getting pain or bleeding often with shots, you may be depositing the insulin into muscle. You should consider using a different site with more fat tissue.)

- The plastic syringes are recommended for one-time use only by the manufacturer. The needle becomes dull after one use and may be more painful by the second or third shot. If they are to be reused, after giving the injection, push the plunger up and down to get rid of any insulin left in the needle. Wipe the needle off with an alcohol swab. Put the cap over the needle and store the syringe and needle in the refrigerator until ready for the next use (to help prevent growth of bacteria).

- Table 2 provides a summary for injecting the insulin.

DIFFERENT AGE CHILDREN AND INSULIN SHOTS

- A young child can help with choosing where the shot will be given (although sites must be rotated) and by holding still.
- Children usually begin to give some of their own shots around age 10.
- It is important that both mom and dad share in giving shots.
- Some age-related issues (see Chapter 18) are summarized below.

Toddlers

- This age group can sometimes be frightened when having to get shots.
- Keep the area where the shot will be given as still as possible. Try to get the child's attention on something else (e.g., television, blowing bubbles, looking at a book, etc.). This will help the child to relax.
- The buttocks are often used first, and later the legs and arms and tummy.
- With the child's permission, the long-acting insulin can be given when the child is asleep.
- The parent must remember when giving their child a shot, they are giving them health.

School age

- The child may help in choosing the area on their body to give the shot.
- Change where the shots are given. Use two or more areas (e.g., abdomen and bottom) and use different sites within the areas (see Figure 2).

Teens

- Many teens give their own shots and do not want help.
- It is still important to give the shots in a place (e.g., the kitchen) where parents can actually see the shot given.

FIGURE 2

Drawing and injecting the insulin

1. Wash your hands!

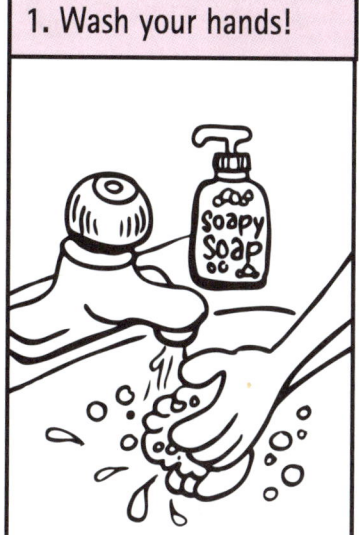

2. Warm and mix (if NPH) insulin.

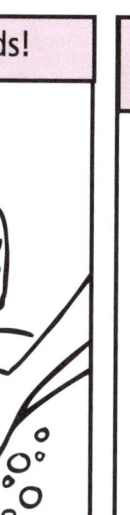

3. Wipe top of insulin bottle with alcohol.

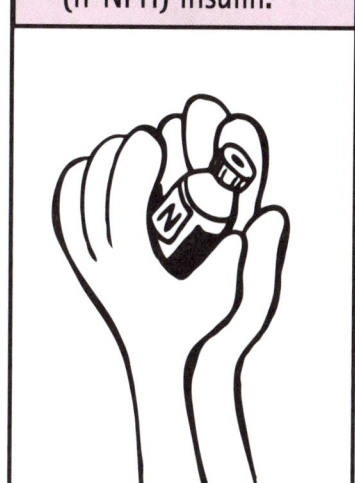

4. Inject air = insulin dose in units. Pull out dose of insulin.

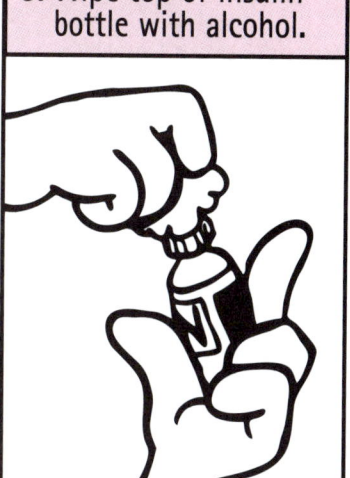

5. Make sure injection site is clean.

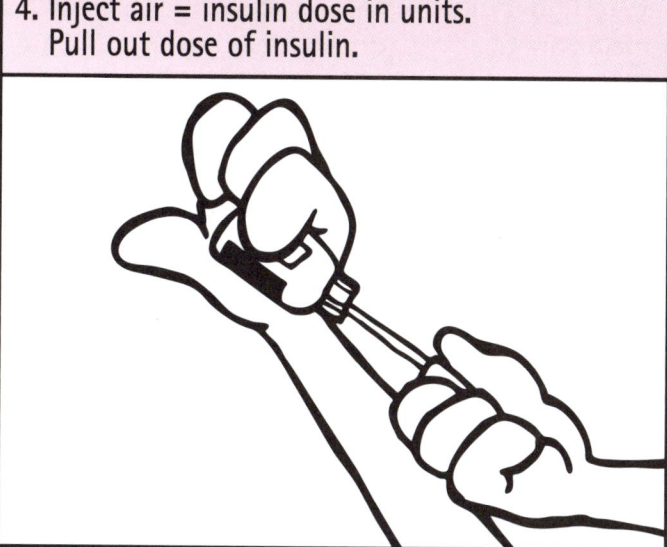

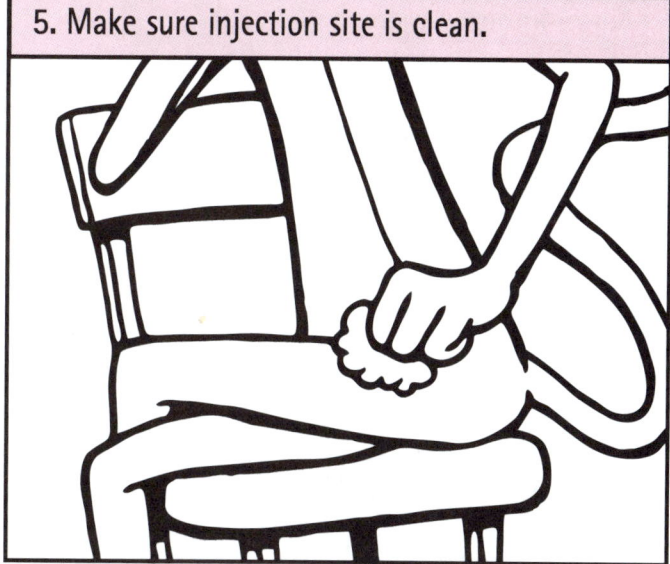

6. Pinch up skin and fat tissue. If using 5/8-inch needle, go in at angle. If using 5/16-inch (short) or the BD Ultra-Fine Nano Needle, can go straight in (assuming adequate subcutaneous fat).

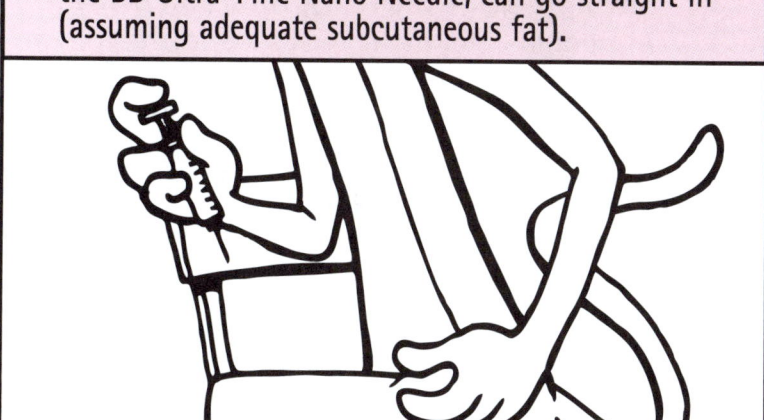

7. Basal insulins (Lantus (Basaglar), Levemir and Tresiba) are best given in the buttocks.

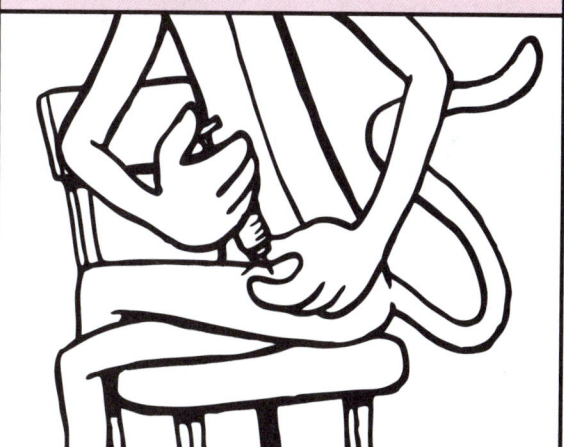

DRAWING UP AND GIVING INSULIN

TABLE 3: Pre-Meal Blood/CGM Sugar and Time to Wait Before Eating

Blood Sugar Level		Time to Wait Before Eating (Minutes) Type of Insulin	
mg/dl	mmol/L	Regular	Humalog/NovoLog/Apidra
above 200	above 11.1	60	30
151-200	8.4-11.1	45	25
80-150	4.5-8.3	30	20
70-80	3.9-4.5	Don't wait (take the shot and start eating)	Don't wait (take the shot and start eating)
<70	<3.9	Treat the low. Take insulin and eat after blood sugar is back up (consider reducing the insulin).	Treat the low. Take insulin and eat after blood sugar is back up (consider reducing the rapid-acting insulin).

- Missing shots (boluses) is a common reason for high blood sugars.
- Parents can stay involved by helping to get the supplies out, and helping to keep records by writing down the blood sugars and insulin doses each day in the log book or by emailing meter or CGM downloads.

WHEN TO INJECT THE INSULIN

Most people now routinely use Humalog/NovoLog/Apidra (rapid-acting) insulin, and it is best to give the shot 20 minutes prior to meals if the blood/CGM glucose level is ≥80 mg/dL (>4.5 mmol/L). When the blood sugar is high, it is wise to wait even longer after the injection to begin eating (Table 3). The rapid-acting insulins peak in 90 minutes, whereas blood/CGM glucose values peak in 60 minutes after food is eaten. It is thus best to get some insulin in 15 to 20 minutes prior to the meal when the blood/CGM glucose value is >80 mg/dL (>4.5 mmol/L). For some, it might be easier to remember to wait the one or two left digits of the glucose value (e.g., 80 = wait 8 minutes; 160 = wait 16 minutes; 320 = wait 32 minutes, etc). An exception is with the toddler or a picky eater who has variable food intake, when it may be better to wait to give the shot until after seeing how much food has been eaten (see Chapters 18 and 19). Higher blood/CGM glucose values after the meals are then exchanged for safety. Figure 2 in Chapter 8 shows the effectiveness of giving insulin 20 minutes prior to the meal.

With Regular insulin, it is best to take the shot 30 to 60 minutes before eating. This allows the Regular insulin to start working at the time food is eaten. It reduces the blood/CGM glucose values in the one or two hours after eating. When the pre-meal blood/CGM glucose level is known, the time can be varied between the shot and eating the meal, as shown in Table 3. It has been our experience that using a time scale such as this can improve blood sugar levels and the HbA1c value (Chapter 14).

One of the advantages of an insulin pump is that it is easy to divide the insulin dose without having to give extra shots. Thus, part of the insulin dose (for high blood sugar correction and the food most likely to be eaten) can be given 20 minutes prior to the meal. By pushing a few buttons, insulin to cover other food eaten can then be given after the meal (See Chapter 28).

DISPOSING OF NEEDLES

It is never recommended to throw any needles or lancets into the trash; someone may get poked and this can spread harmful germs. It is recommended to dispose of sharps into a red biohazard container. An alternative is to place needles into a very thick plastic container such as a bleach bottle or laundry detergent bottle. Once the bottle is full you may recap it tightly and then tape the cap with strong tape such as duct tape to assure the bottle will not open. This can then be put out with your trash.

The BD company provides a **Safe-Clip®** device to clip and store needles. This is a convenient device for traveling. This device holds approximately 1,500 needles, which is about one year's worth of needles.

STORAGE

Ideally, insulin should be stored in the refrigerator and warmed to room temperature prior to giving the shot. Most people keep the bottles they are using at room temperature (except in a very hot climate). It will not be as likely to sting or to cause red spots after injection if it is kept at room temperature. After drawing up insulin that has been in the refrigerator, the filled, capped syringe can be warmed in the closed palm of your hand to avoid stinging. A drawer in the kitchen might be identified for storage of all diabetes supplies. Research has shown that if insulin is stored at room temperature, it loses 1.5 percent of its potency per month (after one month 1 cc U-100 insulin would have 98.5 units of insulin rather than 100 units). For most people, this small change would not make a difference (9.85 units rather than 10.0 units). One of the insulin manufacturers wrote: "**Insulin vials currently in use may be kept at room temperature for 30 days, in a cool place and away from sunlight.**" Insulin will spoil if it gets above 90° or if it freezes.

Insulin bottles (or pens) should not be exposed to extreme temperature changes, such as being left in a car in the hot summer or the cold winter. If NPH insulin has spoiled, sometimes clumps may be seen sticking to the sides of the insulin bottle. That bottle and the accompanying bottle of rapid-acting insulin should not be used if this occurs. Unfortunately, the rapid-acting (clear) insulins have only subtle changes, but they may look cloudy or even slightly yellow. If this is the case the insulin should be thrown away immediately and replaced with new bottles. It may have bacteria (germs) growing in it. We have also suggested throwing away bottles of insulin that have been opened for six weeks or more, even if refrigerated. Families using low dosages of a particular insulin may find it more effective to draw out of 300-unit (3.0 cc) insulin pen cartridges (for Humalog/NovoLog/Apridra, Regular, NPH or basal insulins). If blood/CGM glucose values rise (for no other reason) after the bottle has been open for 30 days or more, throw the bottle away.

INSULIN PENS

Use of insulin pens has increased greatly in recent years. This is related in part to people wanting an easy method to take doses of rapid-acting insulins for high blood sugar corrections or for food intake during the day. Insulin pens provide convenience and accuracy. We typically start patients on insulin pens unless there is a financial or insurance reason not to do so. Most types of insulin are now available in pens. Using a pen is quite easy and is summarized below.

If using only one insulin, and a slightly greater expense is not a problem, we suggest using an insulin pen. However, most nurses initially teach how to use a syringe and vial of insulin (as in Figure 2) in case this becomes necessary in the future. If using two insulins, they cannot be mixed in a pen. Two pen injections would be necessary. Pens are generally easier to use and can be conveniently carried or made available during the day. Some insurance providers cover only certain pens, so this must be considered. It may also be important to know if the pen is marked in half-unit, one-unit, or two-unit increments. Accuracy of low dosages is not a problem, and several studies have shown pens to be more accurate than syringes for administering doses of less than five units. Optimal sized needles for the pen can be ordered by the physician. The giving of the shot is similar to the giving of a shot with a syringe (Table 2).

Use of a pen is summarized below:

- Remove the paper tab from the needle and screw it on the end of the pen.
- Clean the skin where the shot will be given. Rotate sites daily.
- Remove the needle cover.
- Enter 2 to 3 units (by rotating the dial) in the pen as a "priming dose" and with the needle pointed upward into the air, observe that the insulin comes out.
- Dial in the number of units to be given.
- Insert the needle under the skin.
- Inject the insulin slowly. Then count three seconds before removing the needle. (This helps avoid insulin leakage.)
- Rub the injection site gently to close the track of the needle.
- Put the cover back on the needle. (Some say to change the needle with each injection and others say once daily.)

Some care-providers do not recommend reuse of pen needles, as the needle may become dull and cause tissue damage at the injection site. Using a pen results in increased convenience for the person. In addition, people are more apt to cover the food they are eating with insulin, particularly when away from home.

Pens can be divided into two groups. First are those that are pre-filled disposable pens that are discarded after using. Second are permanent pens that hold cartridges of insulin. The cartridge is replaced in the pen after the insulin is used up (or after one month).

A. Disposable Pens

✔ **Lilly Pre-Filled Disposable Pens:**

Lilly disposable pens include the **Humalog KwikPen**™, Humulin NPH, 70/30 NPH/Regular and the Humalog Mix 75/25 or 50/50 KwikPen™. Basaglar ("generic" Lantus) is also available in a disposable pen. All hold 3 mL (300 units) and are readily available. The pens are simple to use and will take any of the needles described below.

✔ **Novo Nordisk NovoLog FlexPen®, the Levemir® FlexTouch® and the TRESIBA® FlexTouch® pens:**

The **NovoLog FlexPen®** is a pre-filled disposable pen for the rapid-acting, short-lasting NovoLog insulin. There is also a NovoLog® Mix 70/30 FlexPen® (70%NPH/30%NovoLog) in a pre-filled disposable pen.

There is a Novo Nordisk pre-filled disposable **Levemir FlexTouch** pen that injects the Levemir insulin by touching the plunger. It is approved for storage at room temperature for 42 days. Dosing has been shown accurate from 1 to 80 units. It holds 3 mL (300 units) of the basal Levemir insulin. NovoFine 30 or 31 gauge needles are used with the pen. The instructions are very similar to the above and are included in the box and on the website (www.novonordiskus.com or www.novologflexpen.com), or talk to your nurse educator.

Tresiba insulin is available using the TRESIBA FlexTouch 3mL disposable U-100 pen or in 10 mL vials. The pen is also available as a U-200 insulin, so make certain you receive the U-100 pen.

✔ **Sanofi-Aventis SoloSTAR® Pens**

Both Lantus (a basal insulin) and Apidra (a rapid-acting, short-lasting) come in 3 cc (300 unit) disposable prefilled insulin pens. The Lantus is a grey-color pen and the Apidra a blue-colored pen (both are clear insulins, so do not confuse).

With any pre-filled insulin pen, the directions above should be followed in giving the injection.

B. Cartridge Pens

The **NovoPen Echo®** is a reusable pen designed for use with PenFill® 3 mL cartridges of the rapid-acting, short-lasting NovoLog insulin. The NovoPen Echo can give half-unit dosing and has a memory for the dose and time of the last injection (of NovoLog). This may be helpful for parents wanting information from the school setting. It also has a variety of fun skins (coverings) available at novologreach.com. It is designed for use with the NovoTwist®, NovoFine® or other Novo Nordisk compatible disposable needles.

The **NovoPen® 3.0** from Novo Nordisk and the BD pen offer the use of cartridges of Regular, NPH, 70/30 NPH/Regular or Humalog/NovoLog insulins. The cartridges contain 3.0 mL of insulin (300 units) and are replaced into the pen when the cartridge is empty. The NovoPen 3.0 delivers a dose of two to 70 units. The BD pen has a maximum dose of 30 units. A colorful pen from Novo Nordisk is called the **NovoPen-Junior®** that can deliver ½-unit doses, when over a minimum dose of 1 unit. It takes the 3 mL insulin cartridges, so it can be used with any Novo Nordisk 3.0 insulin cartridge available.

Lilly provides 3 mL Humalog cartridges for use in their **HumaPen® MEMOIR™** and **HumaPen® LUXURA™ HD** insulin delivery devices. The latter can give half-unit does and has an easily visible window.

The **InPen** (companionmedical.com) is an easy-to-use pen that not only helps calculate doses but also keeps track of injection data. When paired via Bluetooth with the smartphone app, the InPen delivery system keeps tabs on how many units you received at your last injection, when you took it, and other helpful information. It can be particularly helpful in tracking missed injections. The InPen is available for individuals 12 and older undergoing multiple daily subcutaneous injections. It can deliver 0.5 to 30 units of insulin, dialed in half-unit increments. The InPen injector pen is compatible with Lilly Humalog and Novo Nordisk NovoLog U-100 3.0 mL insulin cartridges and single-use detachable and disposable needles (not included). The InPen lasts for one year – no recharging needed. And with options in blue, grey, and pink, you can even add a bit of color to your management plan.

The InPen app is the other half of InPen's smart diabetes management tool. Using information transmitted from the pen, the app can track insulin therapy and calculate doses. The InPen Mobile App is a free download on Apple iOS or android and can share therapy data with your doctor or family.

C. Insulins Readily Available in Pens Include:

- **Lilly:**
  Humalog KwikPen
  Humalog® Mix 75/25® KwikPen™
  Humalog® Mix 50/50® KwikPen™
  Humalog® N KwikPen™
  Humalog® Mix 70/30® KwikPen™
  Humalog® HumaPen Luxura HD™

- **Sanofi:**
  Apidra® SoloSTAR®
  Lantus® SoloSTAR®

- **NovoNordisk:**
  Levemir FlexTouch Pen
  NovoLog FlexPen
  NovoLog Mix 70/30 FlexPen
  NovoPen Echo cartridge (NovoLog) pen

D. Pen Needles Currently Available Include:

Name	Length (mm)	Width (gauge)*
BD Regular™	12.7	29
BD Short™	8	31
BD Ultra-Fine Mini	5	31
BD Nano™	4	32
Novo Fine™	8	30
Novo Fine	6	32
Novo Fine	8	30

*Larger gauge = Less width

The BD Autoshield™ Duo pen needle can attach to any pen and due to the short needle may not require a pinching of the skin. It has a front and back shield to help to help protect from needle sticks. It is not reusable.

INJECTION AIDS

The i-port Advance® and the Insuflon are plastic cannulas very similar to the insertion tube for the insulin pump. However, instead of connecting to a pump, the end is covered and has a port for giving insulin injections. The i-port Advance has a disposable inserter. It can be left under the skin for up to five days (remove sooner if redness develops). EMLA® cream can be applied 30-60 minutes before insertion to diminish pain. All insulins, including Humalog, NovoLog, Apidra, NPH and long-acting insulin may be given through the port. The best place for insertion is the buttocks, followed by the central abdomen. The skin must be pinched if other sites are used. IV Prep™ (Skin Prep™) can be used to help hold the device in place. These are particularly helpful for people with needle fear and for young children receiving multiple daily injections. School aides will sometimes give injections into the device even though they will not inject insulin into the skin. Glucagon can also be given through the device. The pharmacy of one of our families obtains the Insuflon devices through Amerisource Bergen (1-800-523-4020, item #4509725). It can also be ordered from National Diabetic Pharmacies at 1-800-467-8546 and then hit 48965 or 48964. Information on the i-port Advance is available online at www.i-port.com. It is distributed by Medtronic (1-800-646-4633).

PROBLEMS THAT MAY ARISE WITH INSULIN INJECTIONS

- **Hypertrophy (swelling) of Skin (also called lipohypertrophy)**

Swelling of the skin or hypertrophy occurs when too many injections are given in one area over a period of months to years, causing scarring of the fat tissue. Some people like to give shots in the same spot because nerve endings (pain) are dulled after a few injections. You can inject insulin into the body anywhere there is enough fat under the skin. Usually there isn't fat over the joints and bones, so these areas are not used. **If swelling or lumps in an area do occur, you should not give further injections in that area until the swelling is gone.** This may take several months and varies for different people. **The swelling will alter the uptake of insulin.**

- **Skin Dents (atrophy or lipoatrophy)**

You may develop "dents" at the injection site. This is different from skin swelling, and is due to a loss of fat in that place. "Denting" is now rare when human insulin is used. When dents do occur, it is possible to help them go away. To inject into the dented area, pick the skin up at the side of the dent. Slide the needle

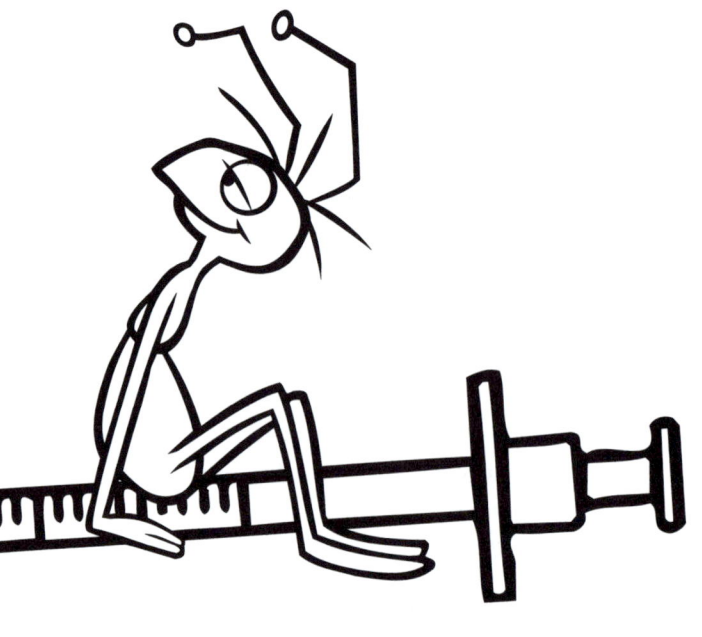

under the dent and inject the insulin. If you inject human insulin four times in a row each week, the dent will gradually go away. This may take several weeks.

- **Plugged Needle**

Occasionally, a small piece of fat or the insulin will plug the end of the needle during the injection. Sometimes it is possible to pull out the needle a little and then push the needle back into a slightly different place. If you still cannot push down the plunger to finish the injection, you will have to pull the needle completely out of the skin. **NOTE VERY PRECISELY THE UNITS OF INSULIN REMAINING IN THE SYRINGE.** After you fill a new syringe with the total insulin dose as originally drawn, discard the amount of insulin you have already injected. Inject the rest into another site.

- **Giving the Wrong Insulin Dose**

"To err is human" is very true. Sometimes the dosages of the rapid-acting and the basal insulin are confused. Similarly, an excess of insulin usually results if the morning insulin dose is accidentally given in the evening. This results in a very long night, as someone must awaken frequently, check blood/CGM glucose levels, and if needed, give extra juice and food. Obviously, if the blood/CGM glucose value is low, more frequent checks will be needed. Glucagon may be required and should be kept nearby.

- **Bleeding After the Injection**

A small capillary blood vessel is probably hit with every injection. Sometimes a drop of blood or a bruise under the skin will be seen after the injection. This will not cause any problem except for the possible loss of some insulin with the blood, but the bruising may be upsetting to some people. As noted earlier in this chapter, place a dry piece of cotton or a clean finger over the injection site and rub gently after removing the needle. This will usually stop any bleeding. Sometimes applying pressure for 30 to 60 seconds will help to reduce bruising. If bruising or blood "leak-back" is happening frequently, you may be injecting into an area with too little fat and depositing the insulin into muscle. This changes the insulin action. Consider giving shots in an area with more fat tissue.

- **Injecting Insulin into Muscle**

If a person is very thin or very muscular, there may be little fat under the skin. Injections may go into the underlying muscle, causing more rapid absorption of insulin and low blood sugar. There may then be less insulin to act later in the day, resulting in high blood sugar. Injections into the muscle are most likely to occur if the syringe is held at a 90° angle to the body or if the skin is not pinched prior to the injection. This is common when a thin person gives their own shot and reaches over to the other arm and injects. Instead, the fat on the arm can be rolled on the back of a chair or on the knee and then the shot given in the rolled fat. Sometimes extra pain will occur when shots go into muscle, but this is not always the case. If injecting into muscle is a problem, it may be wise to pull the skin away from the muscle and insert the needle into the "tent" below (while still holding the pinch of skin). Since the entire pinch is not being held, just the upper tip, the insulin should not "leak-back." This technique can be taught by your diabetes nurse. Occasionally, it may be helpful to give an injection in the presence of your diabetes care-provider to have your injection technique checked. If the patient is newly diagnosed and has very little body fat, the buttocks may be the safest place for injections.

DEFINITIONS

Atrophy (or Lipoatrophy): Areas of fat loss under the skin, which appear as "dents" in the skin. Although they are believed to be due to a form of insulin allergy, they can occur in areas where insulin has never been injected.

Buttocks: The seat; the part of the body that one sits on.

Hypertrophy (or Lipohypertrophy): Areas of swelling of the skin, which occur in places where too many shots are being given. Injecting insulin in areas of hypertrophy may cause altered insulin absorption.

Leak-back: The leaking out of a drop of insulin after the insulin injection is completed. This can be a cause of variation in day-to-day blood/CGM glucose levels.

Needle phobia: The intense fear of needles. Working with a social worker or psychologist on "needle desensitization" may help this, as well as use of injection devices.

QUESTIONS AND ANSWERS FROM NEWSNOTES

Q: I often note that a drop of insulin comes back after I withdraw the needle when giving the morning insulin to my child. Is this of any importance and what can I do to avoid it?

A: We are frequently asked this question. We call this "leak-back." Often this leakage is from the pen and is NOT part of the injected insulin.

Some methods to help avoid any loss are listed below:

1. Injecting the insulin slowly.
2. Letting go of the lift of skin soon after injecting the insulin so that pressure is not forcing the insulin out from under the skin.
3. Making sure the needle is in the full length and that one does not start to pull the needle out until three seconds after the injection is completed.
4. Making sure there is not excessive pressure on the site of injection. For example, if the child is sitting on a chair, he/she should sit on the edge of the chair when injecting in the leg rather than on the back of the chair where the pressure beneath the leg might force the insulin out of the injection site. Having the leg straight rather than bent at the knee may also result in less pressure.
5. Routinely counting for three seconds or longer after the insulin is injected before removing the needle.
6. Rubbing the needle track for two or three seconds as the needle is removed to "close off" the track.
7. If nothing else works, consider drawing 2 units of air into the syringe and letting it rise to the top of the insulin so the air is the last to be inserted (see text, Chapter 9).

If these principles are followed, it is unusual for drops of insulin to "leak-back."

Q: We just gave our son his dinner shot and accidentally gave the morning dose rather than the afternoon dose. What should we do?

A: We hear this question almost every week. The answer is to eat more at dinner and to have a bedtime snack (pizza is particularly effective). In addition, it is wise to set the alarm for every two or three hours, get up, do a blood sugar (or observe CGM value) and give extra juice or food as needed. If the value falls to very low levels (below 70 mg/dL or 3.9 mmol/L), it is necessary to stay up and keep doing the blood sugar levels every 20 or 30 minutes until the value is above 120 mg/dL or 6.7 mmol/L. It is also possible to administer the low-dose glucagon as discussed in Chapter 6. Some families find that having the a.m. and p.m. insulin doses taped to the front of the refrigerator can be a helpful reminder. It may also be a way to communicate or remember recent dosage changes. It is also effective to routinely have a second person check the dose.

CHAPTER 10

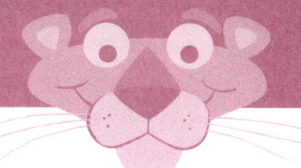

Feelings/Emotional Adjustment at Diabetes Onset

INTRODUCTION

This chapter is about feelings you may experience after learning that you or your child has diabetes. The diagnosis of diabetes is usually a shock and can be overwhelming. Most people are unprepared for this diagnosis. They struggle with why it has happened to them or their child. At diagnosis, families need to focus on their own or their loved one's health and everything that goes into taking care of diabetes. Learning is often difficult when in the middle of an emotional crisis.

The feeling of being overwhelmed is common. Families ask, "How are we going to manage this with work, other children, and other responsibilities?" This feeling decreases with education, time, and talking with others. Parents often find it best when they work together and share responsibilities. This book aims to help provide education for successful management of diabetes with your diabetes care team.

We expect that people and families will experience many different feelings after the diagnosis of diabetes. The emotions felt are common with the onset of any serious medical condition, and are normal during the period of initial diagnosis. People frequently wonder what they could have done to avoid getting diabetes. They think of all the "what ifs?" and try to imagine what they could have done differently. Young adults or parents sometimes blame themselves for eating (or letting their child eat) junk food or for not getting to the doctor right away. Bed-wetting is a common problem in

> **TOPICS:**
> **Psychosocial Adjustment**
>
> **TEACHING OBJECTIVES:**
> The teacher will:
> 1. Describe typical adjustment feelings associated with diagnosis.
> 2. Provide information regarding additional support services.
>
> **LEARNING OBJECTIVES:**
> Learner (parents, child, relative or self) will be able to:
> 1. Recognize feelings of adjustment associated with diagnosis.
> 2. Describe how to access additional support services.

children prior to diagnosis and can cause children to feel ashamed. Some parents feel guilty they didn't recognize the symptoms or because they were critical of their child. It is very important to talk about these feelings in order to adjust and help the medical team better understand how they can assist. Most parents feel grief and worry about how this will affect their family and their child's future. Teens and adults diagnosed with diabetes worry about how it will affect their lifestyle, work and future. In our Clinic, EVERY newly diagnosed family meets with a behavioral health counselor, a clinical social worker, a licensed professional counselor, or a psychologist to help with this process.

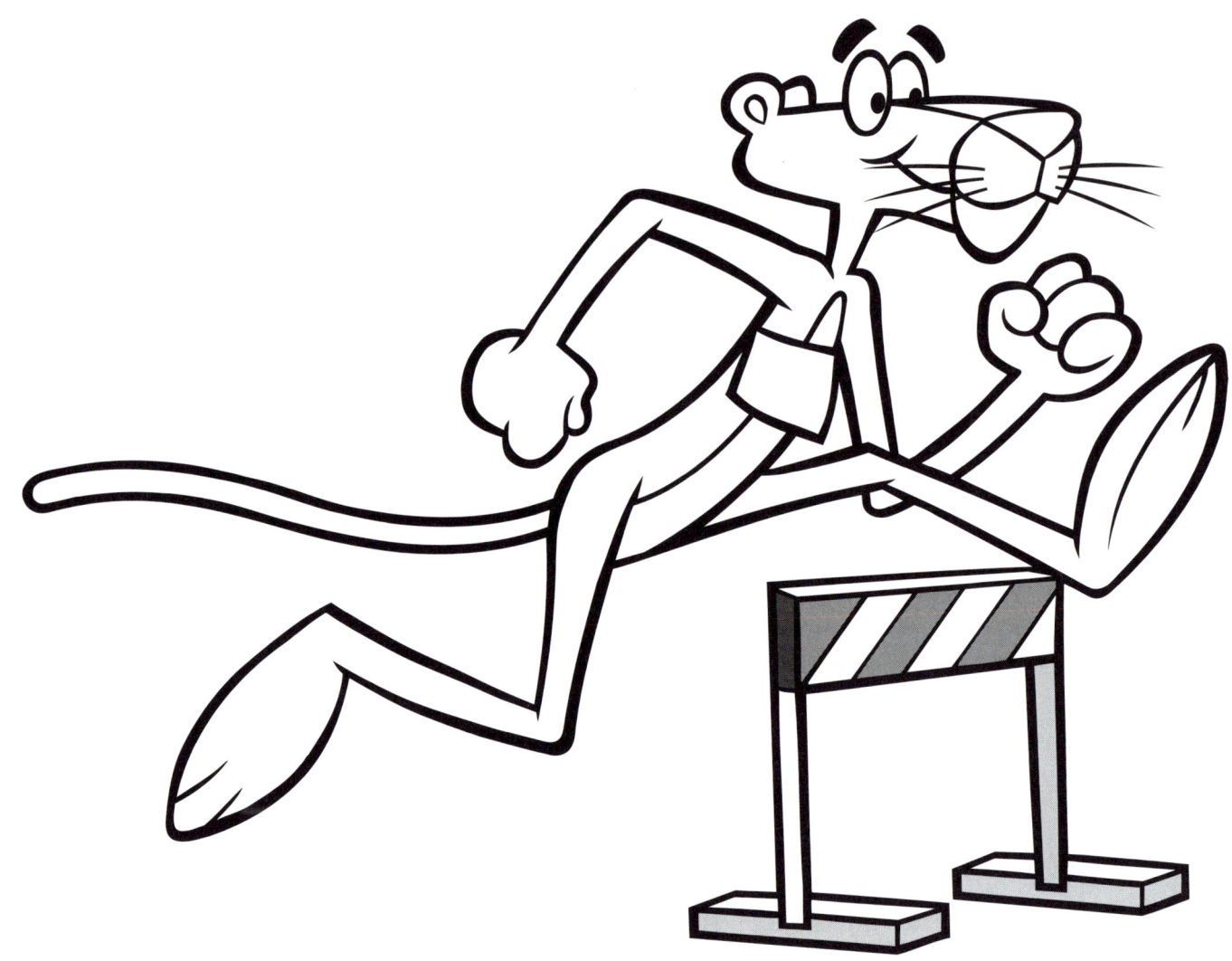

Adjusting to the onset of diabetes can present some emotional hurdles.

Some of the feelings that may be experienced are described below:

CONFUSION AND SHOCK are common feelings for families. Many people describe feeling shocked, scared, upset or even angry that they or their child has been diagnosed with diabetes. They wonder why this has happened, and think, "This can't be real," or "This can't be happening." They worry about whether they will be able to give shots without causing pain, and if they can remember everything that they were taught. Parents may experience a stronger sense of anxiety about their child's well-being and worry more about ordinary separations, like going back to school. All of these feelings are very normal and are important to discuss in order to get information and needed reassurance.

Because of the shock, it is often hard for families to focus on what the medical team is saying about diabetes. Sometimes families will ask to have things repeated. The medical team understands and will go over the information several times. Because of the initial shock, and sometimes lack of sleep, many clinics teach only survival skills (the "basics") for the first day or two. They then go into more depth at future visits.

GRIEF: Talking about grief can help people understand their own feelings as well as how to help their child through this important process. Adults and children react to the diagnosis and handle grief differently. Typically, adults are most upset during the first few days after diagnosis. Children who have been feeling quite sick may actually feel happier and have more energy when insulin is started. It is important to remember that they, too, will need to talk over how they feel about having diabetes and what it means to them. Even very young children get upset, and this may be manifested as changes in behavior.

DENIAL is often expressed in comments such as, "There must be a mistake in the diagnosis." As a result, people may want to seek additional opinions from other doctors. They hope to be told that they or their child doesn't have diabetes. Though initial doubt is a normal reaction, continued denial can make adjustment much more difficult. It can even interfere with medical treatment and education. If denial is very strong, it is important to understand and discuss the reason for this feeling. In some cases, there are complicated reasons and even cultural misunderstandings that can interfere with acceptance of the diagnosis.

For a child to accept his or her diabetes, parents need to accept the reality of diabetes and learn what they must do to care for their child. A child takes important cues from their family and will need their involvement, love, support and care. It is important to have all family members working together to incorporate diabetes into their lives. Though an adult with recently diagnosed diabetes will provide their own care, they will also need love, support and involvement from people important in their lives. This will help them accept the diagnosis of diabetes. Siblings, grandparents, aunts, uncles and spouses (significant others) will all need to work through their feelings about the diagnosis. Support from all family members and friends is crucial when coping with diabetes.

SADNESS: It is common, initially, for parents or siblings to cry, be depressed and feel a loss. Some parents fear that their child's life will never be normal again. The child they previously thought of as healthy will now be "different." If their child has had previous medical experiences or has other medical conditions, people may feel it is terribly unfair that their child has yet another challenge. Adults with newly diagnosed diabetes can also have the very same feelings, fears and concerns about themselves.

Sadness is part of grieving and may be experienced off and on during a family's and patient's lifetime with diabetes. Sometimes this sadness is affected by previous losses or other traumatic experiences and can be quite difficult for a child, parent or affected adult. If feelings of sadness persist and are affecting one's ability to function, it is a good idea to talk with a behavioral health counselor on the diabetes team or in the community to discuss what might be helpful during this difficult time.

ANGER is an emotion that is often difficult or uncomfortable to express. People often feel anger over unexpected circumstances. No one wants to get diabetes, or to have his or her child get diabetes. This anger may be felt or expressed toward doctors, nurses, God, a spouse, and even friends whose children do not have diabetes. Anger can reflect the understandable difficulty in accepting that a loved one must live with a chronic medical condition. Like sadness, anger can persist and not get better. When anger persists, it is very important to talk with a behavioral health counselor.

Children can also feel anger about the many changes in their lives—including pokes, shots, dietary changes, counting carbs, and other diabetes-related daily tasks. They often direct their anger at the parents because they don't yet have the ability to express how they are feeling. Open communication and patience will help children work out their feelings.

FEELINGS/EMOTIONAL ADJUSTMENT AT DIABETES ONSET

ANXIETY is another common feeling. Adults with diabetes may worry about how they will manage normal activities with this new diagnosis. Parents worry about their newly diagnosed child's safety and the extra responsibilities of caring for them. Normal everyday types of separations can take on a new meaning. A parent who previously sent their child to day care or school without concern may suddenly worry about whether their child with diabetes will be safe. The diabetes team will provide a school plan (Chapter 25). Meeting with the school staff will also help. Brothers and sisters may worry about seeing shots and about whether they will get diabetes, too. The child with diabetes may worry about whether their friends will treat them differently. Young adults or parents may wonder how diabetes will affect their or their child's future. These anxieties tend to improve as the family gets practice and experience with diabetes care. If anxieties persist, it is important to discuss these feelings with the diabetes team.

* A special note about anxiety with shots: One of the biggest initial fears for both adults and children is having to give (or get) insulin shots. Nearly everyone has fears about shots. This is normal! Fortunately, newer, smaller syringes and good technique can make shots almost painless. But fear often makes one shaky, nervous and tense. Giving or getting a shot when one is shaky, nervous or tense can be painful. Healthcare-providers can help review the method used. They can also teach relaxation and breathing techniques to help shots be more comfortable (more about this in Chapters 9 and 17). If pain persists, or the process takes more than a few minutes, notify the diabetes team so they can help.

GUILT is something that adults and children often feel. When we don't understand why something has happened, it is easy to blame ourselves. A parent with a family history of diabetes may blame him or herself. This idea occurs even when people have been told that autoimmunity, genetics and other unknown factors are important in causing diabetes. We do not completely understand why someone develops diabetes, but we do know that it is nobody's fault. There is no proven way at this time to prevent it. Earlier diagnosis would not have kept the diabetes from happening or changed the way it is treated.

Children always seek a reason for why something has happened. When we can't provide clear answers, they sometimes develop their own "theories" about why they got diabetes. Children have told us they thought they got diabetes because they "were naughty," "ate candy" or "were not nice to their brother." It is important to reassure them they did nothing to cause their diabetes. These "theories" can sometimes pop up years later. Keeping an open dialogue with children will help work through these times.

ADJUSTING TO DIABETES

The first few weeks or even months after diagnosis may feel like an eternity. The emotional and physical energy needed to manage the many changes resulting from a diagnosis of diabetes can be exhausting. These emotions are normal during the initial period after diagnosis. They may increase and decrease over the first few weeks to months, but tend to improve over time. The good news is that things do get better! As normal household chores, work and school routines are re-established, family members start to settle in with their new diabetes plan. Adults begin to feel more energetic and able to "meet the world" on their terms. Parents are often reassured that their child is feeling better and "back to their old self." Sometimes a child may have spurts in growth after just a few weeks of care. If weight loss occurred prior to diagnosis, appetite may be increased and the weight regained. Everyone begins to feel more confident in new skills, but may still have many questions. These are very important to review with the healthcare team.

As with any chronic medical condition, there will be times when some of the feelings and frustrations will again feel overwhelming. Feelings that arose during the initial diagnosis period may recur at other times in the child's life, including when starting school, spending the night with other friends or family, starting to drive, moving out of the house, and other major life events. Talking with the diabetes team and behavioral health counselors can be helpful during these times. This will be discussed further in Chapter 17.

Making life with diabetes as normal as possible is the major long-term goal. Adjustment over the long term takes time. Communication about feelings within the family is very important, because everyone feels the effects of one member having diabetes. Siblings often feel left out when the child with diabetes needs more attention. It is important to discuss the diagnosis of diabetes with all members of the family, including siblings. Special, dedicated time should be set aside for other siblings as well.

As individuals and families adjust, everyone usually feels more hopeful. People find strengths that they didn't know they had. Parents may seek out connections with other families who have children with diabetes. They may want to volunteer to raise money for research and care or participate in available clinical research studies. The Internet opens up new avenues for information and resources (see websites in back of book). There is a strong worldwide community of families, medical providers and researchers who are very committed to advancing care for people with diabetes and, hopefully, eventually finding a cure. Having hope is a good thing!

DEFINITIONS

Adjustment (adaptation): Gradually learning to live with something (such as the diagnosis of diabetes).

Denial (deny): A refusal to believe something. A person may refuse to believe that he or she has diabetes.

Diagnosis: The process of finding that a person has a disease.

Guilt: A feeling that one caused something to happen.

QUESTIONS AND ANSWERS FROM NEWSNOTES

Q Why is The Pink Panther™ character used in the educational manual, *Understanding Diabetes?*

a Having a family member develop diabetes is often the most traumatic event that has happened to a family. If a child were pictured to demonstrate a side effect, such as hypoglycemia, it might be harder for a family member to accept than a picture of the Pink Panther having a reaction. Also, a bit of humor at this time of intense emotions can often be a big help.

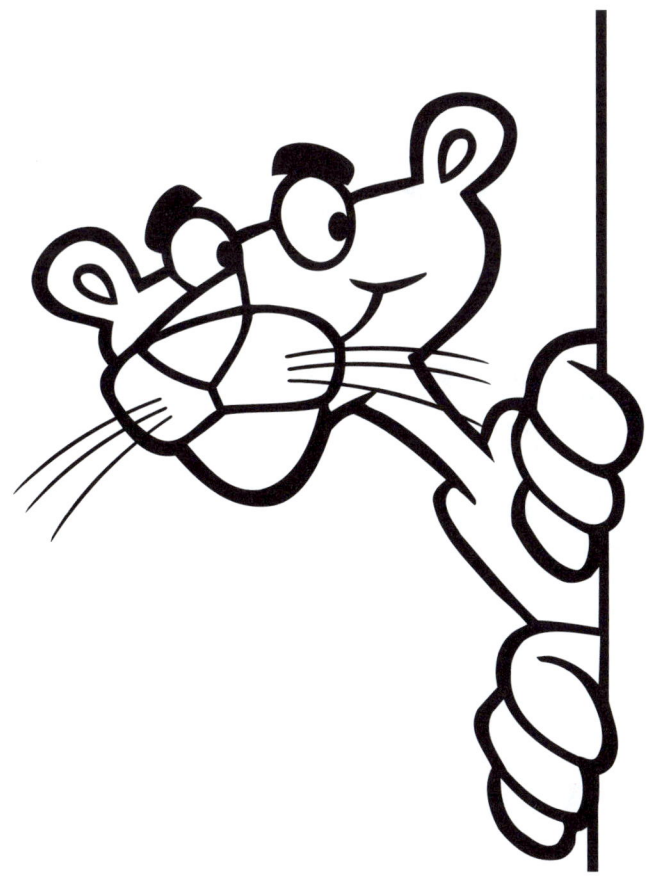

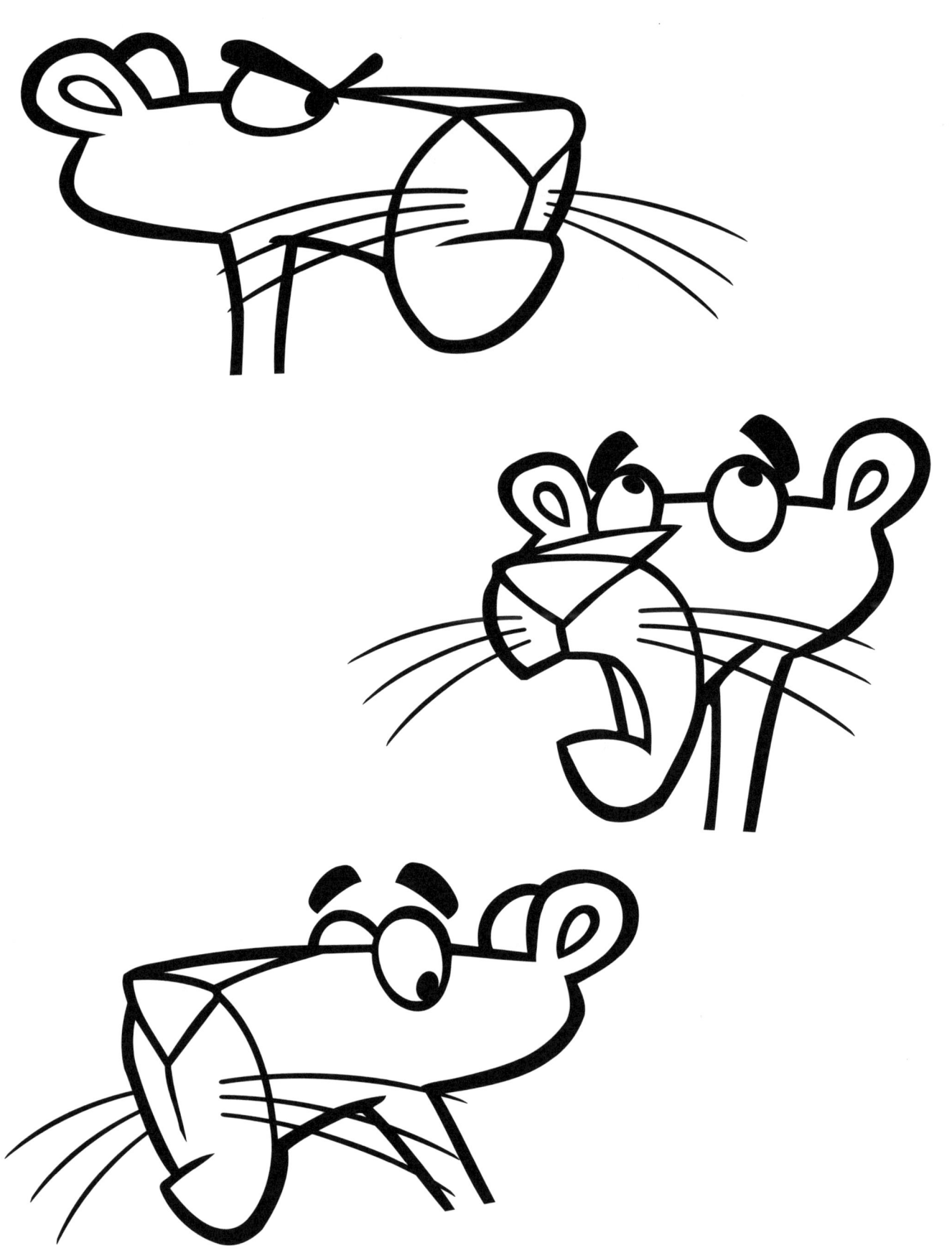

FEELINGS/EMOTIONAL ADJUSTMENT AT DIABETES ONSET

CHAPTER 11

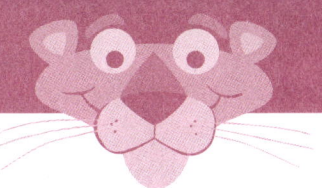

Normal Nutrition

TYPES OF NUTRIENTS

Families of a newly-diagnosed person with diabetes are usually worried about what someone with diabetes should eat. They shouldn't be, as **the ideal diet for someone with diabetes (type 1 or type 2) is really just a healthy diet from which all people would benefit.** This chapter is meant to be a review of normal nutrition, which will help to improve the entire family's nutrition. It will be an introduction to Chapter 12, Food Management and Diabetes. It may also make some of the words used by the dietitian easier to follow.

Foods provide different nutrients necessary for growth and health. If you know about these nutrients, you can help your family eat the right foods. Learning to read food labels will help you to know what you are buying at the grocery store. Portion sizes are also important for a healthy weight. The Dietary Guidelines for Americans is available online at: www.healthierus.gov/dietaryguidelines. Table 1 shows the main recommendations.

There are six major nutrient groups; each will be discussed in detail below:

1. Carbohydrate
2. Protein
3. Fat
4. Vitamins and minerals
5. Water
6. Fiber

TOPICS:
Nutritional Management

TEACHING OBJECTIVES:
The teacher will:
1. Present basic nutritional components including carbohydrates, protein and fat.
2. Introduce the importance of carbohydrate management in diabetes management.
3. Present nutritional guidelines for fat/cholesterol intake and desired blood lipid ranges.
4. Describe current problems with body weight/obesity.

LEARNING OBJECTIVES:
Learner (parents, child, relative or self) will be able to:
1. List three major food components and give an example of each.
2. Explain the effect of carbohydrate intake on blood/CGM glucose levels.
3. Describe a dietary method to lower blood cholesterol/lipid levels.
4. Describe two methods for maintaining a healthy weight.

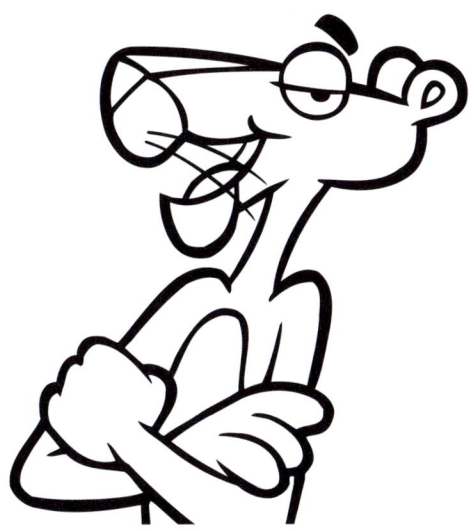

TABLE 1:
Dietary Guidelines (also see Figure 1):

Fruit and Vegetable Intake
5 to 13 servings per day
(2½-6½ cups/day)
Consume enough fruits and vegetables while staying within energy needs: 1-2½ cups of fruit and 1½-4 cups of vegetables per day for a reference 2,000-calorie intake. Make adjustments for various calorie levels.

Fat Intake
Keep total fat between 20 percent and 35 percent of calories, with most fats coming from sources of polyunsaturated and monounsaturated fats such as fish, nuts and vegetable oils; limit solid fats like butter, margarine, shortening and lard, and foods that contain these.

Salt Intake
Consume less than 1,500 mg of sodium per day (3/4 teaspoon of table salt–less for younger children) and include potassium-rich foods such as fruits and vegetables.

Sugar Intake
Choose and prepare foods low in added sugars or caloric sweeteners.

Dairy Intake
3-4 servings per day (3-4 cups per day of fat-free or low-fat milk or equivalent)

Bread, Cereal, Grain Intake
6-11 servings per day of 3-10 ounces
Half of one's intake of grains should be in the form of whole grains.

Protein
2-3 servings per day of 3-7 ounces
2-3 ounces poultry, fish or lean meat 1½ cup cooked dry beans
1 egg = 1 ounce meat
         = 4 ounces or ½ cup tofu

Portion Size
Portion sizes are also important for a healthy weight.

Physical Activity
Engage in 60 minutes of moderate physical activity on most days of the week.
To help manage excess weight, engage in at least 60 minutes of moderate to vigorous activity on most days of the week, while not exceeding calorie requirements.

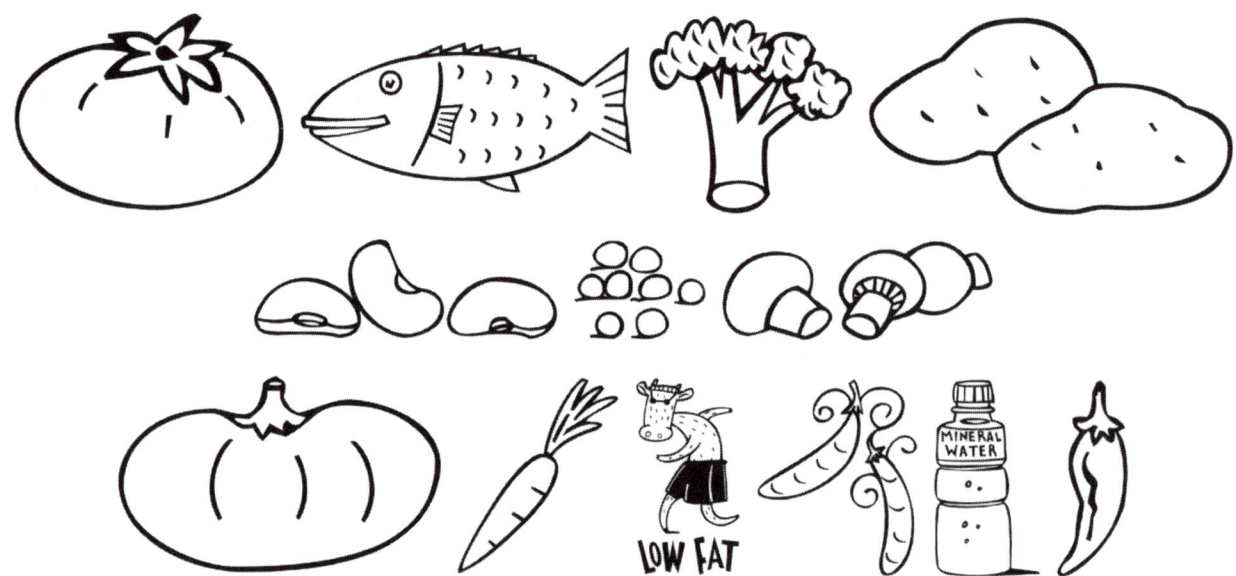

NORMAL NUTRITION

1. Carbohydrate ("carbs")

Carbohydrate is the food source we are most concerned about for people with diabetes. This is because it is the main nutrient that is changed to blood sugar. Carbohydrate is important mainly as an energy source for the body. Each gram of carbohydrate supplies four calories.

It used to be believed that sugar, which is a carbohydrate, was rapidly absorbed while starchy carbohydrates were slowly absorbed. This is an easy concept to explain and to believe, but it is **NOT TRUE**. Research has shown that there is no difference in absorption of a sugar as compared with a starchy carbohydrate. This is because the intestine has such high levels of digestive enzymes that starchy carbohydrate is rapidly broken down to sugar. Thus, **"a carbohydrate is a carbohydrate, is a carbohydrate…"** However, as discussed in Chapter 6, carbs in liquid form are generally absorbed more rapidly than those in solid foods.

Insulin is essential to allow sugar to pass into the cells of the body to be burned for energy. **The balance between all carbohydrate eaten and the insulin dosage is one of the major keys to diabetes management.** These concepts are discussed in detail in the next chapter, Food Management and Diabetes. The Dietary Guidelines for Americans recommends at least 2 cups of fruit and 3 cups of vegetables per day (for 2,000 calories) and cutting back on foods with added sugar.

Some examples of carbohydrate foods are:

- ✔ breads (encourage whole wheat grain)
- ✔ cereals and grains
- ✔ crackers
- ✔ fruits
- ✔ beans (baked, refried, black, kidney, etc.; contain protein also)
- ✔ vegetables
  - starchy (½ cup cooked contains approximately 15g carbohydrate): corn, peas, potatoes and yams, sweet potatoes
  - non-starchy (½ cup cooked contains approximately 5g carbohydrate): green beans, asparagus, broccoli, celery, cabbage, cauliflower and carrots
- ✔ milk and yogurt (contain protein and may also contain fat)
- ✔ most desserts
- ✔ **Sugar-containing drinks such as sugar-soda are a source of "empty calories" and are unhealthy for all. They contribute to obesity and cause high blood sugar levels in people with diabetes.**

Starch: More detailed knowledge about starches and sugars, both of which are carbohydrates, is helpful. Starch is a substance made up of hundreds of sugar units. The sugar from starch is now known to be absorbed as quickly as that from table sugar (when each is taken alone without other foods). Sources of starch are breads, noodles, pasta, rice, cereals and starchy vegetables such as corn, peas, potatoes and legumes.

Sugar: The World Health Organization (WHO) recommends that all people should limit (processed) sugar intake to less than 10 percent of calories. A diet high in sugars contributes to dental cavities and provides few vitamins and minerals. Often high-sugar foods also contain large amounts of fat. A nutritious diet does not contain large amounts of high-sugar foods. There are many different kinds of sugar found in foods. Some sugar is often added to foods as a sweetener and may not be noticed unless labels are read. The names for sugars often end in "—ose."

Some of the common sugars are listed below:

- ✔ **Glucose:** Glucose is the name for the main sugar in our body. When we talk about blood and urine sugar, we really mean glucose. Table sugar is half glucose and half fructose. Corn sugar is primarily glucose. Another name for glucose is dextrose.

✔ **Fructose:** Fructose is sometimes called "fruit sugar" as it is the main type of sugar found in fruits. It is sold in pure granulated form and is a part of many food products. Fructose has the same number of calories per gram as table sugar (sucrose). The liquid form is sweeter than table sugar, but the taste is the same in baked products. Generally, only one-half to one-third the amount of fructose needs to be used to have the same degree of sweetness as table sugar.

"**High-fructose" corn syrup** is different from pure fructose and contains large amounts of sucrose. People with diabetes need to be careful of how much of this is eaten.

✔ **Sucrose or table sugar:** The body breaks down sucrose to glucose and fructose.

Foods high in sucrose and glucose include soft drinks, cake, cookies, pie, candy, and other desserts.

✔ **Lactose or milk sugar:** Lactose is found in milk and yogurt. Children and adolescents should drink three to four 8-oz glasses of milk per day for calcium and vitamin D.

✔ **Syrups:** Corn syrup, corn syrup solids, high fructose syrups, maple syrup, and sugar cane syrup are often added to baked goods. They are all primarily glucose and must be consumed carefully by people with diabetes.

2. Protein

Protein is important for muscle and bone growth. However, eating extra protein does not cause increased muscle growth. Muscles grow only as a result of proper exercise. Foods high in protein include milk, yogurt, meats, fish, chicken, turkey, egg whites, soy, cheese, cottage cheese, beans and nuts. In addition to fish being a good source of protein, the fish oils (fats) are believed to help avoid heart disease (see "Fat" in this chapter). Protein should provide 15-20 percent of the total caloric intake. Protein from animal sources is a complete protein. This means it contains all of the essential building blocks of protein called amino acids.

Adults and teens can receive adequate protein eating only a vegetarian diet, but this is more difficult for growing infants and children. Many people do not realize that protein is also available from non-meat sources. Dried beans, legumes, soy, nuts and seeds are fairly suitable sources of protein.

Most people eat more protein than they need. In a review of three-day diet records from our Clinic, the young men were getting approximately three times, and the young women two times the amount of protein needed. High protein intake usually results in high animal fat intake, which may be unhealthy for the heart. It may also provide an extra stress for some people's kidneys.

It is important to choose low-fat meat and poultry. Low-fat meats may be graded as lean or choice for lower amounts of fat.

Two examples of reducing the fat content of the diet are:

- removing the skin from poultry
- buying lean meats that do not have a lot of visible fat

3. Fat

Fat is an important energy source and is needed for growth. Fat has more than twice the calories (nine calories per gram) than protein or carbohydrate (four calories per gram). Thus, it is more likely to lead to weight gain and obesity. Most effective long-term weight reduction programs emphasize limiting total fat intake. The dietary guidelines recommend that fat should provide only 20-35 percent of total caloric intake. The types of fats found in fish, nuts and vegetable oils are preferred. A major emphasis in nutrition in the past decade has been the reduction of the total daily fat intake. Dietary cholesterol intake should not be excessive. People with high LDL cholesterol levels (Table 2) may benefit from lowering dietary cholesterol to <200 mg/day. Higher-fat and cholesterol intake may lead to increased blood fat levels (cholesterol and triglycerides:

Table 2) and possibly a higher risk for heart disease. Some research shows that teens with diabetes eat close to 40 percent of calories from fat. Fried food eaten in fast-food restaurants is usually very high in fat.

The main fats in the diet are divided into four types:

✔ **monounsaturated:** high in olive and canola oils (best fats)

✔ **polyunsaturated:** most vegetable oils (healthy fats)

✔ **saturated:** mainly animal fats; e.g., meats, cheese, butter (non-healthy fats; may raise LDL cholesterol)

✔ **trans-fats:** hydrogen has been added back to make them trans-fats (worst fats; raises LDL cholesterol)

It is important to eat more of the monounsaturated and polyunsaturated fats than the saturated fats. **Less than seven percent of total calories eaten per day should be from saturated fat.** Increasing the intake of monounsaturated fats (e.g., olive oil and canola oil) can help avoid heart disease.

There are high amounts of polyunsaturated fat in most vegetable oils (coconut and palm are exceptions). Margarines made from vegetable oils are also polyunsaturated. In general, the softer or more liquid a fat is at room temperature, the less saturated it is. For example, liquid margarine (tub margarine) is a better choice than stick margarine, and vegetable oil is better than vegetable shortening.

The saturated fats include most animal fats such as the fat in meats, cheese, milk, butter and lard. Chicken, turkey and fish are lower in saturated fat than beef or pork, particularly when the skin is removed. Chicken, turkey and fish also contain some polyunsaturated fat.

Blood Lipids (fats)

High levels of the two main blood fats (lipids), **cholesterol** and **triglyceride**, can lead to early aging of the large blood vessels (including the coronary blood vessels in the heart). These vessels carry blood to the heart, legs and other body parts. Other risk factors for early aging of large blood vessels are **diabetes, tobacco use, high blood pressure, lack of exercise** and **being overweight**. As people with diabetes already have one risk factor (by having diabetes), they do not need another. Optimal management of glucose levels will help to keep the blood fat levels in the desired ranges. The other risk factors above (in dark print) need to be carefully monitored.

In addition to cholesterol levels, the proteins that carry cholesterol in the blood (lipoproteins) are also important. The **LDL cholesterol** carries the cholesterol into the blood vessel wall. Therefore, this level needs to be low. Some groups are now recommending the value be <70 mg/dL (3.9 mmol/L) rather than

TABLE 2:
Recommended Levels for Lipids and Lipoproteins

Lipid Type	Desired Level **	
Cholesterol	<200 mg/dL	<5.2 mmol/L
LDL Cholesterol*	<100 mg/dL	<2.6 mmol/L
HDL Cholesterol*	>40 mg/dL	>1.0 mmol/L
Triglyceride*	<150 mg/dL	<1.7 mmol/L

* Preferably drawn after fasting overnight. If fasting overnight is not possible, then at least four hours after eating.
** Desired level for a person with diabetes
< = less than   > = greater than

NORMAL NUTRITION

TABLE 3:
Making Food Choices for Fat Content

Food Group (Amount)	Decrease	Instead Choose
Meat, Poultry, & Fish (6-8 oz per day)	Beef, pork, lamb, regular ground beef, fatty cuts, spare ribs, organ meats. Poultry with skin, fried chicken, fried fish, fried shellfish, regular luncheon meat (e.g., bologna, salami, sausage, frankfurters)	Lean beef, pork, lamb (lean cuts), well-trimmed before cooking. Poultry without skin, fish, shellfish, processed meat – prepared from lean meat (e.g., sliced turkey from the deli)
Eggs	Egg yolks: If high blood cholesterol, limit to two per week	Egg whites (two whites can be substituted for whole egg in recipes), cholesterol-free egg substitute
Dairy Products (2-3 servings per day)	Whole milk (fluid, evaporated, condensed), 2% fat milk (low-fat milk), imitation milk, whole milk yogurt, whole milk yogurt beverages, regular cheeses — American, Blue, Brie, Cheddar, Colby, Edam, Monterey Jack, whole-milk Mozzarella, Parmesan, Swiss, cream cheese, Neufchatel cheese	Milk – fat-free, ½%, or 1% fat (fluid, powdered, evaporated) Yogurt – nonfat or low-fat yogurt or yogurt beverages
	Cottage cheese (4% fat)	Low-fat or nonfat varieties of cottage cheese
	Ice cream	Frozen dairy dessert – ice milk, frozen yogurt (low-fat or nonfat), nonfat ice cream
	Cream, half & half, whipped cream, nondairy creamer, sour cream	Low-fat coffee creamer, low-fat or nonfat sour cream
Fats and Oils (≤6-8 teaspoons per day)	Coconut oil, palm kernel oil, palm oils	Polyunsaturated oils – safflower, sunflower, corn, canola*, olive*, peanut
	Butter, lard, shortening, bacon fat, hard margarine	Margarine – made from oils listed above, light or diet margarine, especially soft or liquid forms (e.g., Parkay Squeeze™)

*High in mono-unsaturated fats.

Adapted from Powers, MA; *"Handbook of Diabetes Medical Nutrition Therapy"*, Aspen Publishers, Inc. Gaithersburg, MD, 1996 p. 354.

FIGURE 1

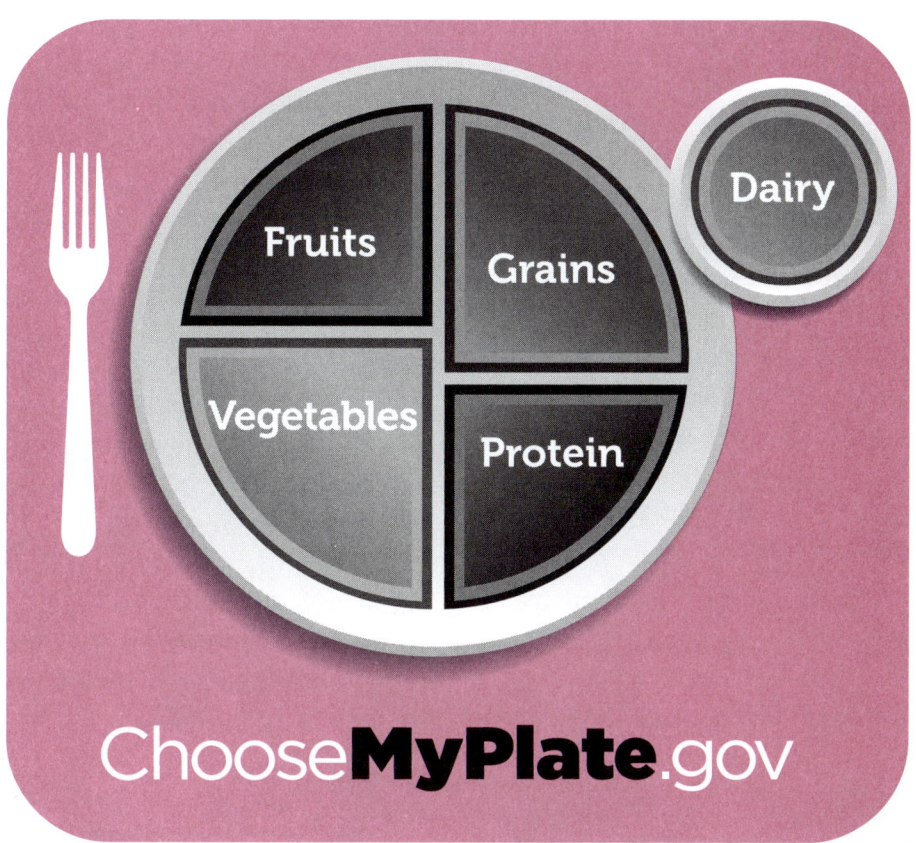

(a helpful website)

Look at the food plate guide to see if you need to:
- eat more whole-grain foods (e.g., whole wheat bread, brown rice, cereals)
- eat more fruits and vegetables
- eat less protein and fat (particularly red meat)

<100 mg/dL (5.5 mmol/L) as shown in Table 2. In general, lower is better. The cholesterol build-up in the blood vessel wall may lead to hardening of the arteries (atherosclerosis) which makes a heart attack more likely to occur. The **HDL cholesterol** carries the cholesterol out of the blood vessel wall. This level should be high. Desired levels for people with diabetes are shown in Table 2.

We recommend a low-fat diet that allows no more than 20 to 35 percent of total calories from fat. We recommend limiting intake of foods that are high in animal (saturated) fats and trans-fats. Suggestions for changes are shown in Table 3. Reduction of total fat, animal (saturated) fat, trans-fats and cholesterol intake are healthy nutrition practices whether a person has diabetes or not. Trans-fats are similar to saturated fatty acids. They both raise blood cholesterol levels. They are found in solid margarines, commercial cookies, crackers and other foods. The dietary guidelines recommend keeping trans-fat intake as low as possible.

Suggestions for healthy nutrition include eating:

- fish and poultry (with the skin removed)
- cold-water fish (e.g., salmon, light tuna), with omega-3 fatty acids, at least twice weekly
- milk with no more than 1 percent fat
- canola, olive, corn, safflower or soy oils should be used for salads and cooking

4. Vitamins and Minerals

These are important for growth, formation of blood cells, healthy skin, good vision, and strong teeth and bones. Fruits and vegetables are rich in vitamins. Minerals are found in milk, meats and vegetables. Calcium is a mineral that is important for the bones and teeth. People who do not drink milk or eat dairy products may need to take a calcium supplement. Many foods (e.g., cereals, waffles) are now fortified with calcium. Children ages 1–3 years need 500 mg of calcium per day, and those who are 4–10 years need 150 mg per day. Most people 10-20 years old need 1,300 mg per day.

Zinc is a mineral that is lost in the urine in proportion to sugar in the urine. Zinc is important for growth. Some children with diabetes may grow better with a zinc supplement.

Sodium is also a mineral, which, in some "salt-sensitive" people, may cause higher blood pressure. It is recommended by the American Heart Association that all people limit their sodium to less than 1,500 mg (approximately 3/4 tsp) per day (less in young children). If blood pressure is elevated, this amount should be even lower. Salt in the food we eat (e.g., chips, hamburgers, hot dogs and convenience foods) is often "hidden" but may be a significant source of salt.

Generally, people who eat a well-balanced diet do not need extra vitamins. If a child does not eat a balanced diet (e.g., not liking yellow or green vegetables), a vitamin supplement may be helpful. Also, vitamins and minerals are often recommended in the month following onset of diabetes as the body rebuilds. In general, "mega" doses of nutrients should be avoided, and the vitamins should not contain more than 100 percent of the recommended daily allowance (RDA). The fat-soluble vitamins (A, D, E and K) are stored in the body, and excessive doses can be harmful. It is now recognized that vitamin D has immune properties. Vitamin D can be synthesized by our own bodies with adequate exposure to sunshine. Low blood levels of vitamin D are quite common due to less time now spent outdoors and the use of sunscreen protection.

5. Water

Water is the most important nutrient for the survival of humans. It makes up much of the blood, the body fluids and the body's transport system. It serves as a coolant, shock absorber, waste remover and has many other important functions. Since the body is made up of about two-thirds water, it is important to drink a lot of it. We recommend at least six 8-oz glasses of liquid per day, including milk and allowed sugar-free drinks. When a person with diabetes is spilling urine ketones, it is important to drink more water and sugar-free liquids. This helps to replace body fluid loss.

6. Fiber

Dietary fiber is the part of plants ("roughage" or "bulk") that is not digested and is not absorbed into the body. Foods vary in the amounts and kinds of fiber they contain. Fiber in the diet supplies bulk (without calories) and roughage, which helps satisfy the appetite and keep the digestive system running smoothly. In people with type 2 diabetes, increased fiber intake has been helpful in slowing the absorption of sugar. Fiber has not been as helpful in lowering blood/CGM glucose levels in people with type 1 diabetes.

Fiber often is divided into two types. The first is **water-soluble fiber**, such as parts of oats and beans, seeds, citrus fruits and apples. These may help lower the blood cholesterol levels. They also may help reduce the blood/CGM glucose levels after meals in people with type 2 diabetes. The other type, **water-insoluble fiber**, such as parts of wheat bran, most grains, nuts and vegetables, helps avoid constipation and may help other digestive disorders. According to the Dietary Guidelines, the minimum intake of fruits and vegetables is "5-a-Day." The Eat 5-a-Day campaign was developed by the Produce for

Better Health Foundation in cooperation with the National Cancer Institute. This includes 2 servings of fruits and at least 3 of vegetables. Make half your plate fruits and vegetables. They have launched a public health initiative: **Fruits and Veggies — More Matters**™. Their website is: www. fruitsandveggiesmatter.gov. The website varies intake by age.

WEIGHT MANAGEMENT

This is also discussed in Chapters 4 and 12, but must now also be addressed as part of normal nutrition. The rate of obesity (a BMI of above 30; see Chapter 12) increased from 14.5 percent in 1999-2000 to 17.3 percent in 2011-2012 in children and teens in the U.S. This means one in six children is obese. Obesity is a major factor related to the cause of type 2 diabetes (Chapter 4). It has gradually become more common in youth who are newly-diagnosed with type 1 diabetes and adds an element of type 2 diabetes (insulin resistance) to the diagnosis of type 1 diabetes.

Reduction of total calorie intake (particularly of high-fat foods) with reduced snacking and smaller helpings is essential.

Foods higher in fat include:

- red meats
- the skin of chicken or turkey
- whole milk
- fats and oils
- processed foods (baked products are cookies and cakes)
- fast foods

Higher intake of vegetables, fruits, and whole grain foods may also help (see Figure 1).

In order to lose weight, **exercise** is also essential (Chapter 13). Most people require 60 minutes of exercise per day in order to lose weight and maintain the loss.

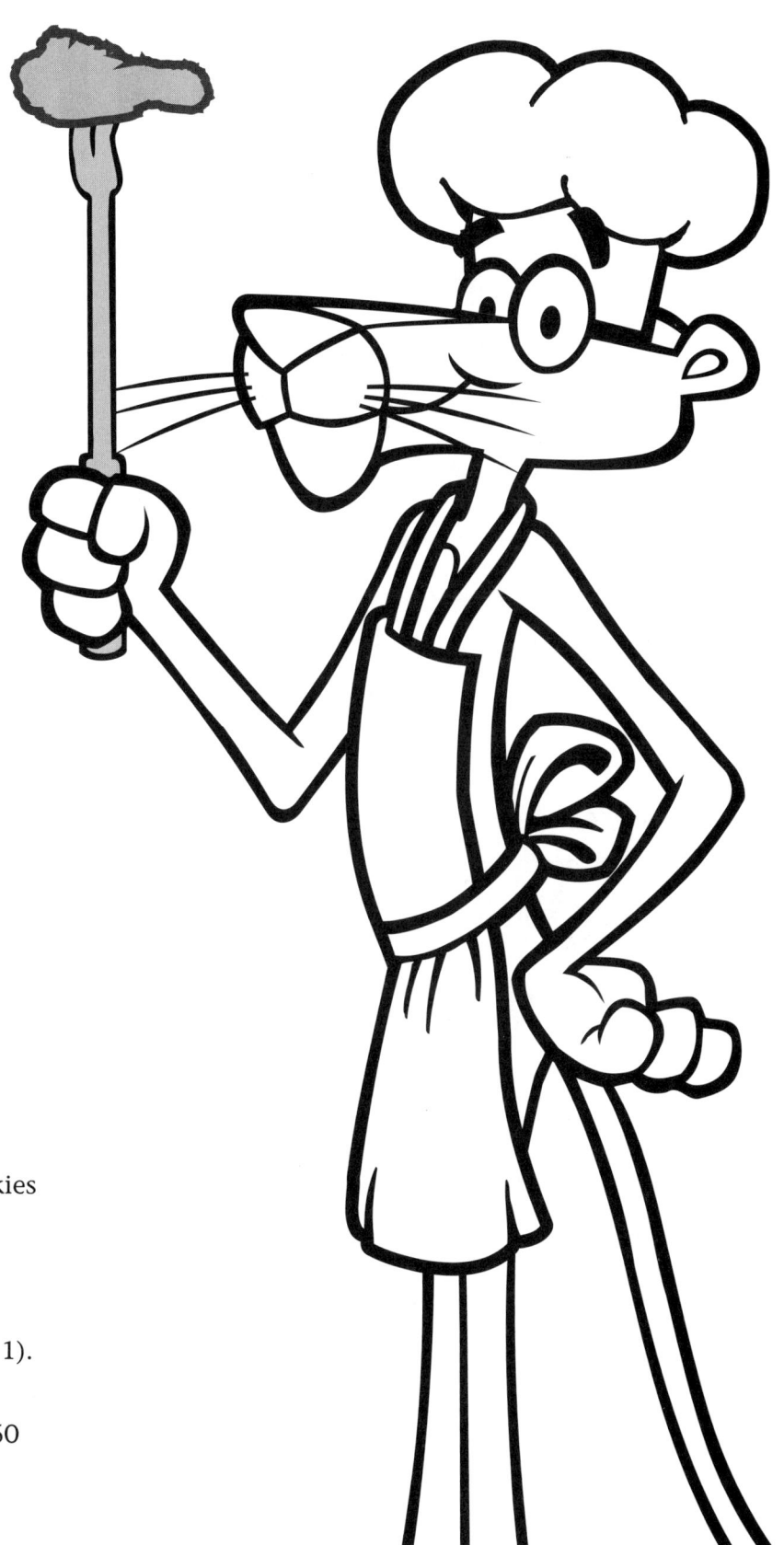

FOOD GROUPS

Foods are often divided into groups or exchanges (see Chapter 12). The common divisions include the milk and yogurt, meat, grains and starchy vegetables, non-starchy vegetables, fruit, and fat groups. At least one-half of the servings of grains for the day should be whole grain. The milk and meat groups are important sources of protein, and the milk group is a major source of calcium and vitamin D. Milk also has carbohydrate. Some of the minerals, such as iron and zinc, are high in the meat groups. Vitamins and fiber are generally highest in the fruit and vegetable groups. Be aware that some foods from each of the food groups should be eaten daily to have a well-balanced diet. The "Plate" method (see Figure 1) of choosing food has been adapted by the U.S. Department of Agriculture Center to provide an easy-to-understand guide for food to eat. They suggest each quarter of your plate have one of the following food groups:

- lean protein
- fruits
- vegetables
- whole-grain carbohydrate foods

Low-fat dairy products can be added (see Figure 1).

Three-day Food Record

It is sometimes helpful to keep a three-day food record. This will help to show if you are eating the right foods. Write down all foods and the amounts you eat for three days, as shown in the Appendix in this chapter. The dietitian can then review the record and suggest changes if needed. Chapter 12 emphasizes the use of food records to evaluate carbohydrate counting. While you are doing the recording, you will need to give accurate information. If you feel you need more help with instructions, ask your dietitian.

SWEETENERS
(Sugars and Sugar-substitutes)

Many foods are now available which contain sweeteners that either do not raise the blood/CGM sugar levels or may cause less of an increase than a similar amount of table sugar. Sweeteners are divided into the nutritive sweeteners (including table sugar), which do provide calories and carbohydrate, and the non-nutritive sweeteners, which essentially provide no calories or carbohydrate.

- **NUTRITIVE SWEETENERS**

✔ **Sugars**
These include all sugars and all sugar-alcohols. Sugars contain 5g of carbohydrate and 20 calories per level teaspoon (5 mL or 5 grams of liquid sugar). The two main sugars used as sweeteners are sucrose (table sugar) and fructose. Both are discussed earlier in this chapter under Carbohydrates, and both cause an increase in blood/CGM sugar levels. **High-fructose corn syrup** is a combination of both fructose and sucrose and raises the blood sugar more than pure fructose. **Agave Nectar** is a syrup refined from a cactus-like plant. It has fructose and glucose in it, but is 140-160 times sweeter than table sugar. Foods sweetened with fruit juices, dates or raisins may have the label "no added sugar." This is misleading, as there is sugar in these food additives.

✔ **Sugar Alcohols**
The sugar alcohols include sorbitol, xylitol, mannitol and others (often ending in "ol"). They provide about 2g of carbohydrate and eight calories per teaspoon. They are more slowly absorbed than sugar, and eating an excessive amount can cause diarrhea. They are often found in "sugar-free" candies and cookies as well as other low carb products.

✔ **Erythritol:** Erythritol is a sugar alcohol that is combined with stevia sweeteners like Truvia™ for bulk and sweetness. It contains zero carbs and calories (less than other sugar alcohols) and does not cause diarrhea as some sugar alcohols do.

✔ **Xylitol:** Xylitol is a sugar alcohol that is found in products like chewing gum and can also be found in a tabletop sweetener called Ideal™. It can be used for baking.

- ## NON-NUTRITIVE SWEETENERS

The non-nutritive (or "artificial") sweeteners do not provide any calories or carbohydrate.

Some currently on the market include:

1. **Saccharin:** Saccharin is 200-700 times sweeter than table sugar. It is found in Sweet'N Low®, other tabletop sweeteners and in some diet drinks.

2. **Aspartame:** Aspartame is 200 times sweeter than table sugar. It is broken down into aspartic acid, methanol and phenylalanine. (Rare patients with a condition called phenylketonuria cannot metabolize phenylalanine and cannot eat foods with this sweetener.) The products that contain aspartame include: Equal®, NutraSweet®, diet pop, sugar-free JELL-O®, Kool-Aid®, ice cream, Crystal Light® and many others. Use in moderation is generally advised (no more than two diet pops per day!).

3. **Acesulfame-Potassium (Ace-K):** Ace-K is 200 times sweeter than table sugar. It is approved for use as a tabletop sweetener and for use in chewing gum, desserts, beverages and other products. It is used in many sugar-free drinks and in other products along with aspartame.

4. **Sucralose:** Sucralose was approved for use in 1998 and is 600 times sweeter than sugar. It is used as a tabletop sweetener (Splenda®) and is found in RC Cola®, diet and sugar-free juices, Log Cabin® Sugar-Free Syrup and many other products.

5. **Stevia:** Stevia is a natural sweetener from the herb Stevia rebaudiana. It is 300 times sweeter than sugar. Stevia leaf and extracts are available as a sweetener in the dietary supplement aisle. In 2008, the FDA approved

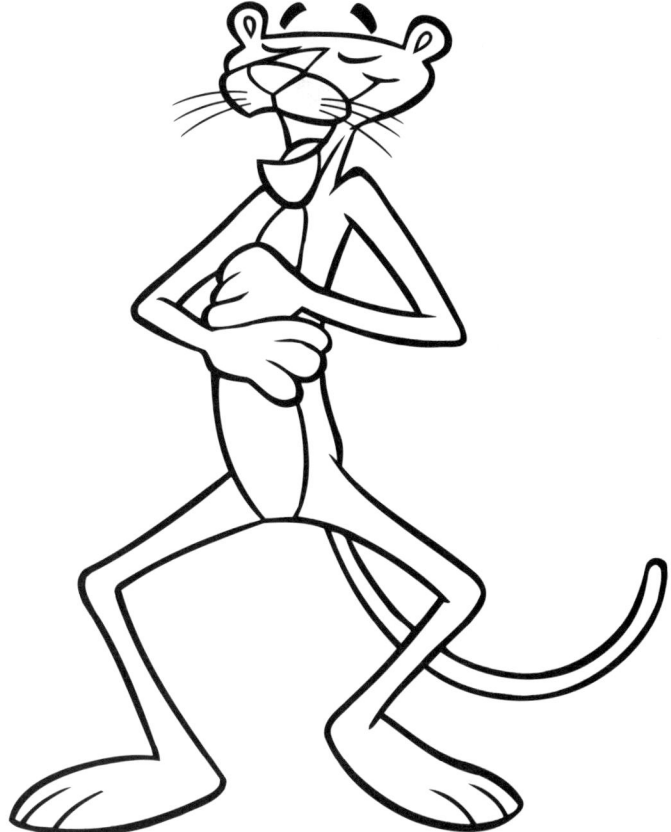

Rebaudioside A (Reb A), a part of the stevia leaf, to be added to food and drinks and as a tabletop sweetener. This part of the stevia leaf can be found in tabletop sweeteners, such as Truvia and Pura Via™.

6. **Neotame:** Approved by the FDA as a general-purpose sweetener and is 30-40 times sweeter than aspartame.

7. **Monk Fruit Extract (luo han guo):** Monk fruit extract is 150 to 300 times sweeter than sucrose. It is approved by the FDA as generally recognized as safe since 2009. It is used with sucralose in a sweetener named Nectresse®.

TABLE 4:
Reading a Nutrition Label

- The serving size is shown at the top. It is important to observe the serving size. (This is often less than the amount people eat. If you eat two cups rather than one, you would need to double all of the amounts listed.) The total calories and the calories from fat per serving are routinely given and are important.

- The total fat includes all types of fat (saturated, polyunsaturated, monounsaturated and trans-fat). The total fat, trans-fat, and saturated fat and cholesterol content are all important in relation to heart disease and it is wise to look for lower fat choices.

- The saturated fats for the entire day should be under 10 percent of the total calories per day. For someone eating 2,000 calories per day, this would mean under 200 calories from saturated fat or under 22g (nine calories per gram).

- † The percent of daily values for fat, carbohydrate and protein are listed on the label based on a 2,000-calorie daily intake.

- More active people will need more calories, in which case these amounts should be figured based on calories actually eaten.

- **One helping of this cereal has 15g of carbohydrate.** If one cup of white milk (any type) is added, then an additional 15 g of carbohydrate must also be added so that there would be a total of 30g of carbohydrate. The sugars include those found naturally in the food (e.g., starches), as well as those added to the food. Both are included in the grams of "Total Carbohydrate." Insulin dosing (Chapter 12) is based on total carbohydrate and not on grams of sugar.

Nutrition Facts		
Serving Size 1.0 Cup (120g)		
Servings Per Container		8
Amount Per Serving		
Calories 130	Calories From Fat 60	
		% Daily Value †
Total Fat 6.5g		10%
Saturated Fat 2.5g		12%
Cholesterol 30mg		10%
Sodium 240mg		10%
Total Carbohydrate 15g		5%
Dietary Fiber 2.5g		10%
Sugars 3g		
Protein 3g		6%
Vitamin A 10%	Vitamin E	5%
Calcium 15%	Iron	5%

†Percent Daily Values are based on a 2,000-calorie diet. Your daily values may be higher or lower depending on your calorie needs:

Calories:	2,000	2,500	3,200
Total Fat (g)	65	80	107
Sat Fat (g)	20	25	36
Cholesterol (mg)	300	300	300
Sodium (mg)	2,400	2,400	2,400
Total Carb (g)	300	375	480
Fiber	25	30	37

Calories per gram:
Fat 9   Carbohydrate 4   Protein 4

Ingredients: Whole wheat, oat bran, raisins, gelatin, malt, flavoring, vitamins, and minerals.

- The recommended daily amounts for cholesterol stay the same for the 24-hour period for the three caloric intakes.

- The ingredients (below) are usually included on the label in order of the amount present.

LABEL READING

Label reading has become easier for people in the U.S. as the law requires labeling of the nutrient content of products. Smart buyers can learn a lot about the foods they consider buying by learning to read labels. The information that can be gained from reading a label is shown in Table 4.

The grams of carbohydrates are listed under "total carbohydrate" on most labels. This value also includes the grams of fiber. Since the body does not completely absorb fiber, half of the grams of fiber can be subtracted from the grams of total carbohydrate to determine the insulin dose if there is more than five grams of fiber. Carbohydrate counting is discussed in detail in the next chapter.

FAST-FOOD RESTAURANTS

It is difficult to eat at fast-food restaurants and not eat foods high in animal fat, calories and salt. Eating at fast-food restaurants often goes against optimal nutrition principles and may be unhealthy for the heart. In addition, meals are usually low in vitamin-containing fruits and vegetables. Some fast-food restaurants are now trying to provide healthier food choices (salads, fruit, milk, leaner meat and deep-frying in vegetable oils rather than animal fat). However, eating at fast-food restaurants should be limited.

ALCOHOL

We hesitate to discuss alcohol under normal nutrition. It is, of course, illegal for children and adolescents to use alcohol prior to reaching the legal drinking age in a particular state or country. We do not condone alcohol use for children or adolescents. However, exposure often begins prior to the legal drinking age. Education is important regardless of the age.

Blood sugars may initially be elevated after drinking alcohol. Beer, for example, contains a fair amount of carbohydrate. However, the more dangerous effect of alcohol is the lowering of the blood/CGM sugar levels (as much as 6-12 hours later). The alcohol blocks the other nutrients stored in the body from being converted to blood sugar.

If alcohol consumption is to occur, some general rules are listed below:

✓ Use alcohol only in moderation. Sip slowly and make one drink last a long time.

✓ Eat (especially carbohydrates) when drinking alcohol. Never drink on an empty stomach.

✓ A low blood sugar is the main worry – and a bedtime snack (solid protein and some carbohydrate) must be taken after drinking in the evening, even if the bedtime blood/CGM glucose level is high.

✓ The next morning, get up at the usual time, do a blood sugar, take insulin, eat breakfast and then go back to bed if you feel ill. "Sleeping in" without eating can result in a low blood sugar.

✓ NEVER drink and drive. Ask a friend who has not been drinking to drive, or call someone to come and get you.

A college student, helping to teach our College Workshop course to newly-graduated high school seniors, had a useful recommendation regarding college parties. He noted that if he had a cup in his hand, no one tried to push further drinks. In contrast, if his hands were empty (no glass), he received a lot of pressure. The answer was to hold the same cup all evening and to just have fun!

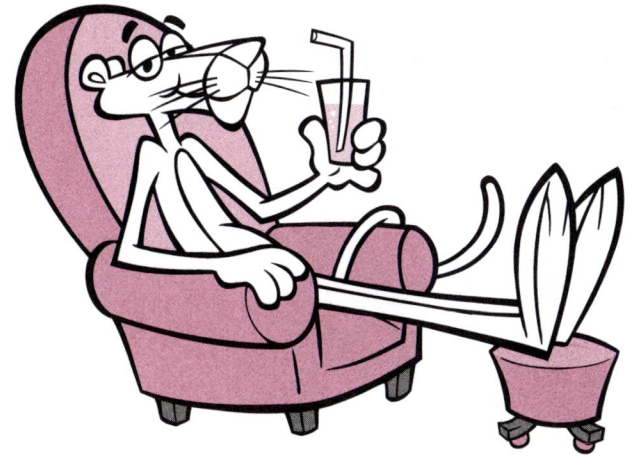

APPENDIX
Three-Day Food Record Form
Instructions for completing food record form:

1. Please write down everything you eat or drink for three days. This includes meals and snacks. Often it's easier to remember what you eat if you record your food intake at the time you eat it.

2. Include the amount (portion size) of food or beverage eaten. Also note the method of preparation (baked, fried, broiled, etc.), as well as any brand names of products (labels can also be enclosed). Use standard measuring cups or spoons. Measure the meat portions in ounces after cooking. If you do not have a scale, you can estimate ounces. The size of a deck of cards is about equal to three ounces of meat.

3. Be sure to include items added to your food, like condiments or sauces (e.g., salad dressing, dips, butter or margarine, or ketchup).

4. Include any supplements you take (vitamin, mineral or protein powders). Write down the name of the supplement, what it contains, and the amount taken. Include a copy of the label, if possible.

5. Please include meal and snack times, blood glucose values, amount and type of insulin, type of food, amount of food, grams of carbohydrate and any activity or exercise. Put a star next to any blood sugar value that is two hours after a meal.

The following is an example of how to complete your food record. Please record what you eat on the forms in this chapter. The forms can then be faxed, mailed or emailed to your diabetes care-provider.

An example for the start of a day follows:

Time	Blood Gluose	Insulin	Food (include amounts)	Carbs	Activity
8:00	170	4H/10N	Cheerios = 1 1/2 Cup	34g	
			Fat-free milk - 1 Cup	12g	
10:00					Jog - 20 min.

NORMAL NUTRITION

Three-Day Food Record Form (copy as needed)

Name: _____

Date: _____

Dietitian: _____

Home #: _____

Cell or Work #: _____

Best time to be reached _____

Insulin-to-Carb ratios (if known)

Breakfast: _____

Lunch: _____

Dinner: _____

Snack: _____

Blood Sugar Correction:

_____

Time	Blood Gluose	Insulin	Food (include amounts)	Carbs	Activity

DEFINITIONS

Artificial sweetener: A very sweet substance (often hundreds of times sweeter than table sugar) used in very small amounts (and thus having almost no calories) to make foods or drinks taste sweet. Several of the non-nutritive sweeteners are described in the text of this chapter.

Calorie: A measurement of the food taken into the body for energy.

Caloric intake: Refers to the energy from foods that are eaten.

Carbohydrate: One of the main energy nutrients. It supplies energy for the body and is further divided into sugars and starches. Carbohydrates are found in all fruits and vegetables, all grain products, dried beans and peas, milk and yogurt.

Dietary carbohydrates include:

- ✔ **Starch:** Carbohydrates such as found in starchy vegetables, pasta, whole grain breads and cereals.
- ✔ **Sugar:** Carbohydrates such as table sugar (see Carbohydrate section).

Cholesterol: A fat present in foods from animals. It is also made in our body. Our blood cholesterol level results from our own body's production (≈ 85 percent) and from the animal products we eat (≈ 15 percent). A high blood cholesterol level (>200 mg/dL) results in a greater risk for heart disease.

Cup (c): A measure of volume of eight ounces or 240 cc (mL). Two cups equal one pint. Four cups equal one quart.

Dextrose: Another name for glucose.

Fat: One of the main energy nutrients. (Types of fats are reviewed in the Fat section.)

Fiber: The parts of plants in food that are not absorbed by the body.

Gram (g): A unit of weight in the metric system; 1,000g is equal to 1 kg. There are 448g in one pound and 28g in 1 oz. Carbohydrate, protein and fat in foods are measured as grams. Information can be obtained from label reading.

Maltitol: A sugar alcohol that is used in foods to give a sweet taste. It usually does provide calories, but doesn't increase the blood sugar as much as sucrose. Too much can cause diarrhea or an upset stomach.

Ounce (oz): A unit of weight equivalent to 28g. It is also equal to 30 cc (or 30 mL) of water.

Protein: One of the main energy nutrients. It is found in meat, eggs, fish, milk, yogurt and, in lesser amounts, in vegetables and other non-meat products (e.g., nuts, seeds, beans, etc.).

Registered Dietitian (R.D.): A person trained to help you with your meal planning and nutrition. He/she has a minimum of a four-year college degree in nutrition or a related area, has completed an internship and has passed a national exam.

Sorbitol: A sugar alcohol that is used in foods to give a sweet taste. It does provide calories, but does not increase the blood sugar as much as sucrose (see text of this chapter).

Tablespoon (Tbsp): A measure of 3 tsp or 15 cc (15 mL). It is equal to 15g (½ oz) of water. There are 16 tablespoons of sugar (sucrose) in one measuring cup.

Teaspoon (tsp): A measure of 5 cc (5 mL). It is also equal to 5g of water.

Triglyceride: One of the two main blood fats. High levels are believed to be related to a greater risk for heart attacks later in life for people with diabetes.

QUESTIONS AND ANSWERS FROM NEWSNOTES

Q: What is fiber and what is its value in the diet?

a: Fiber is generally defined as the part of food that is not broken down by the enzymes in the intestine. Some of the physiological effects of fiber are to prolong the time it takes food to leave the stomach, to shorten the transit of food through the rest of the intestine, to reduce fat absorption and to increase stool weight and bulk.

Although fiber sounds like a blessing for a diabetic diet, it has been more useful in type 2 diabetes than in type 1 diabetes. So many things affect the person with type 1 diabetes, particularly insulin dose and exercise, that altering one part of the diet (fiber) and expecting miraculous changes in glucose levels has not been realistic.

Increasing fiber intake should still be a goal for all children and young adults. The high-fiber foods are mainly vegetables, bran or whole grain cereals, whole grain bread and fruits. At a minimum, according to the Dietary Guidelines, for a 2,000-calorie diet a person should eat 2 cups of fruit and at least 3 of vegetables per day. If, in addition, whole grain breads are eaten (e.g., "whole wheat," not just "wheat"), fiber intake will likely be fine.

Q: What does the food label "low-fat" mean?

a: "Low-fat" on a label means that the food has 3g of fat or less. It does not say anything about whether the fat is a "healthy" fat (e.g., polyunsaturated) or a "bad" fat (e.g., saturated fat, trans-fat). It also does not mean that the amount of fat has been reduced in the food. For example, an apple could be labeled "low-fat" as it has less than 3g of fat normally. In contrast, a food labeled as "reduced-fat" means that one serving of food contains a 25 percent (or more) reduction of fat compared to the usual form of that food. It could still contain a large amount of fat.

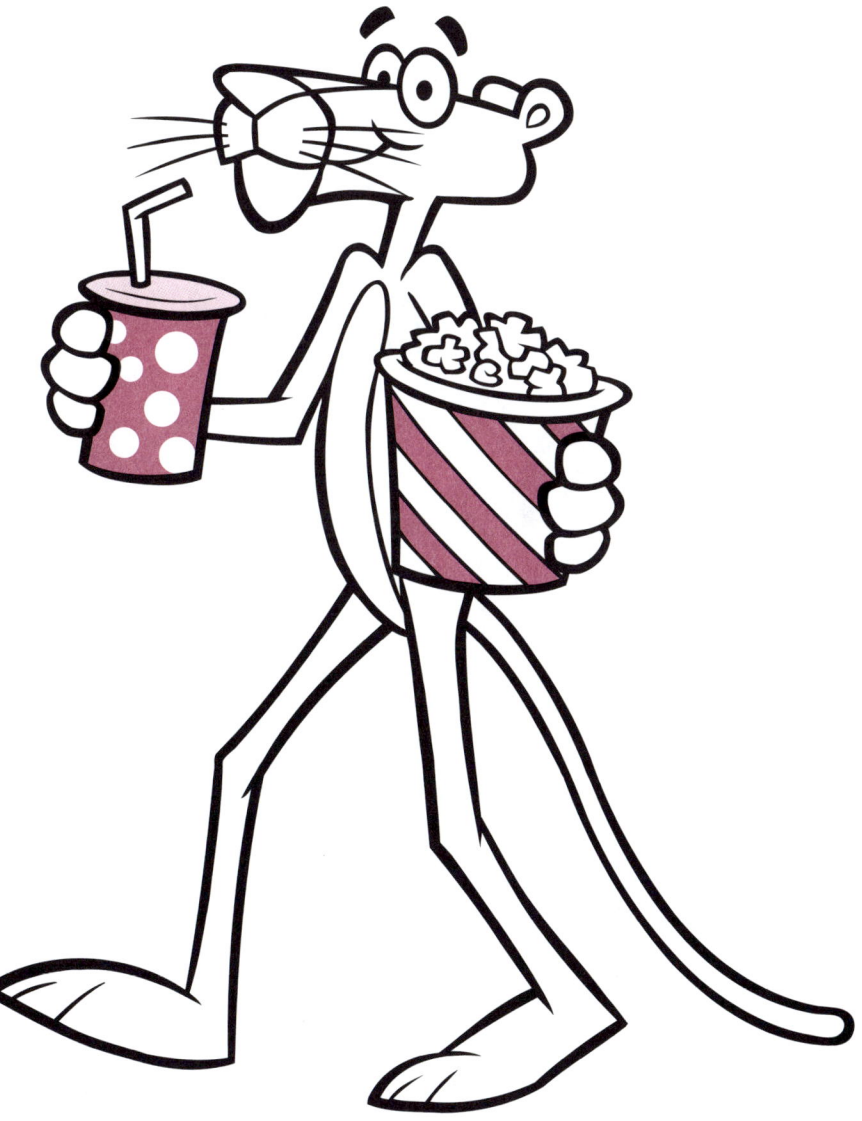

NORMAL NUTRITION

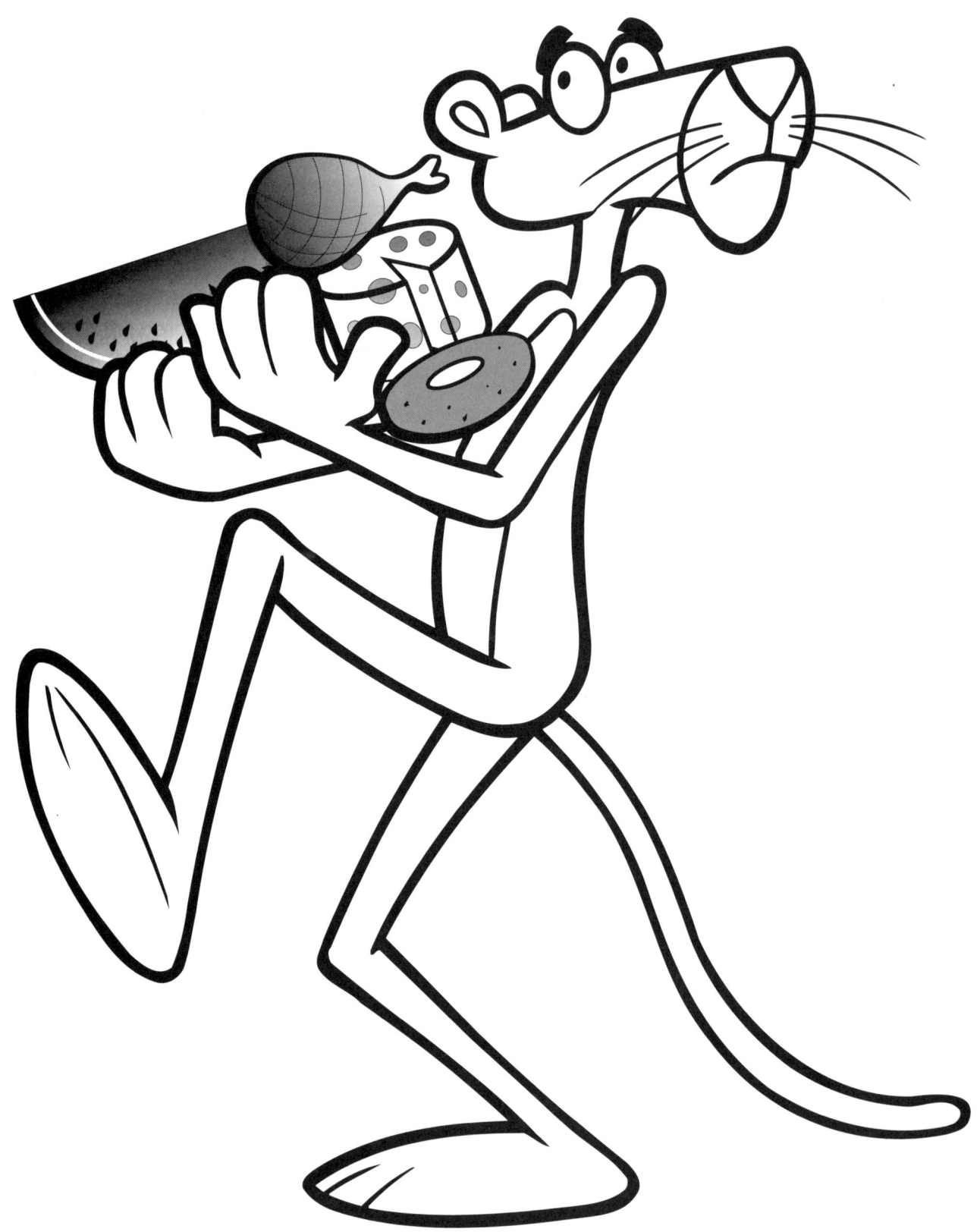

NORMAL NUTRITION

CHAPTER 12
Food Management and Diabetes

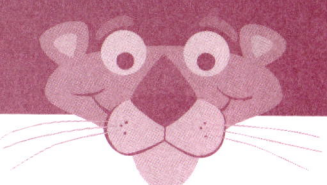

Food (mainly carbohydrate ["carb"]) is one of the major influences on blood/CGM glucose levels in people with diabetes. As discussed in Chapter 2, the body (particularly the liver) also makes sugar (internal sugar), which adds to the blood sugar. Other sugars (external sugars) come from the food we eat. Recommendations for the use of added sugars for people with diabetes have changed. It has gone from complete avoidance to allowing some sugar within the context of a healthy meal plan. As discussed in Chapter 11, the right amount and types of food are essential for normal growth and health. **TYPE 1 (INSULIN-DEPENDENT) DIABETES CANNOT BE TREATED WITH DIET ALONE.** In contrast, type 2 diabetes can sometimes be treated with diet and exercise alone.

OBJECTIVES OF FOOD MANAGEMENT

No matter which of the food plans is used, the objectives of food management are the same:

- to provide general principals related to food management
- to help balance insulin and carb intake in order to keep the blood (or continuous glucose monitor [CGM]) glucose values in the desired range
- to maintain an appropriate weight
- to keep the blood fats (cholesterol and triglycerides) and lipoproteins (LDL and HDL) at desired levels
- to help reduce risk for high blood pressure
- to help avoid long-term diabetes complications
- to help attain normal growth and development for children

> **TOPICS:**
> **Food Management and Diabetes**
>
> **TEACHING OBJECTIVES:**
> The teacher will:
> 1. Present the principles of food management related to diabetes.
> 2. Explain the significance of carbohydrates (carbs) in diabetes management.
> 3. Discuss types of meal planning approaches, including carb counting.
> 4. Present the principles of food management related to body weight.
>
> **LEARNING OBJECTIVES:**
> Learner (parents, child, relative or self) will be able to:
> 1. List three objectives of food management.
> 2. Describe examples of carbohydrate (carb) containing foods and their effect on blood sugar levels.
> 3. Explain the type of food plan you will be using.
> 4. Describe two methods to help maintain a healthy weight.

As in other chapters, the term "blood/CGM glucose" indicates the glucose value can be from either a blood glucose or a CGM.

- to help avoid hypoglycemia
- to improve overall health by maintaining the best possible nutrition

It is amazing how often we hear parents comment, "My child with diabetes is the healthiest in our family BECAUSE HE/SHE EATS THE BEST." Optimal nutrition for a person with diabetes is really just a healthy diet from which **all** people would benefit.

Views on food management for people with diabetes have changed considerably.

According to a Position Statement of the American Diabetes Association (ADA):

"Today there is no one 'diabetic' or 'ADA' diet. The recommended food program can only be defined as a dietary prescription based on nutrition assessment and treatment goals. Medical nutrition therapy for people with diabetes should be individualized, with consideration given to usual eating habits and other lifestyle changes."

There is no evidence that one type of meal plan is any more effective than another. However, it is important to have a meal plan. We believe that all families having a person with diabetes should meet with a dietitian at diagnosis and then at least once yearly. Possible meal plans are discussed below, following the section on Principles of Food Management.

NINE PRINCIPLES OF FOOD MANAGEMENT FOR ALL FOOD PLANS

The nine principles listed below are important in all plans, and the first four will be briefly reviewed.

1. Eat a Well-balanced Meal Plan (Also see Chapter 11)
2. Eat Meals and Snacks Carefully
3. Balance Carb Intake and Insulin Carefully
4. Avoid Over-Treating Low Blood Sugars
5. Reduce Cholesterol, Saturated and Trans-Fat Intake (See Chapter 11)
6. Maintain Appropriate Height and Weight (see Chapter 11)
7. Increase Fiber Intake (see Chapter 11)
8. Avoid Foods High in Salt (see Chapter 11)
9. Avoid Excessive Protein Intake (see Chapter 11)

1. Eat a Well-balanced Meal Plan
(Also see Chapter 11)

A well-balanced meal plan is a step toward optimal health for everyone in the family. It is particularly important in supporting the growth of children. If you understand normal nutrition (Chapter 11), you can help your family have a well-balanced meal plan. Most people have a period of weight loss prior to being diagnosed with diabetes. Starting insulin treatment allows the body to regain weight. Usually the individual's appetite is greatly increased for about one month. The body is returning to its usual growth pattern. The appetite then returns to normal. Most individuals can then self-regulate their caloric intake without a set number of calories being prescribed for each day. Possible meal plans are discussed below under Types of Meal Planning Approaches.

A well-balanced meal plan is currently considered to contain:

- 45-55 percent from carbs
- 15-20 percent of calories from protein
- 20-35 percent from fat

Meals should be balanced and contain:

- a rich source of fruits, vegetables and whole grains. This is generally an area children and teens need to increase. Portion sizes for 15 grams (g) of carbs are given in Table 1.
- a moderate amount of protein such as low-fat milk, fat-free cheeses, reduced-fat yogurt, lean meat, poultry, fish, egg white, nuts and seeds
- a limited amount of fat (especially butter, egg yolk, animal fat, etc.)

TABLE 1:
Suggestions for Snacks: (Foods with 15g of Carbohydrate)

Food Group	Carbohydrate Content	Portion Sizes
Starch/Grains	15g	1 slice bread 1 - 6" tortilla ⅓ - ½ cup cooked pasta 1 small or ½ large (1 oz) bagel ½ hamburger bun ½ cup peas, corn or mashed potato 1 small potato (3 oz) ⅓ cup rice ⅓ cup cooked dried beans
Fruit	15g	1 piece fruit (small) ½ cup canned fruit ½ cup fruit juice ¼ cup dried fruit 1 cup berries or melon
Milk	12g	1 cup skim, 1%, 2% or whole milk 8 oz plain yogurt
These are not exact but are close enough for most people. **NOTE: THIS CHART MAY BE COPIED AS NEEDED.**		

An excess of animal fat may result in higher blood fats and a greater risk for heart disease later in life. A high-protein diet is harmful to the kidneys for people who have either early or advanced kidney damage from diabetes. Working with the dietitian will help assure intake of the recommended balance of foods.

2. Eat Meals and Snacks Carefully

For people following a consistent carb meal plan and using relatively constant insulin dosages (particularly if receiving NPH insulin), it is important to eat meals and snacks at the same time each day. Use of an insulin pump or of multiple daily injections (MDI), usually with Lantus (Basaglar)/Levemir/Tresiba insulin and pre-meal insulin boluses, gives more flexibility. Carb counting (see below) then allows a person to take insulin to match carbs when they are eaten. There can be more flexibility in the timing of meals and snacks as well as in the number of carbs eaten. In general, with the rising incidence of people being overweight or obese, the trend is to use snacks primarily to avoid or treat low blood sugars. Thinking ahead and reducing insulin dosages to avoid lows is often wiser than adding extra snacks.

3. Balance Carb Intake and Insulin Carefully

It is recommended that about half of the food we eat comes from carbs. As insulin must be available to utilize most carbs, it is important to learn to balance your insulin with carb intake. Tables 1, 3 and 4 list the carb contents of different foods. It is known that the rise in blood/CGM glucose levels after eating is dependent upon the total amount of carbs eaten and not the form of carbs.

FOOD MANAGEMENT AND DIABETES

TABLE 2:
Approximate Carb Amounts by Age*

	< 5 years old	5-12 years old	Teens - Adults
Males	30 to 45 grams of carb at each meal	45 to 60 grams of carb at each meal	60 to 75+ grams of carb at each meal
Females	30 to 45 grams of carb at each meal	45 to 60 grams of carb at each meal	45 to 75 grams of carb at each meal

Snacks, if needed, are usually 15 to 20 grams of carb.
Talk to your RD or healthcare professional to help you decide on the amount of carb that is right for your child at each meal and snack.

*Source: Evert, A., Gerken, S. Children with diabetes: birth to adolescence. *On the Cutting Edge.* Summer 2006, Vol. 27, No. 4, 4-8.

We know the most important factors are:

A. how much carbohydrate is eaten
B. when the carbs are eaten
C. with what the carbs are eaten
D. having adequate insulin available when the carbs are eaten.

Each will be discussed in more detail.

A. How much carbohydrate is eaten

Some meals are much higher in carbs than others. For example, at breakfast, a meal of eggs with toast and peanut butter would have fewer carbs than a plate of pancakes with syrup. It is helpful to limit carbs with the breakfast meal, as other factors tend to result in higher blood sugars. Similarly, a meal of meat, vegetables and salad would have fewer carbs than one of spaghetti and garlic bread, or a pizza. Approximate carb intake by age is given in Table 2. More insulin will be required to handle a meal high in carbs compared with one low in carbs.

Avoiding excess sugar is very important in keeping blood sugar levels within targets. Drinks with extra sugar, such as sugar pops and juices, will cause high blood sugars and should be avoided.

B. When the carbs are eaten

Large amounts of carbs should not be consumed between meals unless additional insulin is given. An extreme example is using a regular (sugar) pop (40g of carbs) as a morning or afternoon snack.

One boy with diabetes and other problems brought a can of regular sugar pop (10 tsp sugar, see Table 3) to our Clinic with him, freely admitting that he still drank regular pop. We measured his blood sugar before drinking the pop (180 mg/dL or 10.0 mmol/L) and one hour later (450 mg/dL or 25.0 mmol/L). The liquid sugars cause the fastest rise in the blood sugar. That is why we recommend avoiding intake of any sugary drinks!

When extra carbs are eaten, it is best to take extra rapid-acting insulin. The carb contents of some foods are shown in Tables 3 and 4.

C. With what the carbs are eaten

High-fat meals (e.g., pizza, Chinese food, fast foods) will delay the absorption of carbs, and the blood/CGM glucose levels may stay elevated longer. When this is observed, extra rapid-acting insulin can be given the next time. For people using an insulin pump, the use of a "dual-wave" (see Chapter 28) can be very helpful with a meal high in both fat and carbohydrate. DIFFERENT FOODS AFFECT EACH PERSON DIFFERENTLY. EXPERIENCE IS THE BEST TEACHER.

TABLE 3:
Carbohydrate Content of Foods

Amount of starches/grains that equal 15g carbohydrate

Food	Serving Size
Bagel	½ small or ¼ large (1 oz)
Beans, cooked, dried, canned	½ cup
Bread, white, whole wheat, rye	1 slice (1 oz)
Corn, cooked	½ cup
Crackers	4-6
English muffin	½
Graham crackers	3 squares
Hamburger bun	½ bun
Popcorn	3 cups
Pasta, cooked	⅓-½ cup
Peas, cooked	½ cup
Potato, baked	1 small (3 oz)
Potato, mashed	½ cup
Rice, cooked	⅓ cup
Roll (dinner, hard)	1 small
Squash, winter	1 cup
Tortilla (6" corn or flour)	1

Fruits
15g carbohydrate

Food	Serving Size
Apple, small	1 (4 oz)
Applesauce, unsweetened	½ cup
Banana	1 small (4 oz) or ½ large
Blueberries	¾ cup
Canned fruit, light or juice packed	½ cup
Cantaloupe, melon	1 cup cubed
Cherries, sweet, fresh	12 (3 oz)
Fruit juice	½ cup (4 oz)
Grapefruit, medium	½
Grapes, small	17
Orange, small	1 (6½ oz)
Pear, large, fresh	½ (4 oz)
Raisins	2 Tbsp
Strawberries	1¼ cup whole berries
Watermelon	1¼ cup cubes

Milk/Yogurt
12g carbohydrate

Food	Serving Size
Milk (skim, 1%, 2%, whole)	1 cup (8 oz)
Yogurt (see "Other Carbohydrates" list)	

OTHER CARBS

Food	Serving Size	Carbohydrate (g)
Brownie, small unfrosted	1¼" square, 7/8" high	15g
Cake, unfrosted	2" square	15g
Cake, frosted	2" square	30g
Chicken noodle soup	1 cup (8 oz)	15g
Cookie, sandwich or chocolate chip	2 cookies	15g
Cookie, medium (homemade)	1 cookie	15g
Cupcake, frosted	1 small	30g
Doughnut, plain cake	1 medium (1.5 oz)	20g
Doughnut, glazed	3¾" (2 oz)	30g
French fries, thin	20-25	30g
Granola bar	1	20-25g
Ice cream (regular, light, fat-free)	½ cup	15-20g
Jam or jelly, regular	1 Tbsp	15g
Macaroni and cheese	1 cup (8 oz)	30-45g
Noodle casserole	1 cup (8 oz)	30g
Pie, fruit, 2 crusts	1/6 pie	45g
Poptart, unfrosted	1	35g
Potato chips	9-13 (¾ oz)	15g
Pizza	1 slice (¼ of 12")	30g
Pudding, regular	½ cup (4 oz)	25g
Syrup, light	2 Tbsp	15g
Syrup, regular	1 Tbsp	15g
Tomato soup (made with water)	1 cup (8 oz)	15g
Tortilla chips	9-13 (¾ oz)	15g
Yogurt, light	1 cup (6-8 oz)	15g

The carbohydrate amounts listed on this handout are estimates. If the food you are eating has a food label, check the Nutrition Facts for the accurate amount of carbohydrate in that product.

Measurement Key

3 tsp = 1 Tbsp	4 ounces = ½ cup
4 Tbsp = ¼ cup	8 ounces = 1 cup
5⅓ Tbsp = ⅓ cup	1 cup = ½ pint

Reference: *Choose Your Foods: Exchange Lists for Diabetes*, 2008.

TABLE 4: Sugar Content of Some High-Carbohydrate Foods

Food Item	Size Portion	Sugar Content* Sugar (teaspoons)	"Carb" Choices	Gram Carb
Beverages				
Cola drinks	12 oz can	10	3	50
Root beer	12 oz can	7	2	35
7-Up® *	12 oz can	9	3	45
Grape, orange, apple juice	6 oz can	5	1½	25
Dairy Products				
Sherbet	1 scoop	9	3	45
Ice cream cone	1 scoop	3½	1	17
Chocolate milkshake	10 oz glass	11	4	55
Milk	8 oz glass	3	1	12
Chocolate milk	8 oz glass	9½	3	52
Fruit yogurt	8 oz cup	9	3	45
Cakes and Cookies				
Angel food cake	4 oz piece	7	2	35
Chocolate cake, plain	4 oz piece	6	2	30
Chocolate cake, w/frosting	4 oz piece	10	3	50
Sugar cookie	1	1½	½	10
Oatmeal cookie	1	2	1	10
Donut, plain	1	4	1	20
Donut, glazed	1	6	2	30
Desserts				
JELL-O	½ cup	4½	1½	22
Apple pie	1 slice	7	2	35
Berry pie	1 slice	10	3	50
Chocolate pudding	½ cup	4	1	20
Candies				
Chocolate candy bar	1½ oz	2½	1	12
Chewing gum	1 stick	½	—	2
Fudge	1 oz square	4½	1½	22
Hard candy	1 oz	5	2	25
LIFE-SAVERS	1	⅓	–	1½
Marshmallow	1 piece	1½	½	7
Chocolate cream	1 piece	2	1	10
Miscellaneous				
Jelly	1 Tbsp	3	1	15
Strawberry jam	1 Tbsp	3	1	15
Brown sugar	1 Tbsp	3	1	15
Honey	1 Tbsp	3	1	15
Chocolate sauce	1 Tbsp	3	1	15
Karo Syrup®	1 Tbsp	3	1	15

*3 tsp = 1 Tbsp = 1 carb choice = 15g of carbs

Research on the effects carbs have on blood sugar levels is often studied by giving the carb by itself **(called the "glycemic-index")**. Then, blood/CGM glucose levels are measured to see how much the level rises in comparison to the increase in blood sugar caused by a reference food. However, the effects of other foods are very important, and it is rare that a carb is eaten all by itself. The best way to find out the effect of a given carb is to check the blood sugar, eat the food and/or meal, and check the blood/CGM sugar level again in two to three hours. High-fat intake can delay absorption and can also cause some insulin resistance, making it harder for the insulin to work and requiring extra amounts of insulin.

D. Having adequate insulin activity when the carbs are eaten

Eating extra carbs is possible if extra rapid-acting insulin is added. As discussed in Chapters 8 and 9, if the blood/CGM glucose level is not low, the insulin is ideally taken 20 minutes prior to eating. Measuring the blood/CGM glucose levels two hours after the meal will determine if the insulin dose used and timing were appropriate.

We recommend that extra rapid-acting insulin be given for snacks. Insulin pumps (and insulin pens) can make this easier. Unfortunately, a recent research study found that half of afternoon snacks were not covered with insulin.

It is generally acceptable to allow a person to fit in a sweet food on an "as-needed" basis. Allowing this can help avoid the sneaking of candy or treats. This can be planned for a time when adequate insulin is available. We encourage the entire family to get used to eating foods without a "sugary" taste. To allow for better nutrition, avoid having sweets (Table 4) such as donuts, cookies, cake, candy, etc. in the home. If they are there, they will be hard to avoid. Most have no nutritional value except adding calories. This will result in better nutrition for the entire family.

There are several alternatives for handling holidays and parties where there are a great number of concentrated sweets. Halloween focuses on candy and is a special problem for young children.

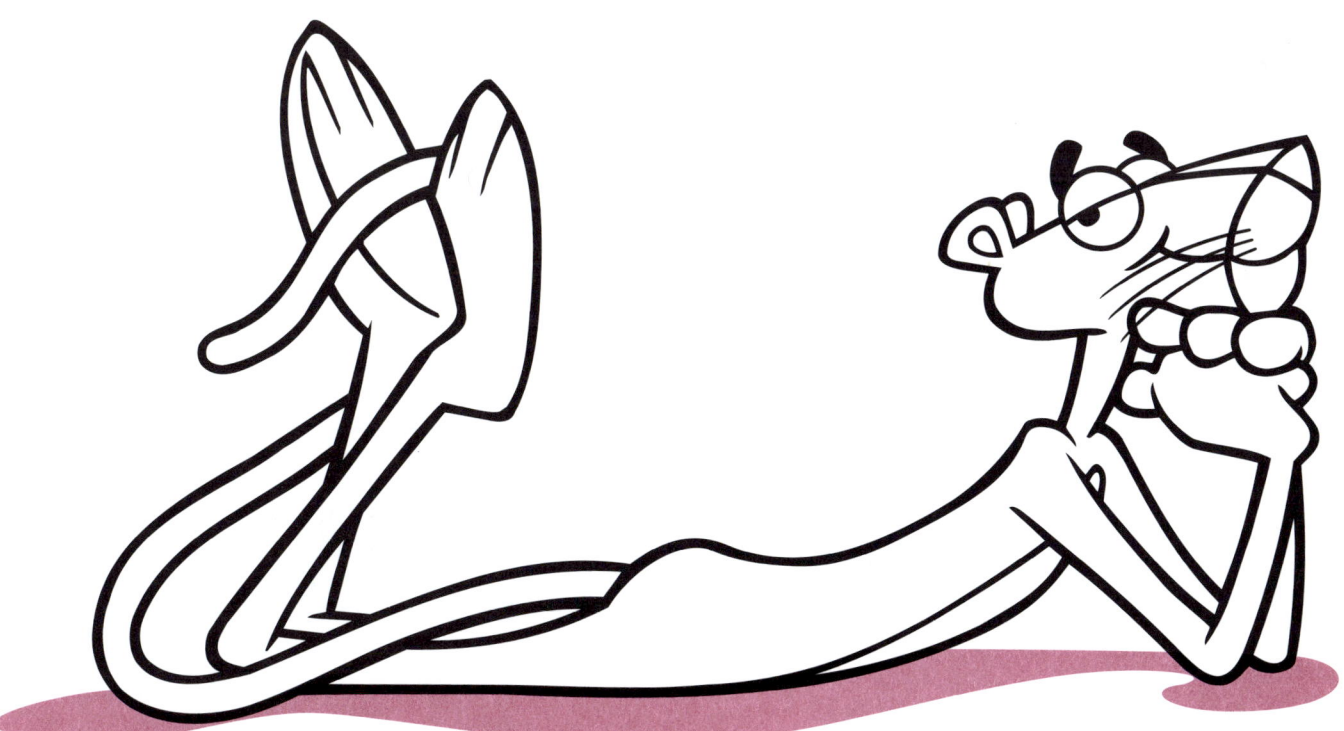

FOOD MANAGEMENT AND DIABETES

> **TABLE 5:**
>
> **The Diabetes and Control Complications Trial (DCCT) found several nutrition factors that contributed to lower HbA1c levels:**
>
> 1. Following some sort of a meal plan
> 2. Avoidance of extra snacks
> 3. Avoidance of over-treatment of low blood sugars (hypoglycemia)
> 4. Prompt treatment of high blood sugars when found
> 5. Adjusting insulin levels for meals

Some suggestions for Halloween trick-or-treating candy:

- The child can select a few for his/her regular treats, and give or throw the rest away. If sweets are to be eaten, it is best to eat them when insulin is working. The dose of rapid-acting insulin for that meal can then be increased.
- Taking the treats to a sick friend or a child in the hospital is a nice option.
- Another option is to "sell" the candy to the parents. The money can then be spent to purchase something the child wants.

It is important not to become upset with a child if he/she does eat extra sweets. The stress of the parent being upset can raise the blood/CGM glucose levels more than the sweets (see Chapter 17 on Family Concerns). Instead, discuss the incident with the child and try to find compromises.

4. Avoid Over-Treating Low Blood Sugars

Avoiding the over-treatment of low blood sugars (hypoglycemia) was one of the factors found in the DCCT to relate to lower HbA1c levels (Table 5). The problem is how to accomplish this. Only a person who has had a truly low blood sugar can know the feeling of being "ravenously hungry" and wanting to eat everything in sight (and so the person does). For many years, people thought "rebounding" to be the cause of the high blood sugar after hypoglycemia. Only in recent years was it realized to be primarily due to excessive eating after the low blood sugar. Chapter 6 discusses the treatment of hypoglycemia.

TYPES OF MEAL PLANNING APPROACHES

Different types of meal planning approaches have been used for people with diabetes for about 4,000 years. They are talked about in an ancient scroll called the "Ebers Papyrus," which was written about 2000 B.C. In 1993 the DCCT showed that people with diabetes who followed a food program had lower HbA1c levels than those who didn't (Table 5). There are now many types of food management plans for people with diabetes. All food management plans require people to pay attention to carbs. Over 90 percent of carbs eaten are converted into glucose (sugar) over the next one to two hours. In contrast, meats (protein) and fat have very little conversion to sugar. Three of the meal planning approaches discussed below pay special attention to carbs.

The approaches used most commonly in our Clinic are:

A. *Consistent (Constant) Carbohydrate (Carb) Meal Plan*

B. *Carbohydrate (Carb) Counting Meal Plan (adjusting insulin for carbs)*

C. *Weight Management Plan (for use by anyone)*

Another approach, the Exchange Meal Plan, is occasionally used for type 2 diabetes. References are given in the back for people wanting more knowledge about this food plan.

*An approach sometimes used for people with type 2 diabetes is the **"Ketogenic ('Keto') Diet."** This involves extreme restriction of carbohydrates and is used for weight loss. For children to receive adequate nutrients and calories for growth, fat intake would be too high and the intake of fruits and vegetables too low. This approach could result in other problems, such as excessive fat accumulation in the liver or more rapid onset of ketoacidosis (Chapter 15). We do not use this food plan for youth with type 1 diabetes, although we do recommend avoidance of high sugar non-nutritive ("junk") foods.*

The clinic healthcare team caring for the person with newly-diagnosed diabetes may prefer one type of meal planning approach over another. It may be unnecessary to read about the other approaches, at least initially. The purpose of all meal plans is to achieve more blood/CGM sugar levels in range. The method that works best for one person may not be the best for someone else.

Any of the meal planning approaches can work. No single approach has been proven better than any other in achieving optimal glucose levels. It is up to each family and healthcare team to eventually decide which works best for them. Some families will switch from one approach to another or combine parts of each to fit their needs. Many families initially use the consistent carb food plan. They then move to adjusting rapid-acting insulin for carbs to be eaten (carb counting) as they gain confidence, knowledge and carb counting skills. It is important to meet with a registered dietitian to develop a meal plan that meets your lifestyle.

CAREFUL MANAGEMENT OF CARB INTAKE MUST BE PART OF ANY OF THE PROGRAMS. It is impossible to eat varying amounts of carbs and keep the blood/CGM glucose values from fluctuating without changing the insulin dosage. Knowing how many carbs are being eaten is important in any meal plan. Tables 3 and 4 may be helpful in providing grams of carbs in various foods.

A. Consistent (Constant) Carbohydrate (Carb) Meal Plan
(see Tables 1-4)

In the consistent carbohydrate meal plan, the amount of insulin (usually two or four shots per day) is kept relatively constant from day to day. This is done to match relatively consistent food intake. **The amount of carbs (types can vary) is kept about the same for each meal and each snack from one day to the next.** Insulin dosages vary primarily with different blood/CGM glucose levels. Often families start with this food plan, and then move to adjusting insulin for carbs as they gain confidence and carb counting skills.

Labels must be read to know the grams (g) of carbs being eaten (see label reading, Chapter 11). The dietitian may give a range of carbs for each meal. This might be 45 to 60g/meal for a pre-teen. A teenage boy might have a range of 75 to 90g/meal. **CONSISTENCY IS THE KEY.** The consistent carb meal plan is formed around the 10 principles discussed earlier in this chapter and is then individualized.

The amount of food eaten at a meal or snack may vary with:

✔ expected (or completed) exercise

✔ insulin taken

✔ blood/CGM glucose level

More carbs may be needed (without increasing insulin) for fun activities such as sports, hiking and biking (see Chapter 22 on "thinking scales"). For work-related activities such as ranching and farming, more carbs may also be needed. However, the normal eating pattern of the child and the family should stay the same as much as possible.

Families often ask, "How much carbohydrate is appropriate for me/my child?" They can count carbs even if insulin adjustments are not being made to match the carb intake. This helps to keep the carbs eaten at each meal consistent. The grams of carbohydrate to be eaten at each meal for each age group can be estimated by looking at Table 4. Families also ask, "How many calories should my child be eating?" Most children under age 14 years need 1,000 calories per day plus 100 calories for each year of age. For example, a five-year-old would need 1,500 calories. Formulas are a guide; each person's calorie and carb needs can be different. We recommend consulting with a dietitian to establish a plan that works for you/your child.

B. Carbohydrate (Carb) Counting Meal Plan (adjusting insulin for carbs)

Adjusting insulin for carbs involves counting the grams of carbs that are to be eaten and adjusting the insulin dose to match. It allows for greater freedom and flexibility in food choices. It is used with both multiple daily insulin injections or with insulin pump therapy. It is not possible to count carbs without learning to read food labels (Chapter 11). The carb counting meal plan is both similar to and different from the consistent carbohydrate meal plan.

Comparison of the Carb Counting to the Consistent Carbohydrate Meal Plan:

Similarity

✔ Both emphasize carb intake and keeping protein and fat relatively consistent. This is helpful as protein may cause a very small increase in blood sugar levels. Similarly, fat decreases the rate of absorption of foods, and glucose levels may remain elevated longer with high fat meals.

Differences

✔ Carb counting presumes that carb intake (and thus insulin dose) will vary, providing more flexibility and greater safety from hypoglycemia.

✔ Carb counting may involve more injections of insulin as extra rapid-acting insulin is taken to cover carbs eaten. Some people take rapid-acting insulin when 15g or more of carbs are consumed, while others cover even lower amounts (5g or 10g) of carbs. This should be discussed with your diabetes team.

Getting Started (Restarted) in Carb Counting

1. **Most people prefer to just think of the number of grams (g) of carbs:**

When using an **I**nsulin to **C**arb ratio (**I/C** ratio) one usually thinks in grams of carbs. An example of an **I/C** ratio is 1 to 15 (1/15). This refers to one unit of insulin per 15g of carbs eaten (or to be eaten). Carb counting was greatly aided by the food labeling laws (Chapter 11). They require the grams of total carbs be given on the label of most every food. The method to determine the I/C ratio(s) is discussed below.

2. **Others prefer to convert each 15g unit to one carb count (choice):**

More detailed quantities of various foods equaling one carb count (e.g., 15g of carb) are given in Tables 1 and 2. The total grams of carbs to be eaten are divided by 15 to get number of carb counts (15g of carbs equals one carb choice or count). The units of rapid-acting insulin are then adjusted at every meal to match the carb counts (units of 15g of carb). The amount of exercise and the blood/CGM glucose level must also be considered in choosing the insulin dose.

3. **Establishing insulin to carbohydrate (I/C) ratios:**

If an I/C ratio has not been used previously, it is possible to "guesstimate" the value by dividing the total units of insulin used per day into 500 ("the rule of 500"). For example, if 33 total units of insulin were taken per day, the I/C ratio would be 1 to 15 (500÷33 = 15). This means the person would take one unit of rapid-acting insulin for every 15g of carbs to be eaten. If 50 units were taken per day, the I/C ratio would be 10 (500÷50 = 10). This means one unit of insulin per 10g of carbs to be eaten. These are only estimates, and steps must then be taken to more accurately determine the I/C ratio. These are:

We ask families to keep precise food, insulin, blood/CGM glucose and activity records for at least three days. (See the Three-Day Food Record Form in the Appendix of Chapter 11.) Using a food scale and/or measuring cup may help assure accuracy of carb estimates.

After completing the food-record form (as accurately as possible), fax/email it to your dietitian for analysis. The dietitian, working with your doctor or nurse, will then make suggestions for I/C ratios. The more blood sugars (or CGM tracings) you can do prior to meals and two hours after meals, the better the advice she/he can give. It is also important to include all doses of insulin or oral meds that were taken.

In calculating the I/C ratio, keep in mind that every person is different in his or her need for rapid-acting insulin. The same person may even need different I/C ratios from one time of day to another.

✔ Some people can use one unit of rapid-acting insulin per 15g of carb (one carb choice) for all meals and snacks. This is an I/C ratio of 1/15.

✔ Another person might need:
  - breakfast – one unit of rapid-acting insulin for each 10g of carb (I/C ratio of 1/10 or 1.5 units per 15g carb. Many people are more insulin resistant in the morning)
  - lunch – one unit of insulin for every 30g of carb (I/C ratio of 1/30 or 0.5 unit per 15g carb)
  - dinner – one unit of insulin per 15g of carb

✔ Table 4 in Chapter 22 provides an example of using the I/C ratio and correction factor for calculating an insulin dose.

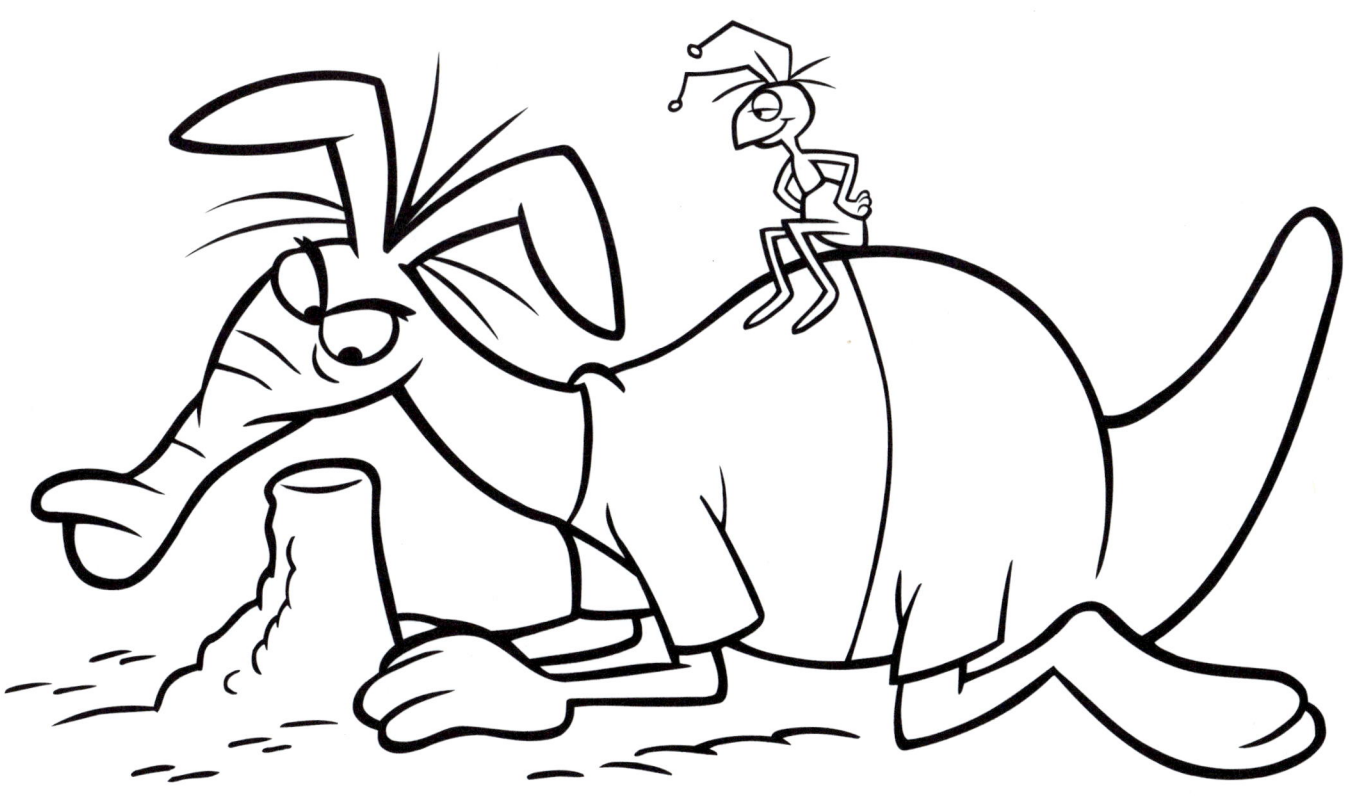

4. **Measuring the accuracy of I/C ratios:**

   The rapid-acting insulin dosages for meals are best adjusted by measuring blood/CGM glucose levels after the meal. When evaluating insulin to determine an I/C ratio, it may be helpful to eat a meal with known grams of carbs (e.g., a frozen meal with carbs on the label). The fat content should be less than 20g, as higher-fat delays stomach emptying and keeps sugar levels up longer. The meal measurements should be done for each of the three daily meals. It is common for I/C ratios to vary at different times of the day for the same person. The ADA recommends that all values after a meal be below 180 mg/dL (10.0 mmol/L). Most people aim for a blood/CGM glucose level below 140 mg/dL (<7.8 mmol/L) two hours after a meal. Others use the ranges suggested by age group in Chapters 7 and 22. You may want to discuss this with your doctor.

   ✔ **If the blood/CGM glucose value is consistently high**, more insulin is needed for the grams of carb in the I/C ratio. An example would be to change from one unit/15g carb to one unit/10g carb.

   ✔ **If the sugar level is below the limit** (often 70 mg/dL [3.9 mmol/L]), a lower amount of insulin is needed. An example would be to change from an I/C ratio of one unit/15g carb to an I/C ratio of one unit/20g carb.

   Call your healthcare-provider if you need help in making adjustments.

5. **Adding the "correction" factor:**

   After calculating the dose of insulin for carb content, the final rapid-acting insulin dose must be adjusted considering a "correction" factor for the blood/CGM glucose level at that time. Exercise and many other factors (illness, stress, menses, etc.) affect blood/CGM glucose levels and should also be considered. The method to calculate "correction" factors is discussed in Chapters 22 and 28. In addition, some people subtract one unit if the blood sugar is below 70 mg/dL (3.9 mmol/L).

6. **Additional carb counting challenges:**

   Some degree of math is obviously necessary for carb counting. However, once the best dosages are determined, the process becomes very automatic. Carb counting is most difficult for combination foods such as soups, casseroles and foods with many ingredients. The grams of carbs can be estimated from the amounts of each of the ingredients.

   It may be necessary to estimate the grams of carbs when eating out. This could be done on the basis of the grams in the same food prepared at home or information available from the restaurant. Obviously, this does not always work (some cooks add more sugar). Doing a blood/CGM glucose level two hours after the meal helps to make a better guess the next time.

   Refer to the carb counting resources at the end of the chapter for help calculating carbs when there are no food labels or when eating out.

7. **Carb counting and insulin pumps:**

   Most people who use an insulin pump use carb counting to determine the bolus of insulin to be taken with any food intake. The person enters the estimated carbs to be eaten, and the pump bolus calculator (using preset information) calculates the insulin dosage. The bolus calculator will calculate the insulin dosage for different I/C ratios that have been entered for different times of the day. Research has shown that people who use insulin pump bolus calculators have lower HbA1c values than do non-users. Use of the InPen™ also allows use of a bolus calculator for people using insulin injections.

8. **Summary of carb counting:**

   Use of carb counting allows people to better observe the relationship between factors affecting the blood/CGM glucose levels and insulin dosage. In some countries, carb counting is done using 10g carb choices. A summary of 15g carb equivalents in foods frequently eaten is given in Tables 1 and 2. Table 3 gives grams of carbs and carb counts for foods that are high in carbs.

FIGURE 1
Body Mass Index (BMI)

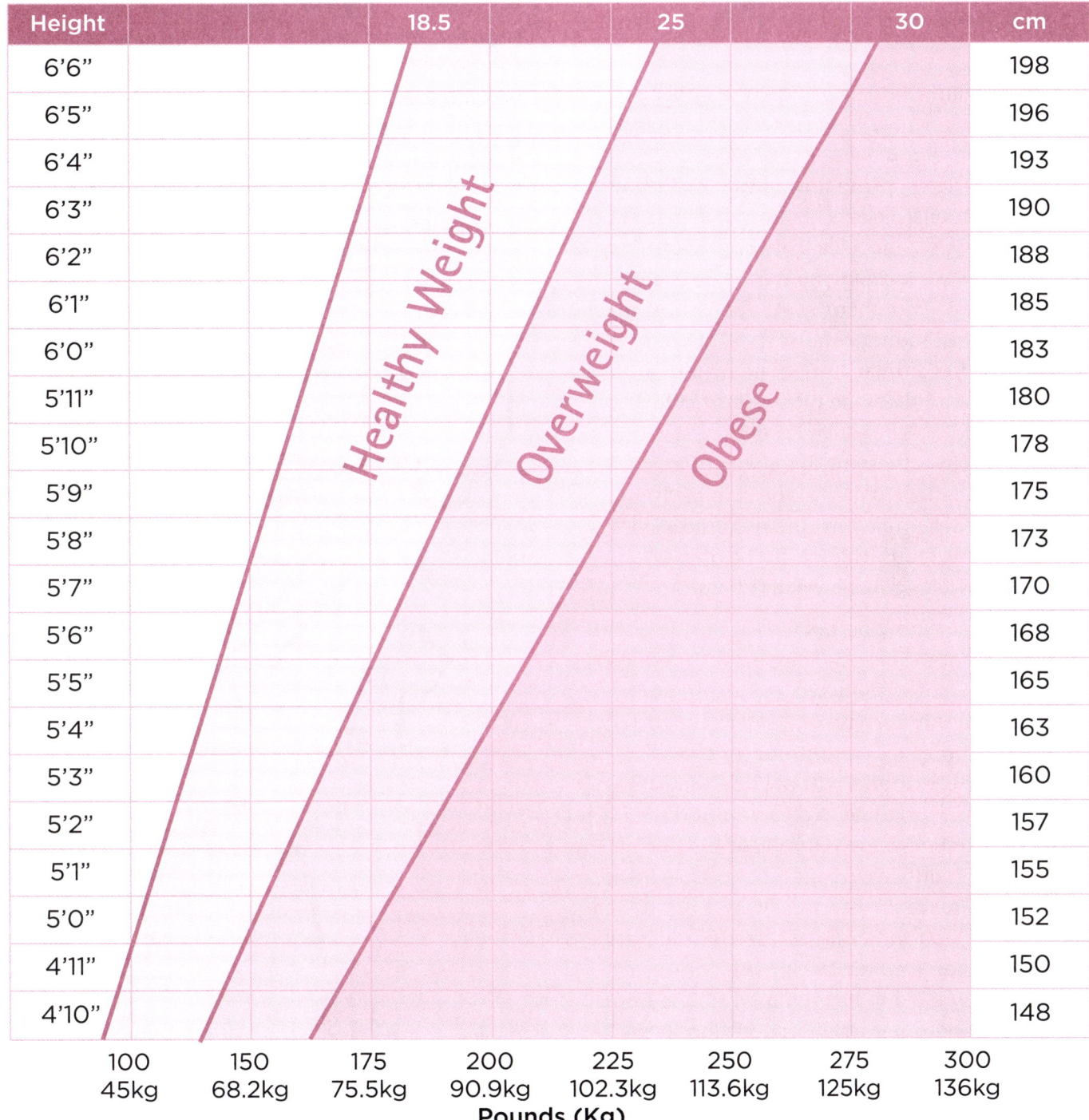

The BMI relates weight to height. To determine your BMI, find your height to the left (inches) or right (centimeters) and track horizontally to where your weight (below) intersects. Your BMI range is then shown at the top. Ratings are:

Less than 18.5 = underweight
18.5-24.9 = normal
25 to 29.9 = overweight
over 30.0 = obese

This Figure was developed for adults and post-pubertal youth (~age 17 years). For children and adolescents, most pediatricians use the BMI percentile. Levels of 85-95 percent indicate **overweight**, whereas values above 95 percent indicate **obesity**. If you are concerned, ask for your child's weight percentile.

FOOD MANAGEMENT AND DIABETES

C. Weight Management Plan

(For people with type 2 or type 1 diabetes, or for anyone)

As noted in Chapter 11, the rate of people being overweight or obese is increasing in all age groups. Approximately one in six children/adolescents are now obese (BMI above 30 – see Figure). This effects management of both type 1 and type 2 diabetes. For people with type 2 diabetes, weight management may be the most important aspect of therapy. All food plans must include weight management. The Choose My Plate guide in Chapter 11 may be helpful. Reduction of total calorie intake (particularly of high-fat foods) with reduced snacks and with smaller helpings is essential for weight loss. High-fat foods include: red meats, the skin of chicken or turkey, whole milk, fats and oil, processed foods and fast foods. Higher intake of vegetables, fruits and whole grains may also help.

Weight loss only occurs if there is a negative energy balance. This can happen with reduced caloric intake or with increased burning of calories through exercise or, preferably, with both. Most every food plan that involves reducing caloric intake will provide weight loss if the person is motivated to stick to it. It is important to find a food plan that the person likes and will adhere to and follow. After initial weight loss, there is often a "leveling-off" of the effect. This is normal, and the person must still follow the plan and not become discouraged. Exercise may need to be increased to one hour per day, six days per week, in addition to the food plan.

Unfortunately, there is no "one-size-fits-all" food plan to achieve weight loss or weight maintenance. Weight loss has been successful with various types of food plans, including a Mediterranean-style food plan. The Mediterranean food plan recommends high intake of fresh fruits and vegetables, with fish, beans and nuts as a protein source (whole eggs limited to once weekly, egg whites more frequently and red meat once or twice monthly). Whole grains are recommended as a major source of carbohydrate. Consider soups and salads and home-prepared nutritious meals! A website to learn more about the Mediterranean food plan is: www.mediterraneanbook.com/the-mediterranean-diet/. An additional resource is from the Academy of Nutrition and Dietetics, www.eatright.org. It can also be helpful to meet with a dietitian who will be able to provide the proper guidance to determine what's best for you.

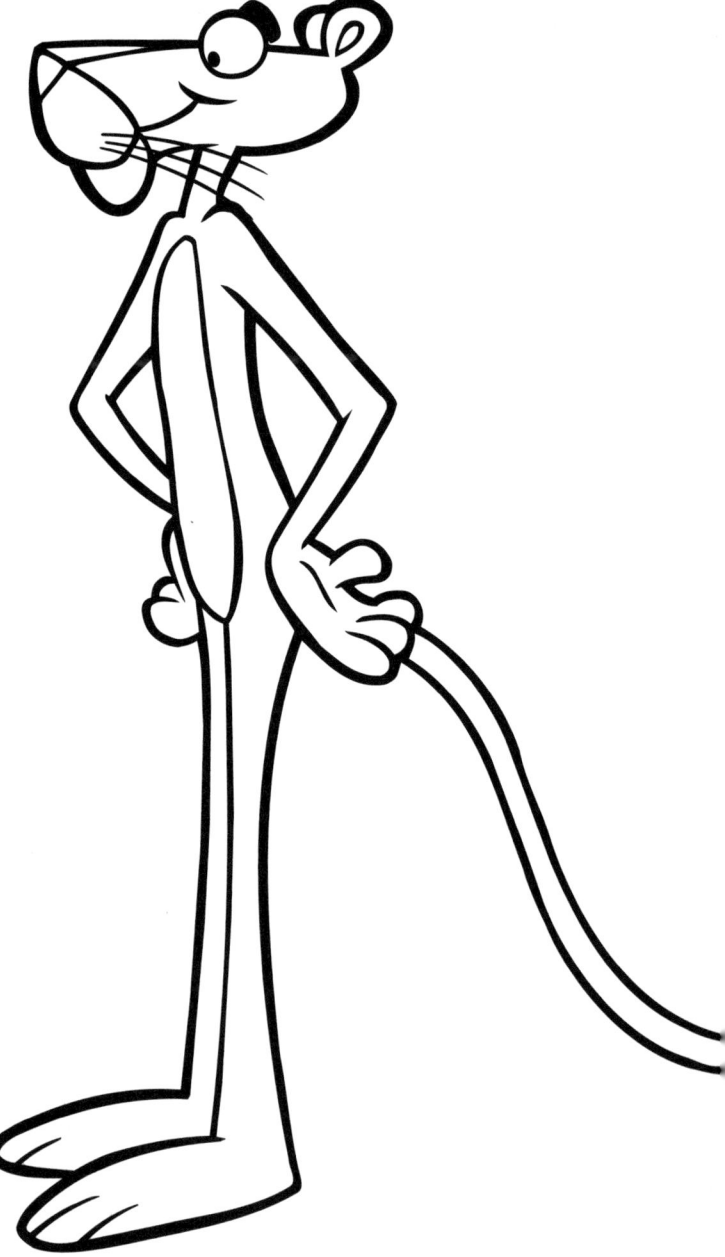

SUMMARY

The key to food management in diabetes is constant thinking and matching insulin to carb intake. The entire family must help with this.

Important points:

- In general, carbs from sugar or from starch will raise the blood/CGM glucose levels about the same amount.
- A person with diabetes can eat almost any food in moderation, if it is worked into the meal plan and the correct amount of insulin is taken at the correct time.
- Nutritious carbohydrates (fruits, vegetables, whole grains) should be encouraged whenever possible.
- Frequent blood/CGM glucose monitoring after meals is encouraged to determine how a given food affects any individual.
- As discussed in other chapters (e.g., Chapter 9), blood/CGM glucose levels are more apt to remain below 180 mg/dL (<10.0 mmol/L) if the Humalog, NovoLog or Apidra is taken 20 minutes prior to the meal.
- Blood sugar monitoring when an insulin reaction occurs is important in avoiding over-treatment of lows. The excessive eating with a hypoglycemic reaction (or just the psychological feeling of hunger) is a major concern in managing blood/CGM glucose levels.

Remember: Food management for people with diabetes does not mean a restrictive diet, but rather a healthy eating plan that family and friends should also follow.

Carbohydrate Counting Resources:

For those wanting more detailed information on carb counting or on carb quantities in foods, there are now entire books written on these subjects. References are included below.

Websites

www.calorieking.com
www.nutritiondata.com (recipe analysis)
www.myfitnesspal.com

Books

1. *"Calories and Carbohydrates"* 16th Edition by Barbara Kraus, Penguin Books
2. *"The Complete Book of Food Counts"* 9th Edition by Corinne Netzer, Dell Publishing
3. *"The Diabetes Carbohydrate and Fat Gram Guide"* 4th Edition by Lee Ann Holzmeister, American Diabetes Association
4. *"Complete Guide to Carb Counting"* 3rd Edition by Hope S Warshaw and Karmeen Kulkarni, American Diabetes Association
5. *The Calorie King® Calorie Fat & Carbohydrate Counter* (Updated Annually) by Allan Borushek, Family Health Publications

Phone and Android Nutrition Applications (free)

Calorie King Food Search App Go Meals: www.gomeals.com

Live Strong: www.livestrong.com/thedailyplate/iphone-calorie-tracker

Lose It!: www.loseit.com

MyNetDiary: www.mynetdiary.com

MyFitnessPal: www.myfitnesspal.com

Fooducate: www.fooducate.com

Spark People: www.sparkpeople.com

Calorie Counter: www.fatsecret.com

Carb Counting with Lenny: www.lenny-diabetes.com/games-n-apps.html

Exchange Meal Plan Resource:

"Choose Your Foods: Food Lists for Diabetes, 2014" is available from the American Diabetes Association at 120 South Riverside Plaza, Suite 2000, Chicago, IL 60606-6995. (1-800-342-2383) www.diabetes.org.

DEFINITIONS

ADA: American Diabetes Association.

"Carb choice": Fifteen-gram equivalent of carbohydrate used to determine the units of rapid-acting insulin to be taken. It is the same as a **"carb count."**

Carbohydrate (carb) counting: A meal plan in which counting the grams of carb to be eaten (and considering the blood sugar level and any planned exercise) is used to adjust the dosage of rapid-acting insulin prior to meals.

Cholesterol: One of the two main blood fats. High levels are related to a greater chance for heart attacks later in life.

Consistent (Constant) carbohydrate diet: A meal plan in which the amount of carb is kept consistent from day to day to match a relatively consistent dose of insulin.

DCCT: Diabetes Control and Complications Trial, which ended in June 1993. It showed that lower HbA1c levels helped to reduce the eye, kidney and nerve complications of diabetes.

Exchange diet: A meal plan in which foods are grouped into one of six food lists having similar nutritional composition. Caloric intake and number of exchanges are set, but foods within a food group can be exchanged with one another.

Glycemic-index: A ranking of foods based on the rise in blood sugar when that food is given alone (with no other food).

Tablespoon (Tbsp): A measure of 15 cc (15 mL) or three teaspoons. It is equal to 15g (½ oz) of water.

Teaspoon (tsp): A measure of 5 cc (5 mL). It is also equal to 5g of water.

Triglyceride: One of the two main blood fats. High levels are believed to be related to a greater risk for heart attacks later in life for people with diabetes.

QUESTIONS AND ANSWERS FROM NEWSNOTES

Q Is there any way to know if the pop received at fast food restaurants, theaters and other places is truly "sugar-free" or the regular sugar-containing pop?

A This question is asked frequently, and the answer is "yes." The Diastix® (the sugar-only part of KetoDiastix), or the distal sugar block on KetoDiastix will change color if there is sugar present. Unfortunately, it is more common for the wrong pop to be served than most people realize, probably in the range of 20 percent of the time (one glass in five). As sugar pop is one of the most concentrated sources of sugar (approximately 10 tsp per can), it usually raises the blood sugar level to the 200-400 mg/dL (11.1-22.2 mmol/L) level. This is especially true if it is consumed without other foods, which slow the absorption of the sugar, or at a time when a rapid-acting insulin is not taken to allow the sugar to enter the cells.

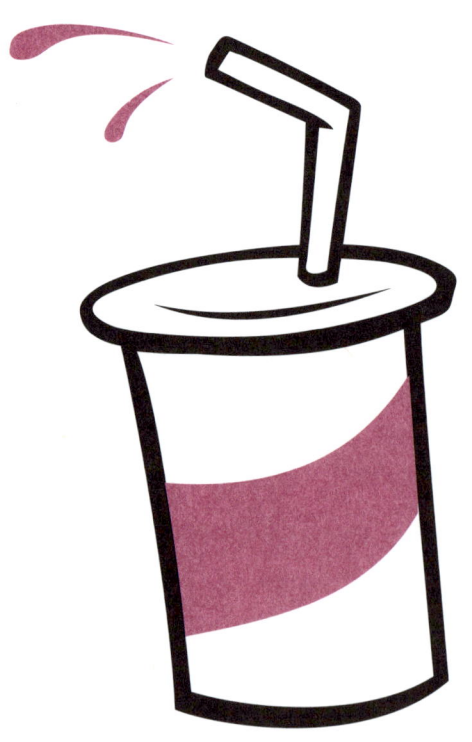

CHAPTER 13

Exercise and Diabetes

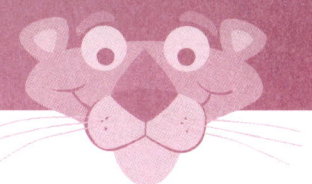

INTRODUCTION

Many of the people with the best-managed diabetes are those who exercise regularly. Exercise should be a normal part of life for everyone. The "Dietary Guidelines for Americans" recommends **60 minutes of moderate to rigorous physical activity per day** to help avoid weight gain and a minimum of 30 minutes a day to reduce the risk of chronic disease (e.g., type 2 diabetes). The American Academy of Pediatrics also recommends **a minimum of 60 minutes of exercise daily for all children and adolescents.** We strongly encourage regular exercise for anyone who has diabetes. Young people from our Clinic have participated in almost every sport: football, baseball, golf, track, swimming, wrestling, dancing, skiing, basketball, soccer, weightlifting, horseback riding, jumping rope, jogging and tennis. In Figure 1 in Chapter 14, Monitoring Diabetes, **EXERCISE** is listed as one of the "Big 4" factors to help attain optimal sugar levels. This is true for people with either type 1 or type 2 diabetes.

Many former and present professional athletes have diabetes. Professional baseball players with diabetes include Bill Gullickson (pitcher) and Ron Santo (third base). Gary Hall, Jr. won four medals (two gold) at the 2000 Olympics and the gold medal in the swimming Free Style at the 2004 Olympics. Adam Morrison played in the NBA. Professional football players include Kenny Duckett (wide receiver), Jonathan Hayes (tight end), Jay Cutler (quarterback) and Jay Leeuwenberg, who was an All-American

> **TOPICS:**
> **Physical Activity, Goal Setting and Problem Solving**
>
> **TEACHING OBJECTIVES:**
> The teacher will:
> 1. Discuss the importance of exercise as a critical component of healthy living.
> 2. Discuss the importance of exercise as a critical component of diabetes management.
> 3. Explain exercise recommendations and precautions for people with type 1 or type 2 diabetes.
>
> **LEARNING OBJECTIVES:**
> Learner (parents, child, relative or self) will be able to:
> 1. List three reasons why exercise is important.
> 2. Develop an exercise plan that includes monitoring of blood sugars, use of snacks and medication adjustments.
> 3. Construct a plan to help avoid hypoglycemia during or following exercise.

offensive lineman for the University of Colorado in the 1990s and then went on to play professional football. Jay spoke about the importance of being "in range" for blood sugars in order to play at his best level in pro football games; he related that he usually did at least 30 blood sugars during a professional football game. In the U.K., Gary Mabbott has type 1 diabetes and is a star football (American soccer) player. Hockey's Bobby Clarke, a former player of the Philadelphia Flyers, developed diabetes at age 15. He won the award for outstanding player in the National Hockey League twice. Billy

TABLE 1:
Why Exercise is Important
(outlined as presented in the text):

- Aerobic exercise lowers blood sugar levels
- Exercise helps people feel better
- Exercise helps maintain proper body weight
- Exercise helps keep the heart rate (pulse) and blood pressure lower
- Exercise helps keep blood fat levels lower
- Exercise improves insulin sensitivity
- Exercise may help maintain normal blood circulation

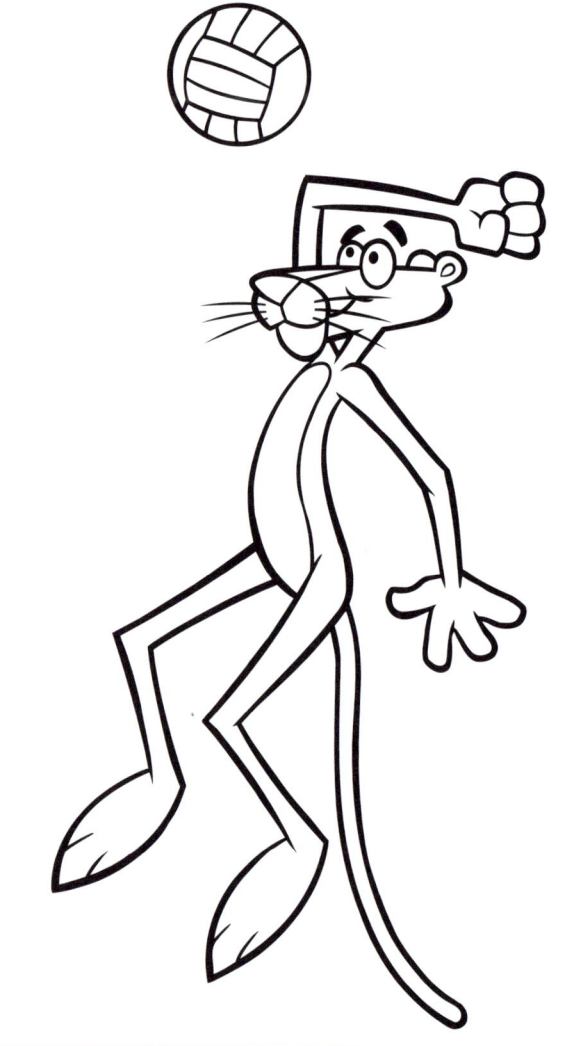

Talbert began playing tennis at age 12, two years after he developed diabetes. He became one of the best tennis players in the world, winning 37 national tournaments and being captain of America's winning Davis Cup Team and a member of the Tennis Hall of Fame. When he was in Denver to instruct youth with diabetes about tennis, we asked Billy why he felt he had no complications after over 40 years with diabetes. He replied, "I have gotten some exercise every day of my life in which it has been possible." These examples are given to show that people with diabetes can participate and excel in athletic activities, just like anyone else.

WHY EXERCISE IS IMPORTANT

Exercise is important and helps people with or without diabetes in the following ways (as outlined in Table 1):

- **Aerobic Exercise Lowers Blood/CGM Glucose Levels:**

Blood/CGM glucose values are usually lower with exercise (Figure 1). The **immediate effect** is likely due to muscles "burning" extra sugar during the exercise. As a result, values tend to be lower during the period of exercise.

There is also a **prolonged effect of exercise** on glucose levels. Following heavy afternoon exercise, blood/CGM glucose values have been shown to be lower throughout the night until the next morning. Figure 1 shows blood sugar (glucose) levels for the same 50 children on a day when they exercised compared to a day without exercise. It may be helpful to think of the exercise as causing increased insulin sensitivity over the next 12 to 16 hours.

As a result of regular exercise, the person is more sensitive to insulin, the insulin can work more efficiently, and a lower daily dose is usually required. Regular exercise and weight loss allow some people with type 2 diabetes to stop insulin injections and to change to oral medication. The old belief that people should

FIGURE 1
The Effect of Exercise on Blood Sugar Levels

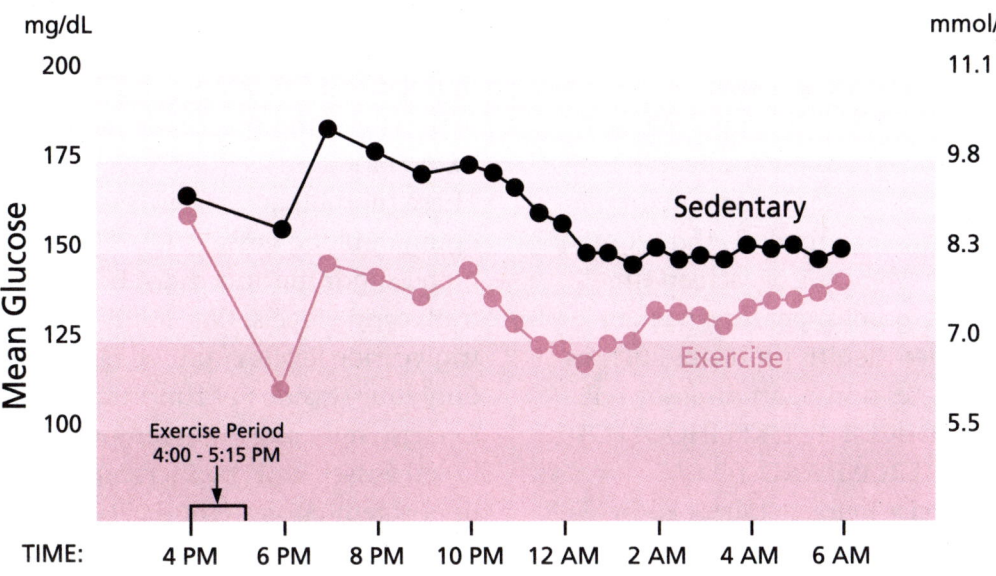

BLOOD SUGARS WITH AND WITHOUT ONE HOUR OF EXERCISE
This Figure presents blood glucose (sugar) levels for the same 50 children with type 1 diabetes on a sedentary day (black circles) and an exercise day (red circles). The one hour of exercise at 4 p.m. resulted in lower blood sugar levels for the next 14 hours (through the night). Insulin doses and food intake were identical for the two days.

(Data compliments of the DirecNet Study Group: J Pediatr 147, 528, 2005)

not exercise if they have high blood/CGM glucose levels is wrong. Exercise usually helps lower the sugar levels. IT IS ONLY WHEN KETONES ARE PRESENT THAT PEOPLE SHOULD NOT EXERCISE.

Some families note a temporary rise in blood sugar levels during or immediately after exercise. This may be due to consuming extra snacks or sugar drinks. It can also be due to adrenaline output with the excitement of exercise or the type of exercise. Non-aerobic exercise (e.g., sprinting) tends to result in more adrenaline output and higher blood/CGM glucose levels than does aerobic exercise.

Examples of anaerobic (or non-aerobic) exercise and aerobic exercise are given in Figure 2. The effect of exercise can differ by person and by intensity of each episode of exercise. Figure 2 was developed by an exercise physiologist (Dr. Michael Riddell, York University, Canada) as a guide to help people with diabetes understand how different activities can have different effects on blood glucose.

• **Exercise Helps People Feel Better**

There is a feeling of "well-being" and pride that comes from being in optimal physical condition. Many people just seem to feel better when they exercise daily. They tend not to tire as easily. Some people even say they are happier.

Teenagers get much of their support from friends. Friends often are made during sports activities. Exercise can give people the opportunity to mix with others. Some people tend to watch TV and eat snacks that raise the blood/CGM glucose levels. Exercise offers a way to avoid this.

- **Exercise Helps Maintain Proper Body Weight**

  Exercise is important, not only for people with diabetes, but for everybody. For thousands of years, people had to hunt for food and were very active. In the last 100 years, modern machines have made it possible for people to live with almost no exercise. The American Academy of Pediatrics recommends that youth have no more than two hours of "screen time" (TV, computer, video games) per day. Lack of activity has led to new health problems such as obesity, type 2 diabetes and heart disease. THE ONLY WAYS TO REDUCE THE LIKELIHOOD OF OBESITY ARE TO EXERCISE AND TO EAT MODERATELY. Exercise helps to burn excess calories. A national study in the U.S. (The Diabetes Prevention Program) showed exercise helped to avoid diabetes in people at high risk for type 2 diabetes. A person who keeps a normal weight is also less likely to have a heart attack later in life. Unfortunately, only around a quarter (25 percent) of youth are meeting exercise goals.

- **Exercise Helps Keep the Heart Rate (pulse) and Blood Pressure Lower**

  The heart is helped by exercise for many reasons. The heart of a person who is in optimal physical shape can do the same work with fewer heartbeats. An average heart rate (pulse) is 80 beats per minute. Many people who exercise regularly will have resting pulse rates in the 60s. Blood pressure tends to be lower in people who exercise. Thus, the heart doesn't have to pump as hard. Lower blood pressure helps reduce the risk of both heart attacks and the eye and kidney complications of diabetes in later life (see Chapter 23 on complications).

- **Exercise Helps Keep Blood Fat Levels Lower**

  We have discussed the importance of reducing cholesterol and saturated (animal) fat in the diet in Chapters 11 and 12. Many people with type 1 and type 2 diabetes have high levels of the blood fats, cholesterol and/or triglycerides. These high blood fat levels can lead to early aging of blood vessels. Exercise and optimal blood sugar management help to reduce blood triglyceride levels. One study showed that triglyceride levels could be reduced greatly after only four sessions of running 40 minutes a day. Exercise may also help remove cholesterol from blood vessel walls by increasing high density lipoprotein-cholesterol (HDL-C, see Chapter 11). HDL-C is considered the "good" cholesterol, and higher levels are better. Lowering the blood fat levels improves the health of blood vessels (including those supplying blood to the heart) and lessens the risk of heart attacks.

- **Exercise Improves Insulin Sensitivity**

  The best way humans can increase insulin sensitivity is by exercising and losing weight. As a result of exercise, the person is more sensitive to insulin and the insulin can work more efficiently. A lower daily insulin dose is often the result. Regular exercise (and weight loss) allows some people with type 2 diabetes to stop insulin injections and change to oral medication. It is now believed many of the beneficial effects of exercise on the risk of heart disease, particularly in type 2 diabetes, are due to improvements in insulin sensitivity. It is important to exercise regularly and vigorously.

- **Exercise May Help Maintain Normal Blood Circulation Later in Life**

  Regular exercise is believed to help maintain normal blood circulation. Data from the Pittsburgh Diabetes Registry showed that when boys with diabetes played in high school sports, they were more likely to keep normal foot circulation in later years. It is likely that the boys who were active in high school were also more apt to be active in later years.

TYPE 2 DIABETES AND EXERCISE

Although exercise is important for all people, it is **essential** for people with type 2 diabetes. It is also important for those people who are at high risk for type 2 diabetes. The Diabetes Prevention Program (DPP) studied 3,234 people with impaired (not diabetic; see Chapter 4) glucose tolerance tests. They were close to having type 2 diabetes. **The DPP showed that 30 minutes of activity per day, five days per week, combined with a low-fat diet reduced the risk of developing type 2 diabetes by over half (58 percent).**

Why don't people with type 2 diabetes or those at high risk get into exercise programs? *Some reasons might be:*

- ✔ psychological/stress/can't find the time
- ✔ started too fast in the past (must start slowly)
- ✔ too painful in the past (forgot warming up and "increasing" gradually)
- ✔ lack of motivation (TV, computer games more fun)
- ✔ not aware of the importance of exercise for optimal health

Whatever the reason, if the person is unable to achieve a lifestyle modification on his or her own, it may be helpful to join a supervised exercise and/or weight loss program. Exercising with friends can be fun and helps people remain committed to exercise. Counseling could be helpful as well. The cost of NOT modifying the lifestyle is just too great!

GETTING STARTED
Which Kinds of Exercise Are Best?

THE BEST EXERCISE IS THE ONE YOU LIKE. Different strokes for different folks! If you hate to jog or swim, but you do it because you are told to, you probably won't exercise regularly. Swimming five days a week in an outdoor pool is fun in the summer, but it may be more difficult to do in the winter. You may need to choose a different exercise such as jumping rope, using a treadmill or riding an exercise bicycle in the winter. Approximate calories used per hour for different types of exercise are shown in Table 2. Some treadmills and exercise bikes give the "calories burned."

Aerobic exercise especially helps heart fitness. Aerobic exercises include most continuous activities (such as jogging, walking, swimming or bicycling) that are done for a period of 30 minutes or longer. Many training programs use machines at health spas that feature continuous aerobic activity rather than short bursts of activity followed by a rest (a non-aerobic activity). When activities such as

TABLE 2:
Calories Per Hour Expended in Common Physical Activities

Moderate Physical Activity for One Hour	Calories Burned Per Hour	Vigorous Physical Activity for One Hour	Calories Burned Per Hour
Hiking	370	Running/jogging (5 mph)	590
Light gardening/yard work	330	Bicycling (>10 mph)	590
Dancing	330	Swimming (slow freestyle laps)	510
Golf (walking and carrying clubs)	330	Aerobics	480
Bicycling (<10 mph)	290	Walking (4.5 mph)	460
Walking (3.5 mph)	280	Heavy yard work (chopping wood)	440
Weight lifting (general light workout)	220	Weight lifting (vigorous effort)	440
Stretching	180	Basketball (vigorous)	440

Source: Adapted from the 2005 *"DGAC Report"* and the *"Dietary Guidelines for Americans,"* 2005

FIGURE 2
Types of "Intense" Activities

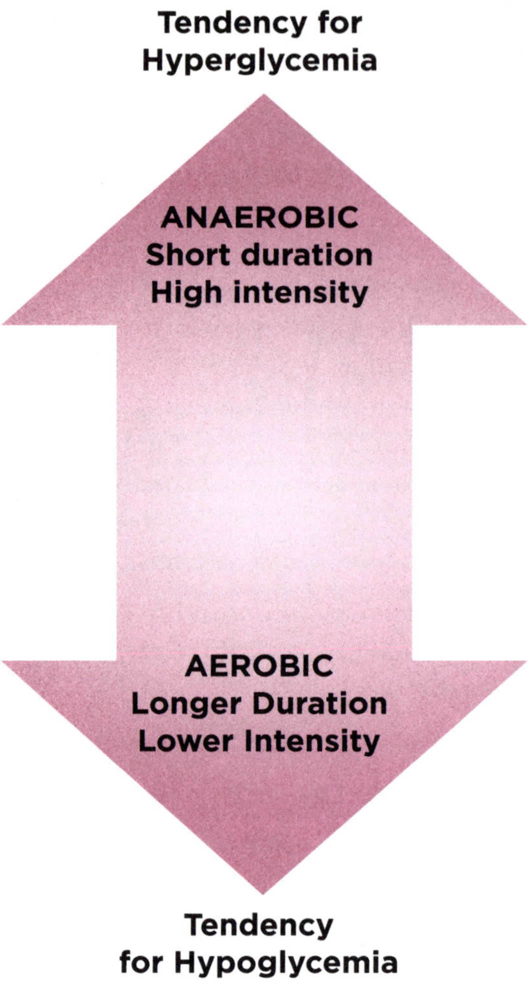

ANAEROBIC:
Weightlifting, tag, weight machines, sprinting, diving, swimming, gymnastics, wrestling, dodge ball, volleyball, ice hockey, track, cycling, basketball, football, tennis, lacrosse, skating

MIXED:
Skiing (slalom & downhill), field hockey, rowing, running (middle distance), cross country skiing, soccer, rugby, golf swings

AEROBIC:
In-line skating, jogging, dancing, cycling, brisk walking uphill, letter carrier, bike courier, gardening, golf

Figure compliments of Dr. Michael Riddell, York University, Canada

Tendency for Hyperglycemia ↑

ANAEROBIC — Short duration, High intensity

AEROBIC — Longer Duration, Lower Intensity

↓ **Tendency for Hypoglycemia**

---

weightlifting are done in short bursts with rests in between, they are considered strength building, not aerobic (see Figure 2).

Boxing is the only activity in which we have asked youth not to participate. The high incidence of eye injuries is not needed by a person who has diabetes (which can also cause eye problems). In addition, the high incidence of brain damage makes boxing dangerous for people with or without diabetes.

When Should I Exercise?

The best time to exercise will vary with your schedule. Think ahead and make changes in insulin doses and snacks to help avoid low blood sugars. Children like to play after school, and most organized sports activities take place at that time. If you take an intermediate-acting insulin at breakfast (e.g., NPH), this is when it is having its main effect, so taking extra care to avoid low blood sugar is important. When possible, pick an exercise time, preferably the same time each day, and adjust the snacks and insulin dose to fit the exercise. Walking after a meal has been shown helpful in lowering post-meal blood sugar levels. YOUR DIABETES MANAGEMENT CAN BE ADJUSTED TO SUIT YOUR LIFESTYLE. YOUR LIFESTYLE DOES NOT HAVE TO BE ADJUSTED TO FIT YOUR DIABETES.

When Should I Not Exercise?

The blood/CGM sugar level must be known and should not be low or excessively high prior to exercise. If blood or urine ketone levels are elevated, exercise can raise the ketone level even higher. Thus, it is not good to exercise when you have ketones. Remember to check ketones before exercising if you are not feeling well or if your blood glucose is >300 mg/dL (>16.7 mmol/L).

How Should I Get Started?

The best way to make exercise a part of everyday living is to begin early in life. Older children may not be as willing to begin a regular exercise program. Exercise should be part of the normal routine. Many people prefer TV or computer games instead of exercise, and the parents may have to encourage exercise. The parents can reward the child with exercise activities such as skating and swimming. It is helpful if the parents can have fun with the child in the activity. Jogging, walking or jumping rope is beneficial for parents too! Whenever a child has a parent's attention and company, the time quickly becomes a reward. A child of any age will often pick up the parents' exercise behaviors. The parents need to set a good example by exercising regularly even if it is not with the child. Exercising with a friend can be fun. Friends can help each other continue the exercise plan.

When beginning a new exercise program, it is always best to START SLOWLY and gradually extend the time and amount of exercise. This will result in fewer sore muscles and a better chance to continue the program. Recommendations for people over 35 years old or who have other risk factors are discussed below under "Age and Exercise."

How Often and How Far?

How often should the person with diabetes exercise? A MINIMUM OF SIXTY MINUTES OF AEROBIC EXERCISE, AT LEAST FIVE TIMES PER WEEK, IS NOW CONSIDERED IDEAL. The more exercise a person gets, the more calories that are "burned." Some people burn more calories with their exercise than others. This is partly related to how hard and how long the person exercises. For example, a person who runs at a rate of seven minutes per mile burns 300 calories in 30 minutes. However, if the person runs at 11 minutes per mile, 200 calories are burned in 30 minutes. If weight loss is one of the goals, it may be necessary to work harder or for a longer period to reach the desired goals. **It is important to remember that all exercise is beneficial, whether it is activity at work or during a specific exercise program.**

It is wise to check the pulse immediately (for 10 seconds, and multiply by six) after stopping the activity. If the pulse is more than 160 beats per minute, the exercise has probably been too strenuous.

EXERCISE AND LOW BLOOD SUGAR (HYPOGLYCEMIA)

Exercise is a known risk factor for hypoglycemia. It is essential to avoid low blood sugar reactions during and after exercise. The DirecNet Study Group found that children were less apt to have low sugars during heavy exercise if their blood/CGM glucose value prior to the exercise was above 180 mg/dL (10.0 mmol/L). The safe level for blood sugar before exercise can be individualized based on experience. Avoiding low sugars can be done in several ways:

✓ **Check blood/CGM glucose values before, during and after the exercise**

The best way to know how any exercise affects a person is to check blood/CGM glucose values before, during (when possible) and after the exercise. The overall effect of activity is usually to lower blood/CGM glucose levels (Table 3). Once a pattern is detected (e.g., "swimming always makes my blood sugar fall" or "softball doesn't seem to affect my blood sugar"), more accurate insulin and food changes can be made. Sometimes blood/CGM glucose values go up with exercise. This may be because of output of the hormones glucagon and adrenaline (epinephrine), which is a normal response in people with or without diabetes. These hormones cause sugar to be released from the liver. If the blood/CGM glucose value is high, a reduced insulin correction (e.g., 50 percent) is sometimes given, knowing that the values will likely decrease. Keeping records is important, so when a similar exercise is done at

TABLE 3:
Insulin Dosing Algorithms for *EXERCISE*

Expected Time of Exercise	Infants *Birth - 2 yrs.*	Preschool *3 - 4 yrs.*	School Age *5 - 9 yrs.*	Pre-Teen *10 - 12 yrs.*	Adolescents/College Age *13 - 25 yrs.*
Before Breakfast	↓ dinner or p.m. N or Lantus / Levemir / Tresiba by ¼ - ½ unit (evening before)	↓ dinner or p.m. N or Lantus / Levemir / Tresiba by ½ unit (evening before)	↓ dinner or p.m. N or Lantus / Levemir / Tresiba by ½ - 1 unit (evening before)	↓ dinner or p.m. N or Lantus / Levemir / Tresiba by 1 unit (evening before)	↓ dinner or p.m. N or Lantus / Levemir / Tresiba by 1 - 2 units (evening before)
Mid-Morning	↓ a.m. RAI or R by ¼ - ½ unit	↓ a.m. RAI or R by ½ unit	↓ a.m. RAI or R by ½ - 1 unit	↓ a.m. RAI or R by 1 unit	↓ a.m. RAI or R by 1 - 2 units
Afternoon	↓ a.m. N or noon RAI or R by ¼ - ½ unit	↓ a.m. N or noon RAI or R by ½ unit	↓ a.m. N or noon RAI or R by ½ - 1 unit	↓ a.m. N or noon RAI or R by 1 unit	↓ a.m. N or noon RAI or R by 1 - 2 units
Evening	↓ dinner RAI or R by ¼ - ½ unit	↓ dinner RAI or R by ½ unit	↓ dinner RAI or R by ½ - 1 unit	↓ dinner RAI or R by 1 unit	↓ dinner RAI or R by 1 - 2 units
All Day	↓ all insulins by 10 - 50%	↓ all insulins by 10 - 50%	↓ all insulins by 10 - 50%	↓ all insulins by 10 - 50%	↓ all insulins by 10 - 50%

↓ = lower, decrease; N = NPH
RAI = Rapid-acting insulin (Humalog, NovoLog or Apidra); R = Regular insulin

FIGURE 3
Percent of Children with Low Blood Sugars
(<70 mg/dL [<3.9 mmol/L]) **During Exercise**

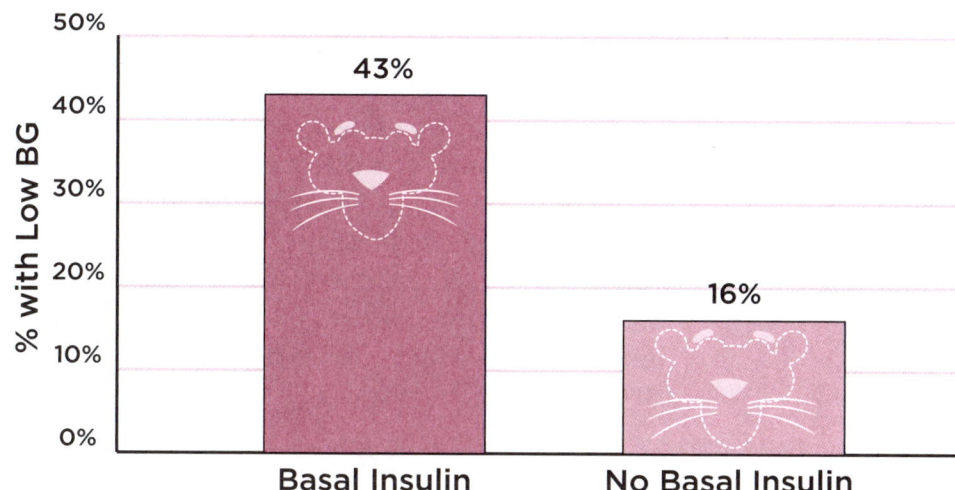

The same 49 children did the same (60 minute) afternoon exercise on two different days, one with basal insulin continued and one with basal insulin stopped. Low blood sugars during the exercise were reduced by almost two-thirds in the group with basal insulin stopped.

a similar time of the day (with the same insulin peaking) and with a similar starting blood/CGM glucose level, the best plans for insulin changes and food can be made.

Some people become frustrated with the "ups and downs" of blood/CGM glucose values during exercise. It is important to remember, **"DIABETES IS A COMPROMISE."** One must put up with the changes in glucose values in return for the better health of the heart, blood vessels and the entire body.

✓ **Eat before heavy exercise**

If you are going to exercise around mealtime, you should eat the meal first. When possible, allow a half-hour for digestion. Liquids such as milk and juices are absorbed most rapidly and generally protect from low blood sugar reactions for the next 30-60 minutes. Solid foods, such as those eaten at mealtime, are digested more slowly and usually provide protection for at least two to three hours. When it is possible to choose the exercise time, try to exercise, even for a short time, after a meal or snack. This will help to reduce the increase in blood sugar levels following the meal. Table 4 gives suggestions for snacks for people who take insulin. Although detailed tables are available matching exercise energy spent with food energy to take in, nothing works better than **EXPERIENCE** and **FREQUENT BLOOD/CGM SUGAR CHECKING**.

✓ **Reduce insulin dosage before and during the exercise (Table 3)**

People who do not have diabetes have very low insulin levels during exercise. To simulate this, it is relatively easy to turn off an insulin pump or to use a (reduced) temporary basal rate during periods of intense exercise. Some people also need to reduce the basal insulin 15, 30 or 60 minutes prior to the exercise. Remember that the activity of rapid-acting insulin peaks 90 minutes after injection.

The DirecNet group found 43 percent of children to have low blood glucose levels during one hour of intense exercise when pump basal insulin rates were continued. In contrast, only 16 percent had low values when the basal insulin rates were discontinued during the same exercise (Figure 3). The ability to quickly alter insulin delivery with exercise is one of the major advantages of insulin pump therapy.

For people using insulin injections the insulin dose can be decreased if you know which insulin is having its main effect during the time of exercise. Suggestions for insulin reductions are shown for people of different ages in Table 3.

If extra morning exercise is planned, you can reduce the morning rapid-acting insulin or Regular insulin. If late afternoon exercise is planned, you can reduce the morning NPH or noon rapid-acting insulin by 10-50 percent. If the activity is in the evening, the dinner rapid-acting insulin is often reduced. Similarly, Lantus/Levemir/Tresiba insulin at dinner or in the evening may be reduced by a few units with heavy exercise days. People reduce insulin by different amounts. **Experience is the best teacher.**

✔ **Change the injection site**

The choice of where you inject the insulin can help in avoiding low blood sugars. Exercise increases blood flow into the part of the body that is moving. The increased blood flow takes up more insulin. When a person with diabetes exercises, the blood insulin level may increase; whereas insulin levels decrease in non-diabetics during exercise. If you inject insulin into an arm or leg that you will use heavily during exercise, your body may absorb the insulin too rapidly. If you are going to run, don't inject insulin into the leg. If you are going to play tennis, avoid the tennis arm. The abdomen is a good site for most strenuous exercise days.

TABLE 4: Extra Food to Cover Exercise*†

Expected length of exercise	Blood sugar level mg/dL	mmol/L	Examples of foods
A. Short (15-30 minutes)†	<80	<4.5	8 oz of sports drink** or 4-6 oz juice**
	80-150	4.5-8.3	A fresh fruit (or any 15 grams carbohydrate**)
	>150	>8.3	None
B. Longer (30-120 minutes)	<80	<4.5	8 oz sports drink** or 4 oz juice plus ½ sandwich
	80-150	4.5-8.3	8 oz sports drink or milk plus fresh fruit
	>150	>8.3	½ sandwich**
C. Longest (2-4 hours)*	<80	<4.5	8 oz sports drink or 4 oz juice, whole sandwich
	80-150	4.5-8.3	Fruit, whole sandwich
	>150	>8.3	Whole sandwich

* Remember to also drink water, sports drink or other fluids (one 8 oz glass for **A**, two 8 oz glasses for **B**, and three 8 oz glasses for **C**) before or during the exercise to avoid dehydration. This Table is for a moderate degree of exercise (e.g., walking, bicycling leisurely, shooting a basketball or mowing the lawn). If heavier exercise (e.g., jogging, bicycle race, basketball game or digging in the garden) is to be done for the same amount of time, then more food may need to be added. Amounts vary for different people, and the best way to learn is to do blood sugars before and after the exercise and keep a record of the blood sugar values (see Table 3).

** Each of these represents 15 grams of carbohydrate, which will last for about 30 minutes of moderate exercise. A sandwich with meat or other protein lasts longer.

† May also need to reduce insulin dosage.

TABLE 5:
Suggestions for Exercising Safely

- Check blood (CGM) glucose values before, during and after exercise to learn the best insulin adjustment for the activity
- Eat before heavy exercise
- Try to have the blood sugar above 180 mg/dL (10.0 mmol/L) before heavy exercise
- Have extra snacks available during exercise; some people use sports drinks, 4-8 oz, for every 30 minutes of vigorous exercise
- Always carry sugar
- Reduce the insulin dose (including the basal and/or pump bolus doses or the rapid-acting insulin shot if within 2-3 hours of the exercise)
- Consider the injection site (the abdomen is usually best)
- Wear an ID bracelet or necklace
- Try to exercise with a friend who knows about low blood sugar reactions
- Make sure coaches know about low blood sugars (see letter at end of this chapter)
- Do not exercise if ketones are present
- Drink plenty of water, especially in hot weather
- If delayed hypoglycemia occurs frequently, the insulin dose should be appropriately reduced
- Have fun!! Find an exercise you enjoy and incorporate it into your daily life.

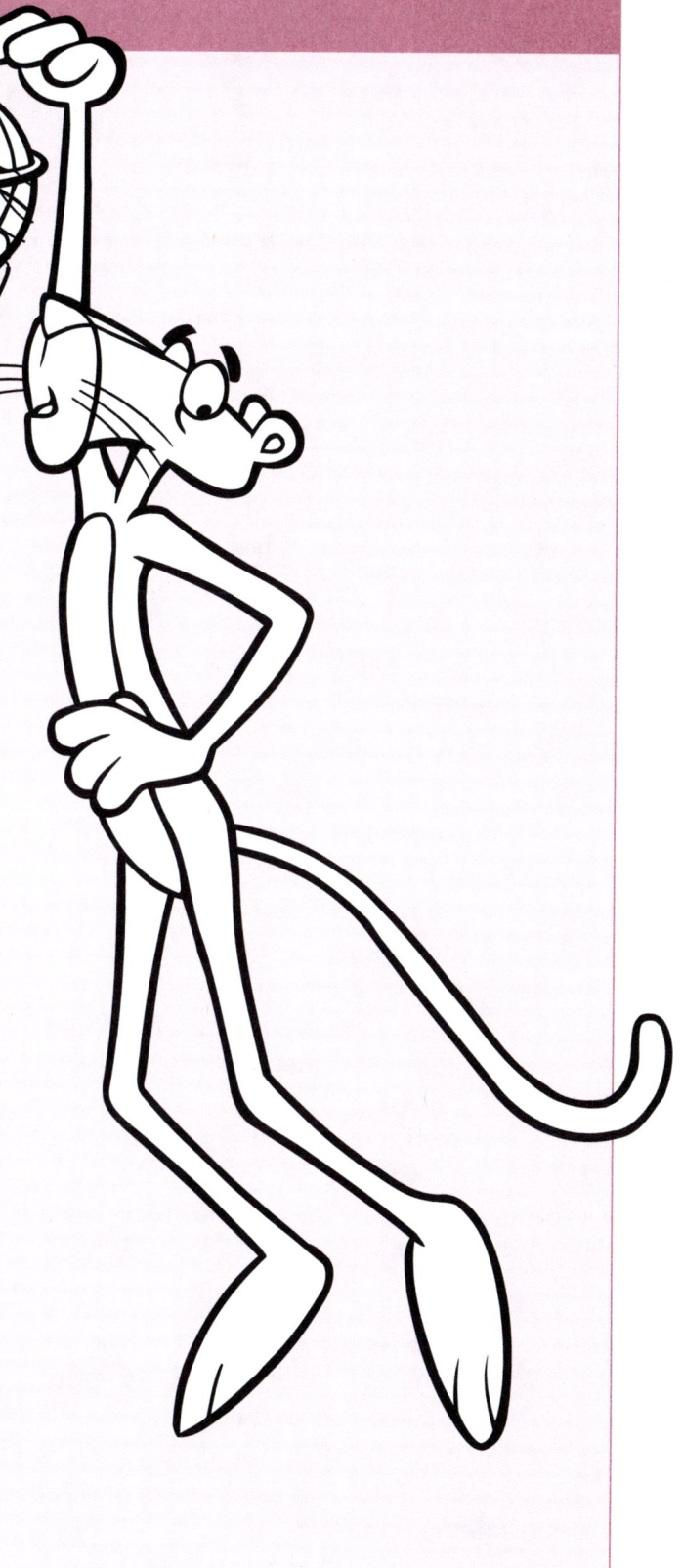

✔ **Make sure others know**

It is important that coaches and teammates are aware of the diabetes. A team manager may be a suitable person to carry extra sugar snacks. It is helpful for the coach to be aware of the diabetes and to know the symptoms and treatment of low blood sugar. A letter is included at the end of this chapter that you are welcome to copy as often as you like to share with coaches. Awareness of diabetes and the care needed to be a successful athlete has improved in part because of "famous" athletes. This chapter and book can help people to better understand the care needed to succeed. Remember that when a low blood sugar occurs during a sporting event, it is important to rest for at least ten minutes to let the blood sugar rise. The coach should be aware of this. Suggestions for exercising safely are summarized in Tables 4 and 5.

✔ **Have extra snacks available before, during and after the exercise**

THE PERSON WITH DIABETES MUST ALWAYS HAVE A SOURCE OF SUGAR AVAILABLE. Parents have sewn pockets in basketball shorts, jogging pants and other clothes to hold three sugar packets, three sugar cubes or three glucose tablets for a possible emergency. Joggers' wallets on shoes work nicely. A sandwich or similar snack should be available nearby, as a sugar packet may last only a few minutes. It is helpful for the coach or instructor to have a tube of instant glucose or some other emergency source of sugar.

It is often difficult to guess the amount of a snack necessary for a particular activity. If the exercise is in the hour after a meal, an extra snack may not be needed. If a person is physically unfit, the blood sugar may drop more rapidly than if the person is physically fit. It is very useful to monitor the blood/CGM glucose values to determine what the correct snack is prior to, during and after the exercise. If the blood/CGM glucose value is low (e.g., below 100 mg/dL or 5.5 mmol/L), a larger snack is needed than when the blood sugar is high. IN FACT, EXERCISING CAN BE A VERY EFFECTIVE WAY TO LOWER A HIGH BLOOD SUGAR (AS LONG AS KETONES ARE NOT PRESENT). The type of snack can be varied depending on the expected length of the activity. IN GENERAL, THE MORE RAPIDLY ABSORBED CARBOHYDRATES SUCH AS JUICE OR SPORTS DRINKS ARE USED FOR SHORT-TERM ACTIVITIES. More food is added, such as crackers or bread, if the activity is to last longer. THE SNACK THAT KEEPS THE BLOOD SUGAR UP THE LONGEST IS ONE THAT INCLUDES PROTEIN AND FAT ALONG WITH THE CARBOHYDRATE. This might be a cheese or meat sandwich with a glass of juice. Snacks that contain fat increase the calories and potential for weight gain. It is wise to check the glucose levels after the activity to help decide what to use for a snack the next time. Extra foods taken during the exercise period can help keep blood/CGM glucose values in the normal range (see Table 4).

It is wise to keep snacks in the glove box of the car (e.g., granola bars) to eat before or after an activity. This is especially important if the distance is great between home and the activity. **ALWAYS CHECK THE BLOOD/CGM GLUCOSE VALUE BEFORE DRIVING.**

Remember, for the best effects of exercise on weight, it is better to reduce insulin for exercise rather than to increase food intake. Table 5 provides a summary for exercising safely.

AVOIDING LOW BLOOD SUGARS AFTER EXERCISE

"DELAYED HYPOGLYCEMIA" refers to low blood/CGM glucose values several hours after the exercise is over. These may occur three to 12 hours after exercise. The 50 youth represented by the lines in Figure 1 had low blood sugar values (<60 mg/dL or <3.3 mmol/L) in 48 percent of the nights after heavy exercise and in 28 percent of nights after no exercise. They did not have a reduction in their insulin during the exercise.

In addition to reducing the insulin during the exercise, the injected or pump basal insulin acting during the night may need to be reduced. We have shown that after a day of heavy exercise **the use of an 80 percent temporary basal insulin rate from 9 p.m. to 3 a.m. can help to avoid delayed hypoglycemia during the night.** The amount and timing of basal insulin rate reduction can be adjusted based on experience.

The artificial pancreas, with automatic suspension of insulin delivery from an insulin pump with a low or predicted low glucose level, can be very helpful in avoiding delayed hypoglycemia occurring during the night. Nighttime is the period of greatest risk for severe lows, as people often do not awaken to alarms. Thus, automatic suspension of insulin delivery while the person is sleeping can be very helpful (Chapter 31).

Some people with type 2 diabetes may also experience delayed hypoglycemia. The result may be a low blood sugar in the middle of the night. It may happen because extra sugar in the blood goes back into storage in the muscle and liver. Hormone changes with sleep (e.g., lower adrenaline levels) may also be important.

INSULIN PUMPS

- Use of an insulin pump and/or CGM makes insulin adjustments easier in order to avoid exercise-related hypoglycemia (see **Reduced Insulin Dosage...** section above).

- Using reduced temporary basal rates before, during and after exercise can be helpful (Figure 3 and Chapter 28).

- Some insulin pump users who disconnect from their pump during exercise can benefit by giving part of their basal insulin as Lantus (Basaglar), Levemir or Tresiba and part via the pump. For example, half of the basal insulin could be given by the pump (50 percent temp basal for 24 hours) and the other half given as a shot of one of the above basal insulins.

NUTRITIONAL SUPPLEMENTS FOR EXERCISE

We frequently have adolescents ask us, "Can I take a protein supplement and/or should I take amino acids?" The answer to these questions is "No." Taking extra protein or amino acid supplements will NOT build muscles and may be harmful to the kidneys. The only way to build muscles is to do the physical exercise necessary to build the muscle mass. The foods to eat are described in Chapter 11. Recent scandals about so-called "performance-enhancing" substances have raised awareness of their dangers and illegality.

HYDRATION AND EXERCISE

Proper hydration (drinking fluids) is essential during exercise. Exercising during hot weather requires special attention. Drinking extra fluids should begin an hour or two before starting to exercise. A general rule is to drink 8 oz of fluids for every 30 minutes of vigorous activity. Liquids such as sports drinks and fruit juices help replace water, salts and carbohydrates. Drinking sports drinks at half-hour intervals in combination with blood/CGM glucose checks during strenuous exercise works well for many people. However, if your blood/CGM glucose level increases above 200 mg/dL (11.1 mmol/L), the sports drink may need to be reduced in amount or diluted. Table 4 recommends suggested fluid amounts for different levels of activity.

AGE AND EXERCISE

Adults are advised to discuss plans to begin a new exercise program with their diabetes care-provider first. As with everyone, starting slowly and gradually increasing the amount of exercise is important. Proper stretching (five to 10 minutes) **BEFORE, DURING** and **AFTER** the exercise will help to avoid cramps and stiffness that may otherwise discourage further exercise.

Having a medical check-up before starting a new exercise program is recommended if you:

- ✔ are over 35 years of age
- ✔ have had type 1 diabetes more than 15 years
- ✔ have had type 2 diabetes more than 10 years
- ✔ have additional risk factors for a heart attack
- ✔ have eye or kidney complications
- ✔ have neuropathy (Chapter 23)

A graded exercise test might also be helpful. The maximum heart rate during exercise should not exceed 220 minus age.

Strenuous activities, including weightlifting and jogging, are discouraged for people who have severe eye changes of diabetes (proliferative retinopathy). This should be discussed with the diabetes eye specialist. Similarly, people with neuropathy should discuss with their diabetes care-provider the pros and cons of exercise. When peripheral neuropathy is severe, weight-bearing exercises should be limited. With both severe eye changes and neuropathy, exercises that involve straining, jarring, or that cause increased pressure on the eyes or feet must be avoided. It is sometimes wise to have a "baseline" electrocardiogram (EKG) done prior to beginning a new exercise program. Other tests are then possible if there are any suggestions of abnormalities. People may ask their diabetes care-provider to review with them the ADA guidelines for exercise that are published each January in the Supplement to "Diabetes Care."

SUMMARY

Exercise is important for all people, but especially for a person with diabetes. Exercise can improve the blood lipids, reduce blood pressure and improve cardiovascular fitness. It is very helpful for weight reduction for people with type 2 diabetes. Choose exercises that you enjoy. If possible, the amount of exercise and the time of day should be fairly CONSISTENT. You can change the diabetes management to fit the exercise. It is not necessary to change the exercise to fit the diabetes. You can plan the exercise after a meal, reduce the insulin dosage or take extra snacks to help avoid low blood/CGM glucose values. YOU SHOULD CARRY A SOURCE OF SUGAR AT ALL TIMES AND YOU SHOULD ALWAYS HAVE A LONGER-LASTING SNACK AVAILABLE NEARBY. Remember, it is wise to THINK AHEAD about what the day's schedule will bring and plan accordingly.

DEFINITIONS

Abdomen: The area around the belly button. The fatty tissue of the abdomen can be used as an injection site.

Adrenaline (epinephrine): The excitatory hormone. This normally increases early in exercise and may result in an initial rise in the blood sugar.

Aerobic: Exercise that uses oxygen at a rate in which the cardiorespiratory system (heart and lungs) can replace the oxygen in the muscles.

Anaerobic: More intense exercise that uses oxygen more quickly than the body can replace it in muscle.

Buttocks (seat): What a person sits on. The fatty tissue of the buttocks can be used as an injection site.

Delayed hypoglycemia: Low blood sugars usually occur 4-12 hours after heavy physical exercise, often during the night. This often occurs as sugar leaves the blood to replace depleted muscle sugar stores.

DPP: The **D**iabetes **P**revention **P**rogram. A study of 3,234 people who were overweight and had impaired (not diabetic) oral glucose tolerance tests. Exercise and weight loss (see this chapter) reduced the development of diabetes by 58 percent.

Glucagon: A hormone (like insulin) that also is made in the islets of the pancreas. It has the opposite effect of insulin and raises the blood sugar.

QUESTIONS AND ANSWERS FROM NEWSNOTES

Q My daughter just started swimming practices every day from 3:30-5:30 p.m. Her pre-dinner blood sugars are over 200 mg/dL (11.1 mmol/L) when she gets home. However, she has awakened at 3 a.m. to 4 a.m. the past two mornings feeling shaky. Is that possible?

a Your daughter has the classic symptoms of "delayed hypoglycemia," which is not uncommon. Her blood sugar is high when she gets home from swimming as she has put out adrenaline (epinephrine), the excitatory hormone, during the exercise. All people, with or without diabetes, normally do this. The adrenaline causes breakdown of stored sugar in the liver (glycogen) to help keep the blood sugar up during the exercise. It is a safety mechanism.

At a later time, the sugar goes back into the muscle – often 4-12 hours later. When this happens, the blood sugar falls and she awakens feeling shaky. This is less likely to happen if the insulin working during the night is decreased. It is often necessary to decrease the dose by as much as 20 percent to avoid delayed hypoglycemia. If using an insulin pump, a temporary basal rate of 80 percent from 9 p.m. to 3 a.m. will help.

Q Our doctor has told us not to reduce the insulin dose on heavy exercise days, but just to eat more food. We were told on ski days to also reduce the insulin dose. We are now confused.

a An important part of managing exercise with diabetes is to avoid low blood sugars or "insulin reactions." Planning ahead is very helpful. Some children can just eat more food and will do fine. We recommend reducing insulin for planned exercise rather than eating more food. Eating extra food may offset some of the benefits of exercise or healthy weight. Often a combination of some reduction in insulin dosage and eating extra snacks turns out to be the best solution.

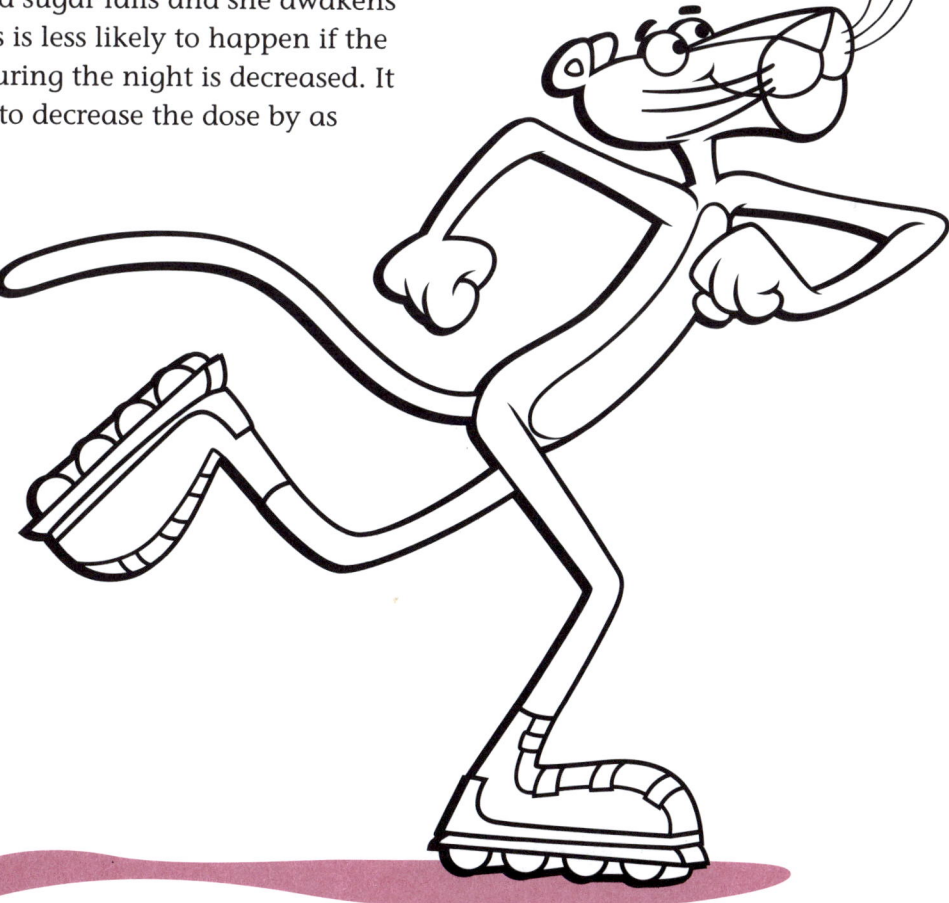

EXERCISE AND DIABETES

Dear Coach,

This letter is on behalf of _____ who is participating in _____ this year. Although we do not want to single out people with diabetes, there are things that you need to be aware of to help _____'s performance and enjoyment of the sport.

Exercise is very important for children and adolescents with diabetes. The overall effect of exercise is to lower blood sugar. We hope _____ will take the right amount of insulin and eat according to the anticipated activity for the day. However, even when these things are done, there may be times, especially with increased activity, when he/she may have an "insulin reaction" (low blood sugar), a condition requiring immediate attention. The symptoms of an insulin reaction include one or more of the following: shakiness, dizziness, sweating, rapid onset of extreme hunger, or tiredness and paleness. Some people complain of double vision and headaches. You may also notice _____'s performance suddenly becomes very poor, or his/her overall mood may change to being very crabby or emotional.

If a low blood sugar occurs, a can of fruit juice, 8 oz of Gatorade®, or two teaspoons of sugar followed in five to 10 minutes by solid food (fruit, cheese and crackers or a sandwich) will help correct this condition. He/She should rest for a minimum of ten minutes to let the blood sugar return to normal. However, some children will still have a headache and may not feel like continuing.

Many people with diabetes will change their insulin dose on days they anticipate a practice or game. The scheduling (or cancellation) of these events ahead of time helps the person (and parents) to be prepared. Again, it is very important for youth with diabetes to be involved in sports. It helps with their diabetes management and allows their insulin to work more effectively. A person with diabetes should not be and does not want to be treated differently because of having diabetes.

Please do not hesitate to call if you need more information or have any concerns. Our phone number is _____.

Sincerely,

(You may copy this letter as often as you wish.)

CHAPTER 14

Monitoring Diabetes

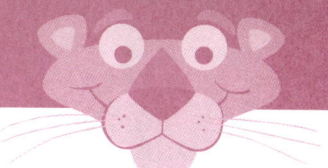

INTRODUCTION

Monitoring diabetes includes following hemoglobin (**HbA1c**) values (see section below) and blood/CGM glucose levels to make certain they are kept within target ranges. The goal is to have blood/CGM glucose levels that more closely approach the normal sugar levels of someone without diabetes. This generally means aiming for 70 percent of values in the desired range for age. In this edition we use blood/CGM glucose values to refer to either blood or CGM (continuous glucose monitor) glucose values.

Monitoring blood/CGM sugar levels is different from monitoring overall diabetes management. The latter might include symptoms of high and low blood sugars (Chapters 2, 6 and 15) and leading a normal life in spite of diabetes (Chapters 10 and 17-20), as well as many other factors. As these are covered elsewhere, they will not be discussed in depth in this chapter. The emphasis will be on aspects of **blood sugar (glucose)** monitoring not included in Chapter 7, and especially on the HbA1c value. Three additional measurements most readily available to CGM users (Chapter 29) are: **Time in Range, Time Below Range**, and **Time Above Range** (see Figure 3).

WHY IS OPTIMAL DIABETES MANAGEMENT IMPORTANT?

The Diabetes Control and Complications Trial (DCCT) proved that, for people with type 1 diabetes, improved sugar levels helped to avoid the eye, kidney and nerve complications of

> **TOPICS:**
> **Monitoring (Sugar, HbA1c)**
>
> **TEACHING OBJECTIVES:**
> The teacher will:
> 1. Discuss the four factors associated with optimal sugar levels.
> 2. Describe the HbA1c and its relationship to blood/CGM glucose levels.
> 3. Describe the blood/CGM glucose "time in range" measurement.
>
> **LEARNING OBJECTIVES:**
> Learner (parents, child, relative or self) will be able to:
> 1. List two factors that can affect sugar levels.
> 2. Explain the HbA1c, your (your child's) current value and the recommended range.
> 3. State the recommended percent of time for blood/CGM glucose values to be in range.

diabetes. The people receiving "**intensive management**" (insulin pumps or 3-4 shots of insulin per day, along with at least four blood sugar checks per day), had lower HbA1c values than people receiving "**conventional management**" (1-2 shots of insulin per day, with 0-2 blood sugar checks per day). The intensive management group was shown to have a much lower risk for the eye, kidney, nerve and cardiovascular (including heart attacks and strokes) complications of diabetes than did the conventional management group. As a result, what was "intensive management" is now the recommended treatment for all people with type 1 diabetes.

FIGURE 1
Four of the Major Influences on Blood Sugar Levels

All four must be in balance for optimal diabetes management. Blood sugars are monitored by daily blood sugar checks or by CGM and by HbA1c levels done every three months.

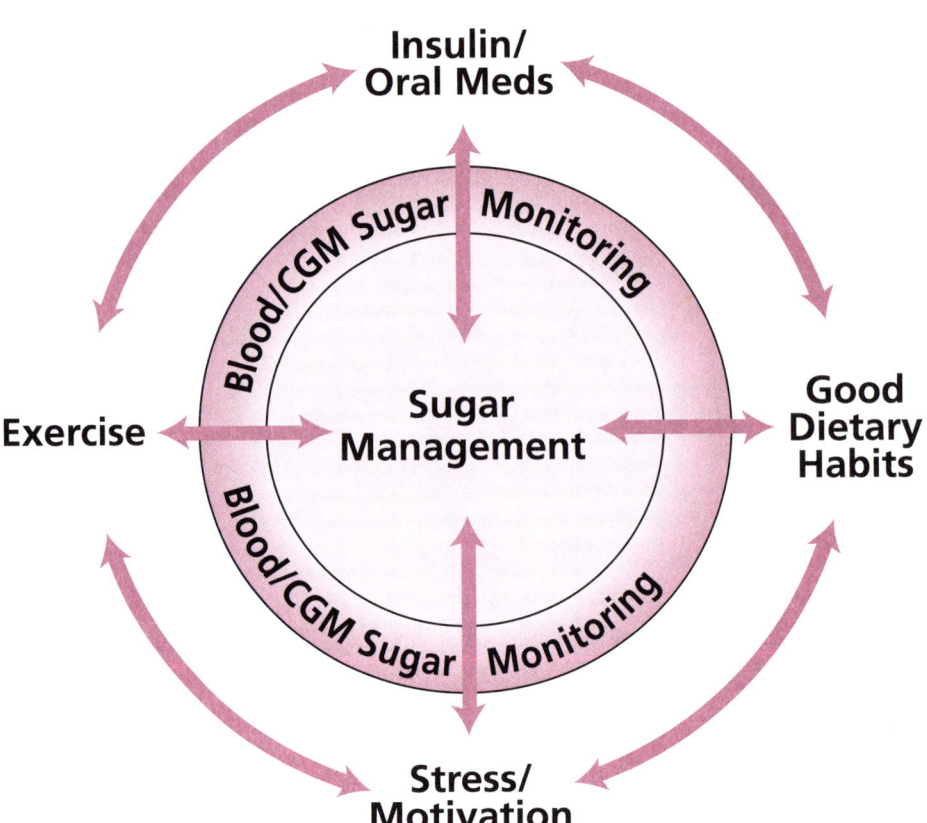

FIGURE 2
Formation of HbA1c

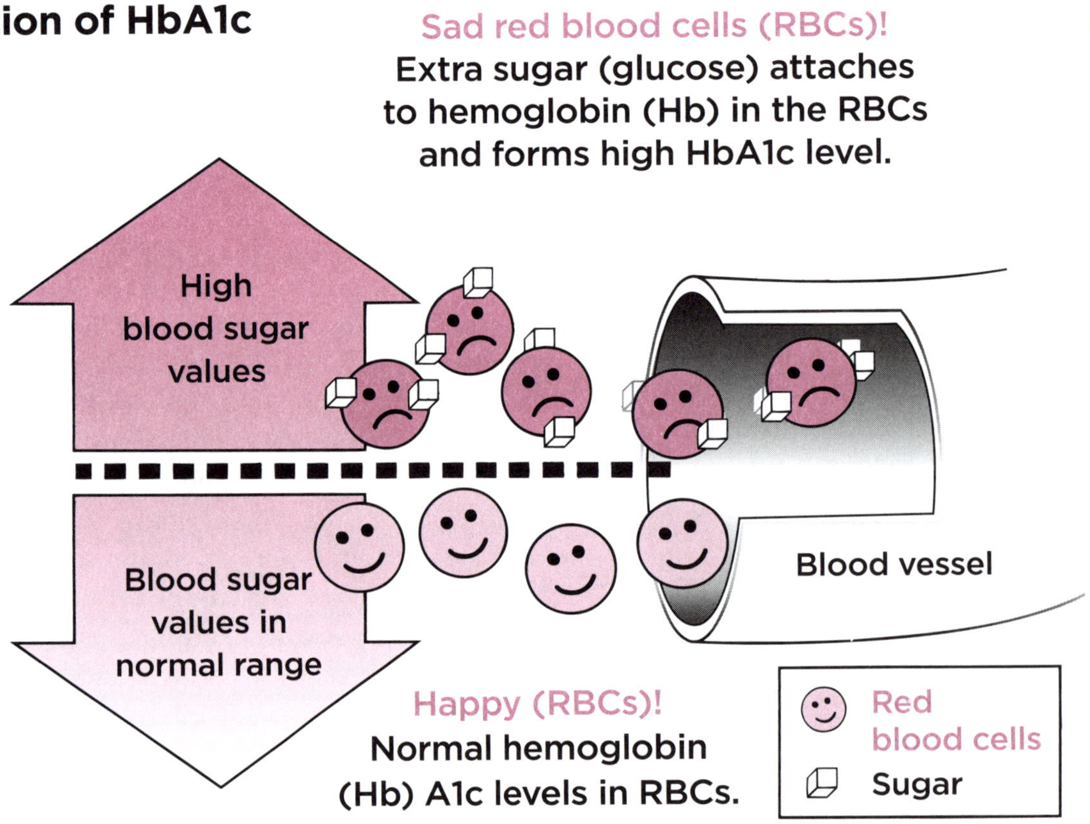

Sad red blood cells (RBCs)! Extra sugar (glucose) attaches to hemoglobin (Hb) in the RBCs and forms high HbA1c level.

Happy (RBCs)! Normal hemoglobin (Hb) A1c levels in RBCs.

Similar studies done in the U.K. and Japan showed optimal sugar levels in people with type 2 diabetes also resulted in a reduction in eye, kidney and nerve complications of diabetes. Some of these studies have also shown a decrease in the risk for heart attacks and strokes with improved sugar levels. However, there is also danger connected with aiming for a very low HbA1c level (e.g., <6.0% [<48 mmol/mol]), as the risk for frequent low blood sugars increases.

FACTORS INFLUENCING DIABETES MANAGEMENT

Optimal blood/CGM sugar levels for people with type 1 or type 2 diabetes are the result of balancing many factors, but especially the following (Figure 1):

1. the correct insulin/oral medicine dosage
2. getting regular exercise
3. having optimal dietary habits
4. using positive ways to cope with stress

Monitoring blood/CGM glucose values assists in maintaining the proper balance between all four factors. Each of these factors is discussed elsewhere in this book in more detail. For people with type 1 diabetes, perhaps the most important of the four is the correct insulin dosage given at the right times. Sugar levels will not improve if the insulin dose is incorrect, even if the other three factors are in balance. It will not help to do extra exercise if the person is not receiving the correct insulin dosage. However, any one of the four factors can result in sub-optimal diabetes management. For example, if the other three factors are normally in balance, but the person decides to regularly drink sugar pop (10 tsp of sugar per can), optimal management will be lost. Similarly, with a lot of stress, the adrenaline (excitatory hormone) levels will be high and will raise the blood/CGM glucose values. Motivation for optimal diabetes care is also often then reduced. Finally, exercise (Chapter 13) is important both for "burning" extra sugar and for making people more sensitive to insulin. Reduced insulin sensitivity is a major factor in type 2 diabetes, so that exercise is essential. Thus, all four of these factors must be in balance to result in the best diabetes management.

The Helmsley Foundation-sponsored T1D Exchange identified six factors that contributed to lower HbA1c levels in children with type 1 diabetes. We added two others at the end of the list. Chapters where these are discussed are shown in parentheses.

- Use of an insulin pump (Chapter 28)
- Doing five or more blood sugars per day (Chapter 7)
- Not missing meal and snack boluses/shots (Chapter 17)
- Using pre-meal timing of insulin boluses/shots (Chapter 8)
- Using higher insulin doses for boluses/shots (Chapter 22)
- Using an I/C ratio (Chapter 12)
- Use of a continuous glucose monitor (CGM, Chapter 29)
- Use of a hybrid artificial pancreas (Chapter 30)

For patients with type 2 diabetes, optimal management also results from a combination of exercise, diet, oral medications (or insulin) and motivation (Figure 1). Little weight will be lost if total food and fat intake are not reduced and an exercise program initiated. If oral medicines (or insulin) are missed, blood/CGM glucose levels will remain high. If the person does not have realistic goals that include motivation, they will not succeed. All must be in balance for optimal diabetes management. The regular monitoring of blood sugar values (Chapter 7) and of HbA1c levels (Chapter 14) is essential to understand the effects of these four influences.

SIGNS AND SYMPTOMS OF HIGH SUGAR LEVELS

It is not always easy to decide whether a person has optimal diabetes management. *Some things that help to reflect management are the following:*

Symptoms of Diabetes

A person who goes to the bathroom very frequently (including getting up two or more times per night), or who is often thirsty, likely has symptoms of high blood and urine sugar. This person usually needs more insulin (or oral medicines), less sugar in the diet and/or more daily exercise.

Occasionally, blurred vision may occur as a symptom of high sugar levels. High sugar levels in the lens of the eye pull water into the lens. This extra fluid makes it difficult for the shape of the lens to change in order to focus for clear vision. The blurred vision usually stops when blood sugar levels improve. After the initial diagnosis, or a period of high blood sugars, people should not be fitted for glasses until blood/CGM glucose levels are stable. If the blurred vision does not improve when blood sugar levels improve, the eye doctor should be contacted.

People with diabetes may have numbness, tingling or pain in the feet. This is due to neuropathy (see Chapter 23), which is related to high sugar levels. The sugar and its by-products can collect in the nerves over a period of years. These complaints may be present at the time of diagnosis for people with type 2 diabetes.

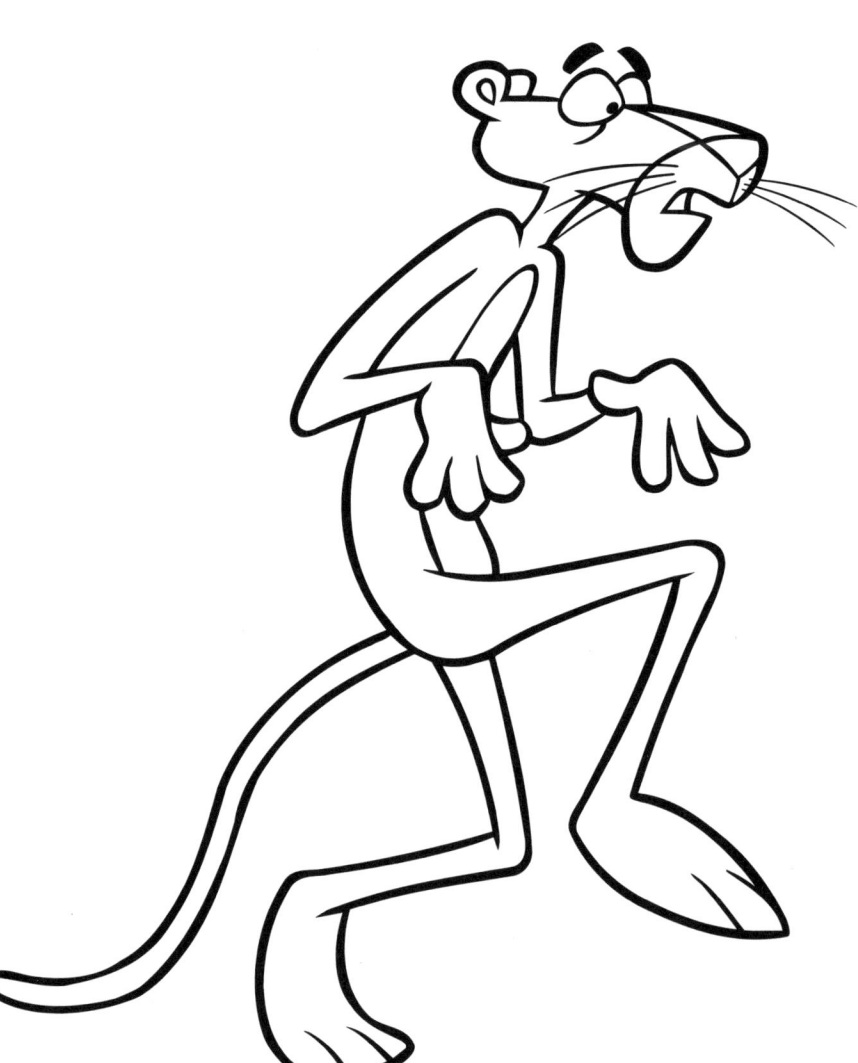

Oral thrush (a yeast infection) may be noticed as a "fuzzy white layer" on the tongue. Vaginal yeast infections are more common in females with diabetes, particularly if the blood/CGM glucose levels have been high. This may be because yeast grows well in a high-sugar environment. When antibiotics are taken for bacterial infections, yeast also tends to grow as the bacteria disappear. If vaginal itching or burning is noticed, the primary care-provider should be contacted.

Physical and Emotional Growth

Children and adolescents who have high blood/CGM glucose levels sometimes have reduced gains in height or weight. One study showed an average growth rate of two inches per year during the adolescent growth spurt when the HbA1c averaged 12.4 percent (112 mmol/mol), but a gain of 3.3 inches per year when the HbA1c averaged 8.4 percent (68 mmol/mol). Research reported from our Clinic showed final adult height was more likely to be taller if HbA1c values were lower during adolescence. Following the height and weight every three months is an important part of the diabetes clinic visit.

Some people just don't feel well when they have high blood/CGM glucose levels. They may be constantly tired, have a poor temper or have any of a variety of symptoms. When improved sugar levels are achieved, they are often surprised to realize how much better they feel. Feeling tired and poorly over a long time does not allow for normal emotional growth.

Sugar levels that do not produce such obvious symptoms may still be too high and result in long-term problems (Chapter 23).

BLOOD/CGM GLUCOSE (SUGAR) MEASUREMENTS

Measuring blood/CGM glucose levels is the best way to monitor diabetes on a day-to-day basis and is discussed in detail in **Chapter 7**. All families with someone with diabetes must have a meter in the home for measuring blood glucose levels. In addition, CGM use is gradually increasing and can be very helpful. Studies have shown that checking blood sugars five to seven times daily (or use of a CGM) and using the results is an important part of diabetes management. The optimal blood/CGM glucose levels vary with the person's age and are given in Chapter 7. Four additional measurements most readily available to CGM users are:

Time in Range: The aim is to have blood/CGM sugar levels in the desired range for age at least 70 percent of the time (Figure 3). With new technology (especially using a CGM or a partial, or hybrid, pancreas), this has been most feasible during the night.

TABLE 1:
Approximate HbA1c and Blood Glucose Correlations

HbA1c %	(mmol/mol)	Blood Glucose (Sugar) Level Mg/dL	mmol/L
12	(108)	345	19.2
11	(97)	310	17.2
10	(86)	275	15.3
9	(75)	240	13.3
8	(64)	205	11.3
7	(53)	170	9.5
6	(42)	135	7.5

This graph shows the approximate relation between average blood sugar levels and the HbA1c. (The HbA1c does not truly reflect "average" blood sugar, as sugar goes onto the molecule when the blood sugar is high but does not come off when the blood sugar is low.)

Taken in part from a production of Partnership to Advance Care and Education (PACE).

FIGURE 3

Time-In-Range has been shown to correlate with HbA1c values (see graph below)

WHAT IS MY TIME-IN-RANGE?

Glucose targets for Type 1 Diabetes are moving away from A1c and toward how much time is spent between 70-180 mg/dL.

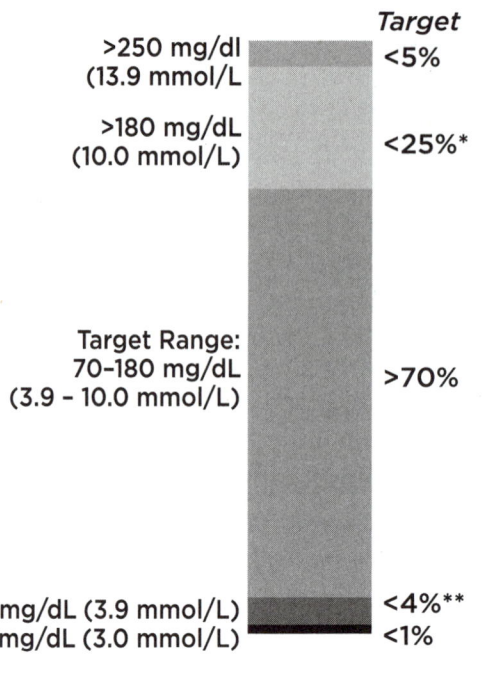

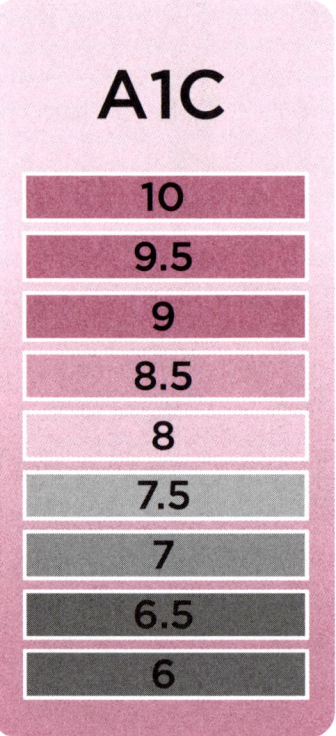

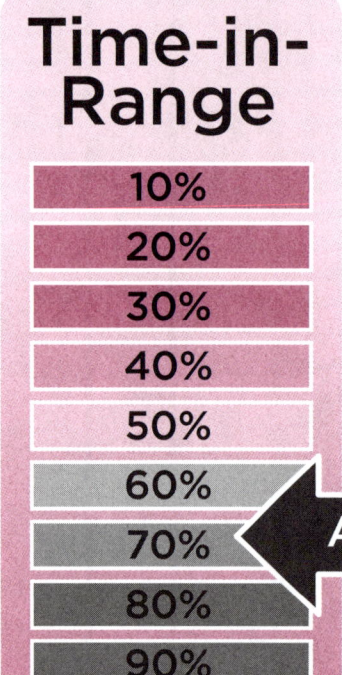

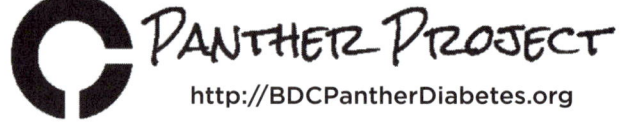

This is called Time-In-Range and is calculated from CGM or fingerstick BGs (if >4 per day).

Time in Range gives a better picture of how often you have high and low glucose levels.

Diabetes Care 2019 Jun;dci190028

PANTHER PROJECT
http://BDCPantherDiabetes.org

Time Below Range: Time spent below 70 mg/dL (3.9 mmol/L) should be less than one hour a day (under four percent of time) as monitored by a CGM (Figure 3). Time below 54 mg/dL (3.0 mmol/L) should be less than 15 minutes (<1 percent of time).

Time Above Range: Time spent at or above 180 mg/dL (10.0 mmol/L) should be less than six hours a day (25 percent of time), and above 250 mg/dL (13.9 mmol/L) less than 1 hour and 15 minutes (5 percent of time) per day, as measured by a CGM (Figure 3).

Blood/CGM Sugar Levels After Meals: Checking blood/CGM sugar levels after meals is important for optimal glucose management. Chapter 8 describes when to inject the pre-meal insulin bolus to help achieve desired values. The American Diabetes Association (ADA) recommends that blood/CGM glucose values be below 180 mg/dL (10.0 mmol/L) at any time after a meal. Some people aim for all two-hour values to be below 140 mg/dL (7.8 mmol/L). It is useful to think of half of the HbA1c value being related to fasting blood/CGM glucose values and the other half related to blood/CGM levels after meals.

MONITORING DIABETES

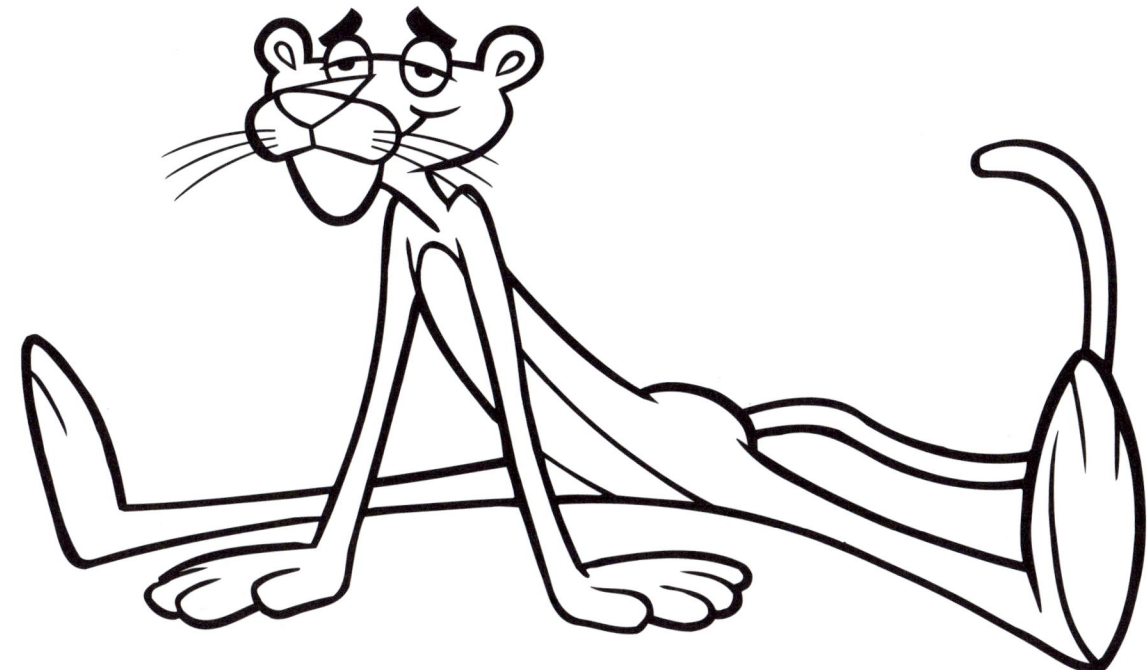

It is important not to be unhappy with blood/CGM glucose results, but instead to always be pleased that the information is available. **We do not use the words "good" and "bad" in this book to describe results. Hopefully, all results will be used as information to help attain better diabetes management.** Blood/CGM glucose monitoring is discussed in detail in Chapter 7.

HEMOGLOBIN A1c (HbA1c)

THE HbA1c VALUE IS A VALUABLE WAY TO MONITOR LONG-TERM BLOOD/CGM GLUCOSE LEVELS. Hemoglobin is the protein in the red blood cells that carries oxygen to the various parts of the body. It was found that the hemoglobin molecule has a secondary property that could be used to monitor sugar levels. If the blood sugar is high, sugar attaches to the hemoglobin (Figure 2) and remains there for the life of the red blood cell (approximately three months). The sugar doesn't come off if a low blood sugar occurs. For the purposes of this book, we will call hemoglobin with sugar attached hemoglobin A1c or HbA1c. The HbA1c reflects how often the blood sugars have been high for every second of the past three months (for the past 7,776,000 seconds). No one could do that many blood sugars. Approximately half of the HbA1c value reflects sugar levels for the past month, whereas the other half reflects sugar levels during the second and third months prior to the value being obtained. **The HbA1c represents the forest while the daily blood/CGM glucose values reflect the trees.** The HbA1c value has been used routinely since the late 1970s and has been called the "answer to a prayer" for people with diabetes and their doctors. Previously there was no way to monitor long-term sugar levels. No one really knew if they were in optimal diabetes management. The HbA1c helped solve that problem.

The HbA1c level can be done at the time of the clinic visit, and the person does not have to be fasting. THE RESULT IS NOT ALTERED BY ANYTHING THE PERSON DOES ON THE DAY IT IS DRAWN. In contrast, the blood sugar level can be affected by eating, exercise habits, emotions, etc. The main disadvantage of the HbA1c is that an illness may make the level go up quickly (by as much as one to two points). After the illness, the HbA1c value comes down much more slowly. Table 1 shows an approximate relation between the HbA1c level and the average blood/CGM glucose level over the past three months.

MONITORING DIABETES

Most diabetes clinics now use a micro-method for doing the HbA1c, so it can be done on a finger-stick and not require a venous blood draw. It is also important to be able to get the result back in a few minutes, so the health team can discuss the result and future goals with the person/family. The DirecNet research group showed that the DCA 2000 instrument, which fulfills all of these goals, was also very accurate. Other clinics have patients go to the lab in advance to have the result available at the time of the clinic visit.

The ADA (American Diabetes Association) recommendations for HbA1c levels for children in the U.S. changed in 2014. **The goal for children of all ages was changed to now aim for levels below 7.5% (<58 mmol/L).** With improvements in management, such as basal and rapid-acting/short-lasting insulins, insulin pumps and continuous glucose monitors (CGMs), it was deemed safe to lower goals for young children. In addition, data from Austria and Germany (where 75 percent of preschoolers with diabetes use insulin pumps) suggested that the lower HbA1c goal resulted in lower HbA1c values without increasing the number of episodes of severe hypoglycemia. Having a higher HbA1c (in the U.S.) was not associated with fewer episodes of severe hypoglycemia. Preschoolers in the U.S., with higher mean HbA1c levels than in Austria/Germany, had a higher incidence of diabetic ketoacidosis (DKA; Chapter 15). It is hoped that aiming for lower HbA1c levels in the U.S. will decrease episodes of DKA. **The ADA recommends that the HbA1c goal for adults ≥ age 18 years be below 7.0% (53 mmol/mol).**

The ADA Standards of Care (see Chapter 21) recommends that the HbA1c be done every three months for a person with diabetes. IT IS THE ONLY WAY TO KNOW HOW A PERSON WITH DIABETES IS DOING EVERY SECOND OF THE DAY. **It is currently estimated that for every percentage point reduction in HbA1c levels, there is a 35 percent reduction in the likelihood of eye, kidney and nerve damage (Chapter 23). It is thus very important in relation to diabetes complications. The ADA desired ranges are achievable, and families should continue to strive to reach these goals.**

GLUCOSE VARIABILITY

There is now evidence that excessive glucose variability (sugar levels bouncing up and down) relates to some diabetes complications (particularly cardiovascular). This has only been possible to measure in recent years as people began to use continuous glucose monitors (CGMs). The use of CGMs is discussed in Chapter 29.

The use of the CGM trend graphs, which can easily be seen on the receiver/pump screen, give an indication of frequent swings up and down of sugar levels. The standard deviation (SD) is a measurement of glucose variability and is obtained with the retrospective download of the CGM. Recommended values are discussed in Chapter 17 of the Pump and CGM book (ordering information in the back).

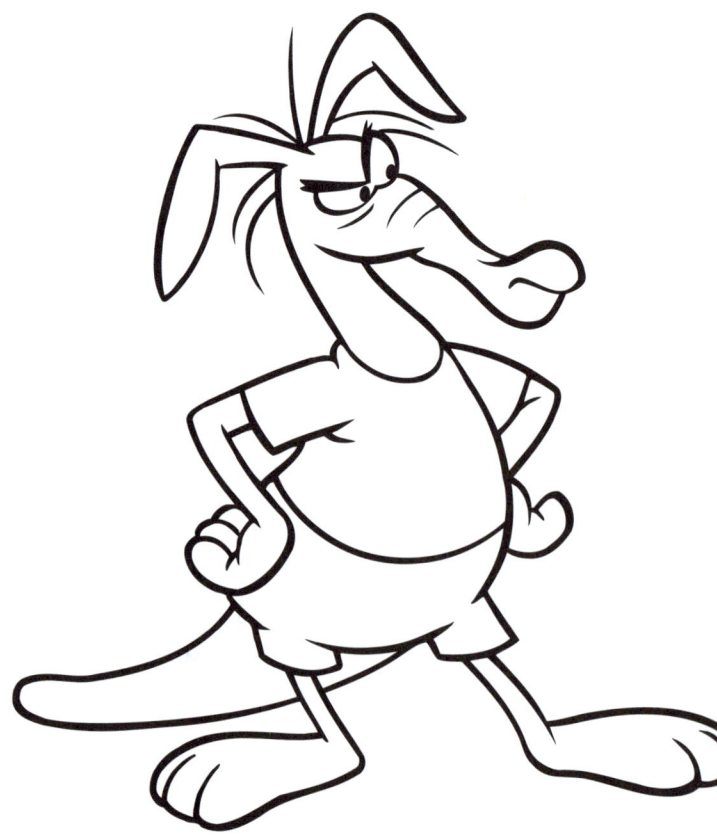

DEFINITIONS

ADA: American Diabetes Association

Bacteria: Microscopic (only able to be seen with a microscope) agents that cause infections such as "strep throat."

DCCT: The Diabetes Control and Complications Trial. A very large research trial, which showed that lower HbA1c levels reduced the likelihood of eye, kidney and nerve problems in people over age 13 years with type 1 diabetes.

Emotions: How one feels psychologically (e.g., happy, sad).

Hemoglobin A1c (HbA1c): Hemoglobin protein in the red blood cells with sugar attached to it. This is used as a measure of sugar levels over the previous three months.

Lens: The structure in the front of the eye that changes to allow the eye to focus on near or distant objects (see picture in Chapter 23).

Symptoms: The complaints of a person; how they are feeling.

Yeast: A fungus that grows more readily when blood sugar levels are high and can cause an infection.

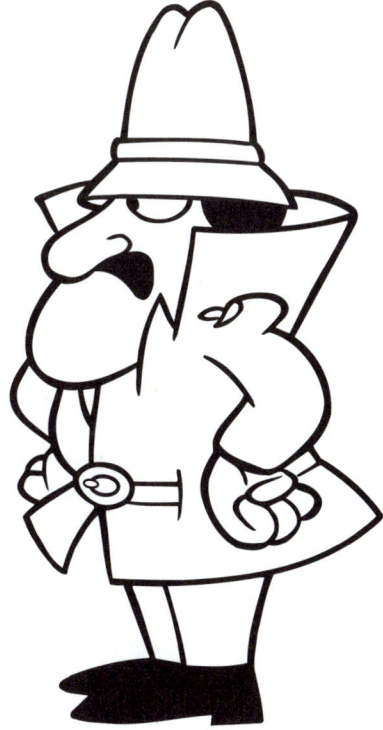

QUESTIONS AND ANSWERS FROM NEWSNOTES

Q Does the hemoglobin A1c really give the average blood/CGM glucose value over the past three months?

A No. It reflects how often the blood sugars have been high over the past three months. When the blood sugar is high, the sugar attaches to body proteins, including the red blood cell hemoglobin, and then stays attached to the hemoglobin (as HbA1c) until the red blood cell is replaced 2-3 months later. To represent the "average blood sugar," the sugar molecule would also have to detach from the protein when the blood sugar is low. This does not happen. Thus, the value only reflects how often the blood sugar has been high. The HbA1c should be measured every three months on all people with diabetes. The data in Table 1 gives an example of how average blood glucose levels over the past three months are related to HbA1c. Remember that there can be some variation in this relationship in each person.

Q Changes in our daughter's insulin dose have confused my wife and me. Initially she was on a low insulin dose, which you increased after reviewing her blood sugars and seeing that her HbA1c was high. Her HbA1c level came down, and now her insulin dose is coming back down again. This doesn't make sense to us.

A This is quite common. For someone whose liver is making sugar at a very high rate, it takes very little (stress, infection, etc.) to make even more sugar and it may take a lot of insulin to get the liver's sugar production machinery turned off. This may also be the case for a newly-diagnosed person.

However, once the liver's pathways for making sugar are turned off, it may not take as much insulin to keep them turned off. This may be part of the reason for the "honeymoon" period in the newly diagnosed person. Also, once sugar production is reduced, stress and infections will not have as great an effect.

TABLE 1: The Two Emergencies of Diabetes

	Low Blood Sugar (Chapter 6) (Hypoglycemia or Insulin Reaction)		**Ketoacidosis** (Chapter 15) (Acidosis or DKA)	
Due to:	Low blood sugar		Presence of ketones	
Speed of onset:	Fast – within minutes		Slow – in hours or days	
Causes:	Too little food Too little insulin Too much exercise without food Missing or being late for meals/snacks Excitement in young children		Too little insulin Not giving insulin Infections/Illness Traumatic body stress Pump insertions malfunctioning	
Blood sugar:	Low (below 60 mg/dL or 3.3 mmol/L)		Usually high (over 240 mg/dL or 13.3 mmol/L)	
Ketones:	Usually none in the urine or blood		Usually moderate/large in the urine or blood ketones over 0.6 mmol/L	
	SYMPTOMS	**TREATMENT**	**SYMPTOMS**	**TREATMENT**
Mild:	Hunger, shaky, sweaty, nervous	Give juice or milk. Wait 10 minutes and then give solid food.	Thirst, frequent urination, sweet breath, small or moderate urine ketones or blood ketones less than 1.0 mmol/L.	Give lots of fluids and Humalog/NovoLog/Apidra or Regular insulin every two or three hours.
Moderate:	Headache, unexpected behavior changes, impaired or double vision, confusion, drowsiness, weakness or difficulty talking.	Give instant glucose or a fast-acting sugar, juice or sugar pop (4 oz.). After 10 minutes, give solid food.	Dry mouth, nausea, stomach cramps, vomiting, moderate or large urine ketones or blood ketones between 1.0 and 3.0 mmol/L.	Continued contact with healthcare provider. Give lots of fluids. Give Humalog/NovoLog/Apidra or Regular insulin every two to three hours. Give Zofran (a tablet) or Phenergan medication (suppository or topical cream) if vomiting occurs.*
Severe:	Loss of consciousness or seizures.	Give glucagon into muscle or fat. Check blood sugar. Intranasal glucagon (Baqsimi) is an acceptable alternative	Labored deep breathing, extreme weakness, confusion and eventually unconsciousness (coma), large urine ketones or blood ketones above 3.0 mmol/L.	If no response, call paramedic (911) or go to E.R. May need intravenous fluids and insulin.

*Note: If these medications are given, a helper must assist to make sure blood sugar and ketones are checked frequently, as the patient will be sleepy.

CHAPTER 15

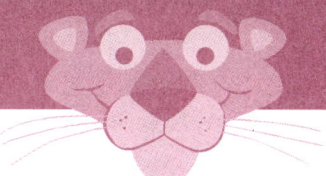

Ketones and Diabetic Ketoacidosis (DKA)

DIABETIC KETOACIDOSIS (DKA)

The two most common emergencies in diabetes are severe low blood sugars (hypoglycemia, discussed in Chapter 6) and diabetic ketoacidosis (DKA, or acidosis). When ketones build up in the blood, a person can develop DKA (Figure 1). Acidosis is most common with type 1 diabetes, but it can also occur with type 2 diabetes. Severe hypoglycemia is more common than DKA, although episodes of DKA are more dangerous. Table 1 may be helpful in differentiating hypoglycemia versus DKA. The measurement of urine or blood ketones is very easy and is discussed in Chapter 5.

When people with known diabetes are referred to our Center, the most common knowledge deficits are:

- ✔ not understanding the dangers of ketone build-up
- ✔ not knowing when to measure ketones
- ✔ not having the supplies in their home or on trips to measure for ketones
- ✔ not knowing what to do when ketones are present

Because DKA is not a common event, families may not remember their initial training and need regular review of this information at follow-up clinic visits. Having the tools to recognize and treat ketones helps to avoid a serious and potentially life-threatening episode of DKA.

> **TOPICS:**
> **Avoid, Detect and Treat Acute Complications (Ketones and Acidosis)**
>
> **TEACHING OBJECTIVES:**
> The teacher will:
> 1. Describe causes of ketone production.
> 2. Present signs and symptoms of having ketones.
> 3. Discuss treatment plan for detecting and eliminating ketones.
>
> **LEARNING OBJECTIVES:**
> Learner (parents, child, relative or self) will be able to:
> 1. List two causes of ketones.
> 2. Describe two symptoms of having ketones.
> 3. Explain two methods to help avoid ketones.

WHY IS IT IMPORTANT TO AVOID DEVELOPING DKA?

Acidosis is the cause of 85 percent of hospitalizations of children with known diabetes. It is a very dangerous condition and can cause brain injury or coma, complications of severe dehydration, or in rare cases death. The good news is that DKA can usually be avoided if people follow the instructions in this chapter. "Large" urine or elevated blood ketones are usually present for at least four hours before a person develops DKA. Early recognition and treatment can help to avoid more severe illness. It is essential for families to read thoroughly the section later in this chapter on Reducing the Likelihood of Acidosis.

FIGURE 1

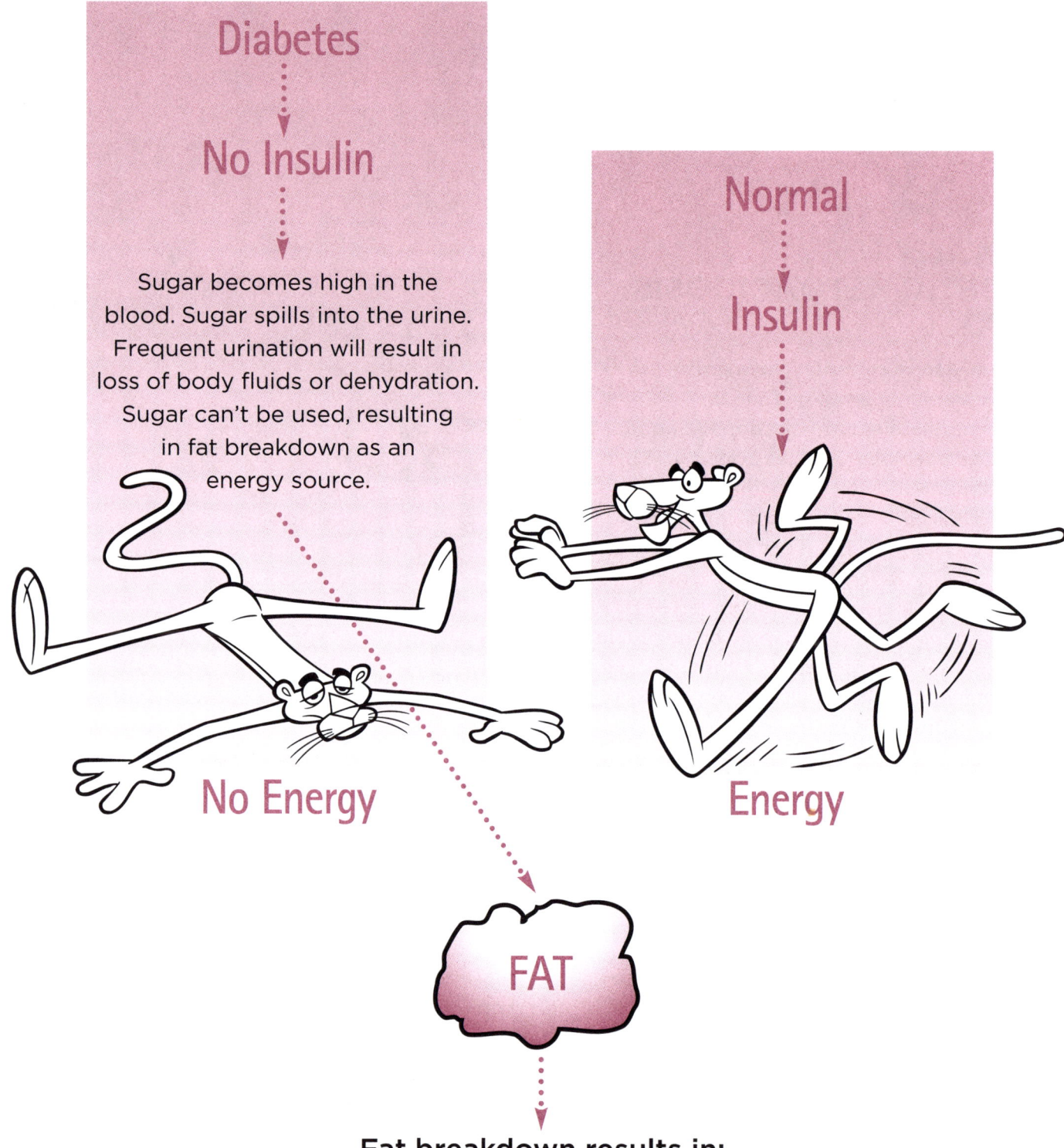

Fat breakdown results in:

1. Weight loss

2. Ketones, which are a breakdown product of fat, appear in the blood and urine

3. Too many ketones in the body ➝ DKA

CAUSES OF DKA:

Acidosis (DKA) occurs because not enough insulin is available. Three (of the many) functions of insulin are to:

1. allow sugar from food to pass from the blood into the cells to use for energy, or to store in the liver
2. stop breakdown of fat, and of liver glycogen (stored sugar), to use for energy
3. turn off the body's machinery for breaking down fat to make ketones

Ketones are normally produced when the body is in a starvation state. When there is little or no insulin, the body responds as if it is starving, and the above three functions do not occur. Instead of storing energy, the body begins to break down fats for energy, and as a result, produces ketones. Ketones (and acidosis) are not caused by high blood/CGM glucose levels; ketones are caused because **there is not enough insulin.**

Ketones are acids. In small amounts, they do not cause problems. However, if the body produces more and more ketones, the blood becomes more acid, leading to development of acidosis.

Ketones may start with trace or small levels in the blood and urine and gradually build up to moderate and large levels. Once ketones reach the large level, they may start to build up in the body tissues. The longer someone has large ketones, the more likely they will build up in the body, resulting in acidosis. Ketones are easier to reverse if treated early. High ketones require a lot of insulin to turn off the machinery for making ketones. Thus, the early detection and reversal by giving extra insulin is critical.

The three main causes for excess ketones are summarized in Table 2 and below.

TABLE 2:
Main Causes of Acidosis

1. Not enough insulin given:
- Missed insulin injections
- Needing increased doses
- Giving spoiled insulin
- A pump insertion coming out or not functioning (Chapter 28)

2. More insulin needed:
- Illnesses/Infections
- Traumatic stresses on the body (particularly type 2 diabetes)

3. Very low carbohydrate intake or excess sugar lost:
- Vomiting illnesses with prolonged fast
- Very low carbohydrate (ketogenic) diet
- A medicine (e.g., SGLT inhibitor) masking hyperglycemia

---

1. **Not getting required insulin:**

   - *Forgetting to take an insulin shot (bolus) or, for people with type 2 diabetes, insulin or oral medicine.*

   - *Needing increased doses.* This could happen in a person coming out of the "honeymoon" period who has not had insulin dosages increased, or in a child who has grown or had hormone changes that result in increased insulin needs.

   - *Giving "spoiled" insulin, usually from the insulin getting too hot (over 90°F, 32° C) or freezing.*

   - *A pump insertion coming out or not functioning (Chapter 28):* As pumps use only rapid-acting insulins, ketones start to be made 3-4 hours after an insertion malfunctions. Sometimes when changing a pump site or because of activity, the canula (tubing) gets a kink or bend. Even though the site may look fine from the outside, insulin will not be delivered correctly.

2. **Needing more insulin than usual:**
   - *Illnesses/infections:* During illness, hormones and immune responses can make the body insulin resistant. This means more insulin than usual is needed for the body to use energy.
   - *Traumatic stresses on the body (particularly with type 2 diabetes):* People with type 2 diabetes sometimes get ketones during an illness. However, other body stressors such as surgery or a heart attack may also result in ketone production. This can make the body insulin resistant and can lead to even more ketone production.
3. **Very low carbohydrate intake or excess sugar loss:** If the body does not get enough carbohydrates from the diet, the body will break down fat, resulting in ketones. Some medicines (e.g., SGLT inhibitors) may cause excessive urine sugar output. In these situations, ketones can be present without significant elevation in blood/CGM glucose levels.
   - *Illnesses which cause vomiting:* During vomiting illness, a person may eat very little. Over an extended time, this can lead to ketone production.
   - *Very low carbohydrate (also known as "ketogenic") diets:* People who avoid carbohydrates for an extended time cause the body to break down fats to make energy and ketones. In people with diabetes, ketone production can more easily lead to ketoacidosis.

SYMPTOMS OF ACIDOSIS (DKA)

In any of the above cases, fat is broken down. Ketones are made from the fat. *Acidosis usually comes on slowly, over several hours, and has the following symptoms:*

- ✔ upset stomach and/or stomach pain
- ✔ muscle aches or cramps
- ✔ nausea and vomiting (if it persists, may need to go to emergency room)
- ✔ sweet (fruity) odor to the breath
- ✔ drowsiness or confusion
- ✔ deep, rapid breathing (indicates need to go to emergency room)
- ✔ if not treated, coma (loss of consciousness)

Because blood/CGM glucose levels are frequently high in DKA, symptoms also can include:

- ✔ thirst and frequent urination
- ✔ dry mouth from dehydration
- ✔ blurry vision

The blood/CGM glucose levels are usually high with large ketones and acidosis because not enough insulin is available. The high blood sugar causes sugar to pass into the urine (see Chapter 2), and the person must go to the bathroom a lot (**frequent urination**). The body may lose too much water and become too dry (**dehydration**). The tongue may feel dry and furry. Drinking lots of fluids may help prevent this. The main treatment, however, is taking extra insulin to shut off the body's machinery for making sugar and ketones.

On occasion, it may be difficult to know whether a person is having difficulty with low blood sugar or with acidosis. Measuring the blood sugar and ketones will help identify the correct problem. Table 1 may also be helpful in thinking about the two problems.

REDUCING THE LIKELIHOOD OF ACIDOSIS

Acidosis is the cause of 85 percent of admissions to the hospital for someone with known diabetes. Most of these admissions could be avoided if the problem were identified and treated earlier. The simple instructions outlined in Table 3 will help avoid most cases of acidosis. **It is a good idea to review this chapter at least once a year, especially during cold and flu season.** Families may forget the importance of checking urine or blood ketones during any illness. Some people with diabetes who still make some of their own insulin, or who are in optimal diabetes management, will have the "machinery" (enzymes) for making the ketones be "turned off." As a result, they may go several years and never have urine or blood ketones with an illness. As they grow older and a few more islet cells are lost, or they outgrow their remaining islets, they may suddenly find ketones develop more easily.

The important message is ALWAYS to remember to check for ketones anytime a person with diabetes is ill. You must also check for ketones anytime the blood/CGM glucose level is above 240 mg/dL (>13.3 mmol/L) fasting or above 300 mg/dL (>16.7 mmol/L) on two occasions (approximately 1 hour apart) during the day.

The avoidance of DKA is based on being able to detect changes early. Knowing when ketones are increasing in the urine or blood, but before the ketones build up to high levels in the body, is important.

Reducing the likelihood of DKA – the person with diabetes or the family:

✔ must have a method in the home to check urine or blood ketones (see Chapter 5)

✔ must remember to check for urine or blood ketones anytime the person is sick (even with vomiting only one time and even if other family members are sick too)

TABLE 3: Helping to Avoid Ketoacidosis
Check urine or blood ketones with any illness (even an upset stomach or vomiting one time) or anytime the blood sugar is above 300 mg/dL (16.7 mmol/L) for more than an hour.
Call the diabetes care-provider immediately (night or day) if moderate or large urine ketones or blood ketones above 1.0 mmol/L are found.
Take extra insulin (after checking the blood sugar and urine or blood ketones). Take Humalog/NovoLog/Apidra every two hours, or Regular insulin every three hours, until the urine ketones are small or less or the blood ketones are below 0.6 mmol/L.
If the blood sugar falls below 150 mg/dL (8.3 mmol/L) and urine or blood ketones are still present, drink juice (preferably orange as it replaces potassium, although apple juice is suitable), Pedialyte® or sips of sugary soda pop to keep the blood sugar up, so that more insulin can be given to turn off the ketone production.
Drink lots of fluids to help wash out the ketones.

✔ needs to check ketones if the blood/CGM glucose level is high (e.g., above 300 mg/dL [16.7 mmol/L] twice, at least 1 hour apart

✔ must check for ketones with a pump infusion set failure

✔ should call the diabetes care-provider immediately (see Table 1, Chapter 16) if moderate or large urine ketones or blood ketones >1.0 mmol/L are present

✔ needs to give extra rapid-acting insulin (Humalog/NovoLog/Apidra) every two hours, or Regular insulin every three hours, until the urine or blood ketones have decreased (give by shot if using an insulin pump [in case tubing is kinked]; see Chapter 28).

✓ must drink lots of fluids to wash the ketones out of the body and to prevent dehydration

A low blood sugar can sometimes be present with acidosis, so urine ketones must be checked with every illness, even if the blood/CGM glucose level is not elevated. A summary of instructions to help avoid DKA is in Table 3.

TREATMENT OF ELEVATED KETONES

Extra Insulin (Table 4)

When ketone production becomes total body acidosis, it is usually because the large amount of ketones has been present for four to 12 hours. This can happen because the urine or blood ketones have not been checked or no extra insulin has been given. Insulin shuts off ketone production. Extra insulin must be given if someone has moderate or large urine ketones or blood ketones above 0.6 mmol/L. The dose of extra insulin varies for different people, and the diabetes care-provider can help decide on a safe dose. The insulin dose must be given by a shot if using an insulin pump (not a pump bolus).

General Guidelines When Giving Extra Insulin

The blood/CGM glucose level should always be checked before each insulin injection.

For **moderate** urine ketones or blood ketones between 0.6 and 1.5 mmol/L, the extra dose is usually in the range of 5-10 percent of the total daily dose (see Table 4). Others use the correction insulin dose for the blood sugar at the time. The extra dose is given as Humalog/NovoLog/Apidra every two hours or Regular insulin every three hours.

For **large** urine ketones or blood ketones above 1.5 mmol/L, if possible, the diabetes care-

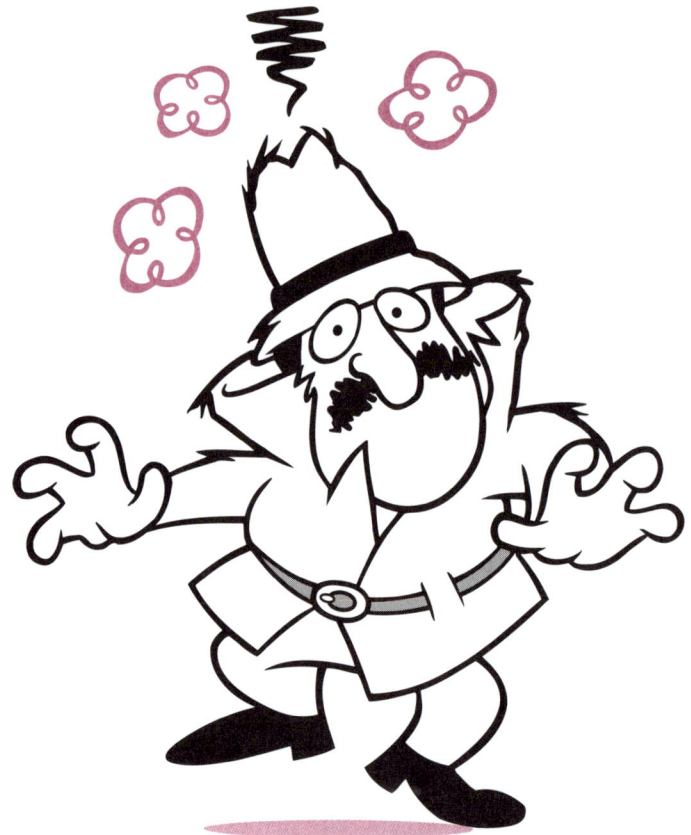

provider should be contacted to help choose the insulin dose. If not possible, the dose of extra insulin is usually 10-20 percent of the total daily dose. Others use an insulin dose which is double the correction factor for the blood sugar level. This extra insulin is given as Humalog/NovoLog/Apidra every two hours or Regular insulin every three hours.

The extra insulin may seem like a large dose, but ketones block the normal sensitivity of the body to insulin. Although every person is different, dosages in these ranges are usually needed.

It is important to keep giving extra insulin until the ketones are cleared (less than 0.6 mmol/L in the blood or trace/small on urine test strips). Sometimes this may require giving additional carbohydrates in order to keep the blood glucose from going low with the additional insulin.

If the blood/CGM glucose level drops below 150 mg/dL (8.3 mmol/L):

TABLE 4: Ketone Levels* in Blood or Urine and a Suggested Dose of Rapid-Acting or Regular Insulin

Urine	Blood (mmol/L)	Dose of H/NL/AP every 2 hours or Dose of Regular every 3 hours
Trace/Small	≤1.0	Give "correction" factor for blood sugar
Moderate – Large	1.1 – 1.5	Give "correction" factor plus 10 percent of total daily insulin dose**
Large	>1.5	Give "correction" factor plus 20 percent of total daily insulin dose**
Very Large	>3.0	May need to go to emergency room if blood ketones above 3.0 mmol/L or persistent vomiting

* The blood and urine ketone results do not always agree exactly and the above correlations are estimates. The blood ketone result reflects the ketone level at the exact time the test is done. If the urine has been in the bladder for some time, then the urine ketone result may not tell the current status.

** Calculate the total daily insulin dose by adding up all insulin taken in a 24-hour period (rapid-acting plus intermediate-acting plus long-acting) or by looking at insulin pump history for total daily dose over previous week.

- It may be necessary to sip juice or another sugary drink. This is done to bring the blood sugar back up before giving the next insulin injection.
- Remember, the extra insulin and fluids are being given to clear the urine or blood ketones.

Extra Fluids

In addition to taking extra insulin, drinking fluids (e.g., water and fruit juices) is important in the avoidance of acidosis. These liquids replace the fluid lost in the urine and help prevent dehydration. They also help to wash the ketones out of the body. The juices also replace some of the salts that are lost in the urine. Orange juice and bananas are particularly suitable for replacing the potassium that is lost. As discussed in the next chapter, Sick Day Management (Chapter 16), medications (Zofran or Phenergan) are used by some providers if vomiting is a problem. The main side effect of Zofran is headaches. Sleepiness may also be a problem, and another person must help to make sure repeat checks are done every two hours.

A person who is experiencing ketoacidosis should not be left alone in case his or her condition worsens. If acidosis is being treated at home for more than four hours without improvement or if condition worsens, you should call the diabetes care-provider immediately (night or day) or go to the hospital for evaluation. When severe acidosis has been present for many hours, coma (loss of consciousness) can follow. This is dangerous. It is much better to avoid severe acidosis than to have to treat it with IV fluids and a hospital admission. Intravenous lines are usually put in both arms (and sometimes the feet). A constant heart-monitoring machine is attached to the person. The hospital admission is usually in an intensive care unit, which is scary for everyone.

Avoiding acidosis is generally possible when the directions in Table 3 are followed. When it does occur, it is usually because these directions were not followed.

DEFINITIONS

Acetone: One of the main ketones that build up in the urine, blood and body during acidosis. It is sometimes used (incorrectly) to refer to all ketones.

Acidosis (diabetic ketoacidosis or DKA): This occurs when there are too many acids in the blood. For people with diabetes, acidosis can happen when not enough insulin is available and ketones (which are acids) are produced. Blood/CGM glucose levels are usually high at this time. Moderate or large ketones are present in the urine or blood and then build up in the body. The ketones make the body fluids more acidic, resulting in total body acidosis.

Beta hydroxybutyrate (ß-OH butyrate): The most important of the three main ketones (along with acetone and acetoacetic acid). It is the ketone that is measured by the blood ketone meter.

Dehydration: Loss of the body fluids. The tongue and skin are usually very dry, and the eyes look sunken. Babies have less than half the usual number of wet diapers.

Ketoacidosis: See Acidosis (diabetic ketoacidosis or DKA) above.

Ketones: Fat breakdown products that initially spill into the urine and later build up in the blood when there is not enough insulin. The main ketones are beta hydroxybutyrate, acetone and acetoacetic acid. Many people can smell a sweet odor on the breath, similar to nail polish remover (acetone). The fat breakdown products cause acidosis (or ketoacidosis).

Potassium: One of the salts (along with sodium) lost in the urine when ketones are spilled in the urine. Orange juice and bananas contain a lot of potassium and are best to give if urine ketones are present.

QUESTIONS AND ANSWERS FROM NEWSNOTES

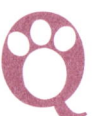**Will my child develop ketoacidosis and need to go to the hospital whenever he or she is ill?**

No, not necessarily. Most hospitalizations due to ketoacidosis can be avoided with family education and by following instructions for early intervention.

Sometimes during an illness the body needs extra energy, and it responds by breaking down fats into ketones. As the ketones build up following the fat breakdown, ketoacidosis eventually results. The most frequent symptoms are a stomachache and, eventually, vomiting. Deep breathing is a late sign and indicates a need to go to an emergency room.

Families can check for ketones at home with urine or blood. The bottles of urine strips expire six months after they have been opened. Checking for ketones should be done ANY TIME THE PERSON IS FEELING ILL. Also, check ketones if the blood/CGM glucose level is above 300 mg/dL (>16.7 mmol/L) for more than an hour. If moderate/large urine ketones are found or blood ketones are above 1.0 mmol/L, the healthcare-provider should be called immediately. Calling the healthcare-provider may be necessary every 2-3 hours for dosages of Humalog/NovoLog/Apidra or Regular insulin. After the ketones have decreased to small amounts or have gone away, the extra injections can be stopped.

On any given day, five to 10 children are being treated by telephone for elevated ketones by our staff. This happens especially during the flu season. Fortunately, hospital admissions have gone down dramatically as a result of early treatment and are now infrequent.

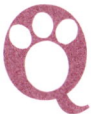 **Why does someone feel sick when the ketones are moderate or large in the urine or >0.6 mmol/L in the blood?**

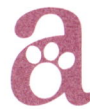 There are at least three parts to the answer to this question:

1. The body's acid-base (pH) balance is finely tuned (a bit on the basic side at 7.35-7.45). Acids and bases are difficult to explain. An example of a base is soap, and examples of acids are lemons and vinegar. Ketones (which are acids) make the body fluids more acidic as they start to build up. As the body becomes more acidic, many of the body's functions can no longer work as they should. If left untreated, death will eventually follow.

2. The second reason a person feels ill is because of a potassium and sodium imbalance. These are important body salts that are lost with ketones going out in the urine. Potassium is important for the movement of the intestine (moving food through). If too much potassium is lost, this movement decreases or stops. When this happens, an upset stomach and vomiting can occur. We often recommend orange juice (high in potassium) and apple juice in addition to water when someone has urine or blood ketones. Drinking lots of liquids helps to keep hydrated and to flush out the ketones.

3. Poor hydration is a third reason for feeling ill. Usually, high blood sugar happens together with ketones, resulting in frequent urination. This can lead to dehydration. Our bodies are 60 percent water. If even 10 percent of body weight is lost as water, it is possible to be very sick. Fluids can also be lost in large amounts with the flu (vomiting and diarrhea). If fluid is being lost in large amounts from both the kidneys (frequent urination) and from vomiting and/or diarrhea, dehydration can occur even more rapidly. Children under the age of five can become dehydrated in less than four hours. They are more likely to require IV fluid treatment sooner than older children.

KETONES AND DIABETIC KETOACIDOSIS (DKA)

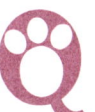 **What is cerebral edema and how does it relate to diabetic ketoacidosis (DKA)?**

Cerebral edema refers to swelling of the brain, which is a rare complication of DKA. The cause is not fully understood, and when it does occur, it can cause brain damage or be fatal.

Part of the reason it is so rare relates to the now relative infrequency of DKA. Our families are asked to check urine or blood ketones with every illness or high blood/CGM glucose level. If using a CGM, the alarm can be set to warn the person/family when the value is high. They are asked to call when urine ketones are moderate or large or the blood ketone level is >1.0 mmol/L. Extra shots of Humalog/NovoLog/Apidra or Regular insulin are then given to reverse the ketones before DKA occurs. Stopping ketone formation early reduces the likelihood of a case of DKA resulting in cerebral edema. It is better to avoid DKA than to deal with its bad effects. Unfortunately, cerebral edema is more common in newly diagnosed children when the ketones have built up over a longer time period.

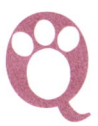 **Our son has had diabetes for over two years. Every time he has gotten sick we have checked for urine ketones. The results have always been negative or trace. Can we stop checking now?**

The answer is NO! This is often the case for someone who still makes some of their own insulin and/or someone who is in excellent sugar control. The machinery for making ketones from fat is so completely turned off that it doesn't get turned on by the illness. Unfortunately, as your son's insulin production declines or he outgrows his remaining insulin production, he will probably suddenly have ketones with an illness. One never knows when this will occur. Thus, the only answer is to keep checking the urine ketones at least twice each day with each illness.

TABLE 1:
Sick Day Guidelines

When calling a diabetes health provider please give:

1. Name and age of the person with diabetes about whom you are calling:
   _____

2. About how long the person has had diabetes: _____

3. Name of the diabetes doctor and when last seen: _____
   _____

4. Present problem: _____

5. Blood/CGM glucose results: _____

6. Urine or blood ketone results: _____

7. Injection of pump therapy: _____

8. Time and dose of last insulin given: _____

9. Any noticed weight loss: _____

10. Other types and dosage of medications usually given:
    _____
    _____

11. Phone number of the person calling: _____

12. Phone number of the pharmacy where prescriptions can be called:
    _____

This information can be photocopied and used on sick days.

CHAPTER 16

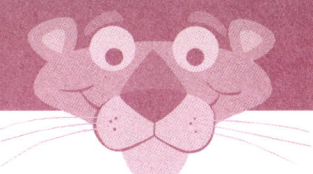

Sick Day and Surgery Management

SICK DAY MANAGEMENT

The purpose of this chapter is to discuss the essential steps to take when a person with diabetes becomes ill or undergoes surgery. In general, the person whose blood/CGM glucose values are mostly within target range can be just as healthy as anyone who does not have diabetes. When a person with diabetes does become ill, more attention and effort needs to be given to their diabetes management (otherwise there is a significant risk that the illness can become severe and require hospitalization). It is, therefore, extremely important for all persons with diabetes and their families to learn all there is to know about sick day and surgery management. We recommend that you review this information annually.

WHAT YOU NEED TO KNOW

When you get sick, the first thing you must do is to gather the information you need. This will help you decide if you need assistance from health professionals. They will always want to know this information. Key information about you and your illness can be filled into the form in Table 1 and then used to guide your conversation with your health care provider. (This form can be photocopied and used on sick days.) Table 2 has a list of important things to remember during illness and Table 3 will help you decide when to call for help or emergency care.

- **Present Problem:** Vomiting, diarrhea, fever, cold, congestion and cough, earache, sore throat, stomachache, labored breathing, chest pain or other concerning discomforts.

> **TOPICS:**
> **Prevention, Detection and Treatment of Acute Complications (with illness)**
>
> **TEACHING OBJECTIVES:**
> The teacher will:
> 1. Discuss the information needed when the person with diabetes becomes ill.
> 2. Distinguish treatment plans for small, moderate and large ketones.
> 3. Indicate the appropriate time to call a healthcare-provider for assistance with illness or planned surgery.
>
> **LEARNING OBJECTIVES:**
> Learner (parents, child, relative or self) will be able to:
> 1. List three areas of care that must receive special consideration when the person with diabetes is ill.
> 2. State treatment plans for small, moderate and large ketones.
> 3. Identify the appropriate time to call the healthcare-provider for assistance with illness or planned surgery.

If vomiting or diarrhea is present, note the number of times and when the episodes happen. It is also important to note if there have been any recent illnesses in other family members or close friends. This will help you decide if this is a similar illness.

- **Fever** does not generally occur with diabetes-related problems. Fever is usually a sign of an infection. However, infections can be present without a fever. It is helpful to take the temperature before calling the doctor to discuss an illness. If a fever is present, it may be important to call your primary care-provider. Sick people usually don't feel like doing much. If you are still active, it is usually a positive sign.

- **Blood/CGM Glucose Values:** As noted in Chapters 7 and 15, you must check even more blood sugars than usual on sick days. Parents, spouses, or friends should know how to accurately measure blood sugars (or observe CGM values) in case you are feeling too sick. **THE BLOOD SUGAR LEVEL MUST ALWAYS BE CHECKED BEFORE CALLING YOUR DIABETES CARE-PROVIDER.**

- **Ketones:** DON'T FORGET, URINE OR BLOOD KETONES MUST ALWAYS BE CHECKED PRIOR TO CALLING, **AND AT LEAST TWICE DAILY IF A PERSON DOESN'T FEEL WELL** (see Table 2). This is necessary even if the blood sugar is normal!

Ketones must always be checked if fasting blood/CGM glucose levels are >240 mg/dL (>13.3 mmol/L). During the day, blood/CGM glucose levels that are above 300 mg/dL (>16.7 mmol/L) two times in a row (about one hour apart) indicate a need to check ketones. **However, with an illness, ketones can be present even when the blood/CGM glucose level is lower.** Thus, be prepared to check ketones during an illness even though the blood/CGM glucose level is in range. This is also necessary if the person is on a medicine called an SGLT-2 inhibitor.

- As explained in Chapter 5, to check urine ketones, dip the beige end of the strip into a small amount of urine, shake off the excess urine, and time for **exactly 15 seconds**. Keep small paper cups in the bathroom to collect the urine sample. The urine can be left in the cup so that another person can confirm the results (and to make sure it was actually

TABLE 2:
Sick Day Plan

- Many illnesses can be managed at home, see Table 3 for list of signs and symptoms that should prompt emergency care.

- **Always check ketones with any illness. Even if the blood/CGM sugar is low, check for ketones at least twice daily every day you are sick. Call your healthcare-provider if urine ketones are moderate/large or blood ketones are above 1.0 mmol/L (see Chapters 5 and 15). Re-check every 2 hours until ketones are below these levels.**

- **It is particularly important to check ketones if you vomit even ONCE! Ketones can cause vomiting. If you vomit more than three times, call your diabetes care-provider.**

- **Always take some insulin. Never skip a dose entirely. Call your diabetes care-provider if you don't know how much to take.**

- **If using an insulin pump, if ketones are moderate or large, change pump site and give all corrections by injections until ketones are negative.**

- **If able to eat, drink water or sugar-free fluid; otherwise use fluids as in Table 4 according to blood/CGM glucose. DO NOT give extra insulin for the carbohydrates in the fluid. For sugary fluid examples, see Table 5.**

- **During illness, give 1 oz. of fluid per year of age per hour (example: for a 10-year-old, give 10 ounces per hour).**

> **TABLE 3:**
> # Sick Day Management: When to Call for Emergency Care
>
> - **If you have vomited more than three times and can keep nothing in your stomach,** and urine or blood ketones are not elevated, call your primary care physician. If help is needed with an insulin dose, call your diabetes care-provider.
>
> - **If moderate or large urine ketones or blood ketones (above 1.0 mmol/L) are present,** call your diabetes care-provider (see Table 1).
>
> - **If you have difficulty breathing or have rapid or deep breathing,** you need to go to an emergency room. This usually indicates severe acidosis (ketoacidosis; Chapter 15).
>
> - **If there is any unusual behavior such as confusion, slurred speech, double vision, inability to move or talk, or jerking,** check the blood/CGM sugar level. If the value is low, give sugar or instant glucose. Glucagon (Chapter 6) must be given if the person is unconscious or if a convulsion (seizure) occurs. The healthcare-provider should be contacted if a severe reaction occurs. In case of a convulsion or loss of consciousness, it may be necessary to call the paramedics or to go to an emergency room. Have an emergency number posted by the phone.

done). Always use a new strip for double checking results.

Make certain the Ketostix bottle has not been opened for longer than six months. The strips in the Ketostix bottle lose their sensitivity six months after opening. Others check the blood ketone level (Chapter 5) using the Precision Xtra meter, especially if the urine ketone measurement is moderate or large. This gives a more precise measurement of an increased ketone level at that moment. **Remember to always check ketones before calling your diabetes care-provider if you need help with sick day management.**

- **Signs of low blood sugar or of acidosis:** These conditions were discussed in Chapters 6 and 15, respectively. Deep, labored breathing or continual vomiting can be signs of acidosis. It is critical that a person with these symptoms be seen in an emergency room as soon as possible.

- **Eating and drinking:** It is important to know how well the person is taking liquids and/or eating. Use a 1-liter water bottle to help keep track of how much liquid has been consumed. One way to determine if you are becoming dehydrated is to look at your tongue in the mirror. If the tongue is dry (dehydrated), intravenous fluids may need to be given in the emergency room. Be cautious with children five years old and younger, as they can become dehydrated in 4-6 hours. If trips to the bathroom occur only 1-2 times per day, or if there are half the usual number of diapers, dehydration is likely present. Call the healthcare-provider if fluids can't be increased. See Table 4 for guidance on what type of fluid and how much to give.

- **Insulin dosage:** You should know the usual insulin dose and when it was last taken. Were any doses skipped or forgotten? Could the insulin have been in high heat or frozen and thus spoiled? Finally, if you have had a similar illness in the past, it is helpful for the doctor or nurse to know how much extra Humalog/NovoLog/Apidra or Regular insulin was given at that time. Did the dose seem to work? If the morning, noon or evening insulin dose has not yet been given and you have moderate or large ketones, call the diabetes care-provider before you give the injection. Extra rapid-acting insulin will probably be needed.

TABLE 4:
Plan for Fluid and Insulin Based on Blood/CGM Sugar and Ketone Levels

Blood Glucose	Type of fluid	Ketones*	Plan
<100 mg/dL (<5.5 mmol/L)	¾ sugary fluid + ¼ water	Any	→ Need to get glucose level up before giving more insulin → Consider low dose glucagon (see text) if blood sugar <70 mg/dL (3.9 mmol/L) and unable to take food or sugars.
100-180 mg/dL (5.5-10.0 mmol/L)	½ sugary fluid + ½ water	Negative or small ketones	→ Give normal correction dose, recheck in 4 hours.
		Moderate or large ketones	→ Give normal correction dose + extra for ketones: add 5% of total daily insulin**, recheck in 2 hours.
181-250 mg/dL (10.0 -13.9 mmol/L)	¼ sugary fluid + ¾ water	Negative or small ketones	→ Give normal correction dose, recheck in 4 hours.
		Moderate or large ketones	→ Give normal correction dose + extra for ketones: add 10% of total daily insulin **, recheck in 2 hours.
251-400 mg/dL (13.9-22.2 mmol/L)	¼ sugary fluid + ¾ water	Negative or small ketones	→ Give normal correction dose, recheck in 4 hours.
		Moderate ketones	→ Give normal correction dose + extra for ketones: add 10% of total daily insulin **, recheck in 2 hours.
		Large ketones	→ Give normal correction dose + extra for ketones: add 20% of total daily insulin **, recheck in 2 hours.
>400 mg/dL (>22.2 mmol/L)	¼ sugary fluid + ¾ water	Negative or small ketones	→ Give normal correction dose, recheck in 4 hours.
		Moderate or large ketones	→ Give normal correction dose + extra for ketones: add 20% of total daily insulin **, recheck in 2 hours.

* If ketones are negative or small, give normal correction dose for blood glucose.
**Total daily insulin is the amount of basal insulin added to the amount of insulin given for boluses throughout a typical day. On an insulin pump, you can find this under the pump history section.

Fortunately, with use of basal insulin therapy (given as injection or by pump), people have less fear of low blood/CGM glucose levels from a peak insulin (NPH) when they can't eat. The basal insulin should be continued during the illness, although the dose may need to be adjusted.

- **Oral medications:** If the person is taking metformin (Glucophage) or other non-insulin diabetes medications and having vomiting, diarrhea, difficulty breathing or any serious illness, **the medicine must be stopped.** If you need help, call the healthcare-provider AFTER checking the blood sugar and ketone levels.

- **Body weight:** It is helpful to know the last weight from a clinic visit (within three months) and the present weight (if you have a scale). This will help the doctor choose the right amount of insulin and also know how much weight you may have lost.

CHANGING THE INSULIN DOSAGE FOR ILLNESS

It is important to remember that SOME INSULIN MUST ALWAYS BE GIVEN EACH DAY (Table 2). You cannot skip taking at least some insulin just because you are sick and/or vomiting. Sometimes the basal insulin (by pump or injection) is all that is needed. During illness the body requires more energy to help fight the infection or virus. Hormones in the body other than insulin increase with illnesses and raise the blood/CGM glucose levels. More insulin is needed to allow the body to burn extra sugar for energy when the blood/CGM sugar is high, and ketones will also increase insulin needs. It is usually only the rapid-acting insulin that is increased. See Table 4 for guidance on how much extra insulin to give during illness.

If the blood sugar is low, the rapid-acting insulin may instead be reduced or omitted until blood/CGM sugars increase (see Table 4). If using an insulin pump, a temporary basal rate increase or decrease may be helpful. Remember, even if the blood sugar is low during illness, ketones may still be present. Ketones are formed from the breakdown of fat to provide the body with the extra energy it needs during the illness. When this is the case, it is important to eat carbohydrates to eliminate the formation of ketones. More insulin can be taken once the blood/CGM glucose level is back up.

When **vomiting** is occurring and the blood sugar is low or normal, sips of regular pop, sugar popsicles, honey or other "high-sugar" liquids may help raise the blood/CGM glucose levels. A low-dose of glucagon (see below) may also help. Once the blood sugar is up, insulin is needed to stop ketone production (if ketones are still present). Table 5 gives other suggestions for the management of vomiting.

Supplemental Rapid-Acting (Humalog, NovoLog, Apidra) or Regular Insulin

- If urine ketones are negative or small, or below 0.6 mmol/L in the blood, extra insulin can be based on the blood sugar level alone. Most people have a "correction factor" for high blood/CGM glucose levels already established (Chapter 22). For example, a common formula is to give 1 unit of rapid-acting insulin for every 50 mg/dL (2.8 mmol/L) of blood sugar above 150 mg/dL (8.3 mmol/L), but this will vary by person.

- If urine ketones are moderate or large, or above 1.0 mmol/L in the blood, and the blood/CGM glucose level is high, then use the sick day plan in Table 4 to calculate extra insulin needed.

These dosages are in addition to your usual daily dose. When possible, you should call the diabetes care-provider to get help with the dose. You will need to repeat the giving of rapid-acting insulin every 2 hours if moderate or large urine ketones are still present (or blood ketones above 1.0 mmol/L). For people using an insulin pump, this must be done using an insulin syringe. If the glucose level is lower than 150 mg/dL (8.3 mmol/L) it may be necessary to first give sips of a high sugar drink, glucose tablets, honey (greater than one year old) or other high-sugar-containing foods.

GENERAL GUIDELINES: SICK DAY MANAGEMENT
(see Tables 1 to 6)

To review, the body requires more energy during an illness. More insulin allows more sugar to pass into cells, providing more energy to fight the infection. **Some insulin is always needed.**

Important things to remember are:

- **Ketones:** Always check for ketones if you feel ill. Always check for ketones if the

TABLE 5:
Management of Vomiting (➔ ONLY FOR Negative or Small Ketones)

- Avoid solid foods until the vomiting has stopped.

- If vomiting is frequent, many physicians recommend giving oral Zofran or a Phenergan suppository (or patch) to reduce vomiting and waiting to give fluids for an hour until the medicine is working. Zofran is a newer oral medication, with fewer side effects, which dissolves in the mouth. The Phenergan gel requires composition by a Prescription Compounding Center of America (or equivalent). The usual dose for a teen is 50 mg in 1 cc. The gel is rubbed into the skin while wearing a rubber glove, and is then covered with plastic wrap. Preteens usually get 25 mg (1/2 cc). The dose can be repeated in four hours. The main side effect of the Phenergan is sleepiness. **If using these medications, make sure another person is available to remind you to recheck the blood sugar and ketones in two hours.** The medicines cause sleepiness, and the person might need help. Some doctors do not prescribe these medications because of this concern.

- Sometimes the blood/CGM sugar can be low (<70 mg/dL or <3.9 mmol/L) and the person cannot keep any food down. Glucagon can be mixed and given just like insulin – using an insulin syringe (see Low-Dose Glucagon below). The dose is one unit per year of age up to a maximum of 15 units. If the blood sugar is not higher in 20-30 minutes, the same dose can be repeated.

- Gradually start liquids (sugar pop [soda], juice, Pedialyte, water, etc.; see Table 6) in small amounts. Juices (especially orange) replace the salts that are lost with vomiting or diarrhea. Pedialyte popsicles are also available. Start with a tablespoon of liquid every 10-20 minutes. If the blood sugar is below 100 mg/dL (<5.5 mmol/L), sugar pop can be given. For the child five years of age and over, sucking on a piece of hard candy often works well. If the blood sugar is above 180 mg/dL (>10.0 mmol/L), do not give pop with sugar in it. If there is no further vomiting, gradually increase the amount of fluid. If vomiting restarts, it may again be necessary to rest the stomach for another hour and then restart the small amounts of fluids. A repeat suppository or topical Phenergan dose or Zofran tablet can be given after three or four hours. Dairy products should not be used until the person is able to drink fluids and eat crackers and soup without vomiting.

- After a few hours without vomiting, gradually return to a normal diet. Soups are often suggested to start with, and they provide needed nutrients.

---

blood/CGM glucose level is over 240 mg/dL (>13.3 mmol/L) fasting or over 300 mg/dL (>16.7 mmol/L) two times in a row (about one hour apart) during the day.

- **Vomiting:** If you are vomiting and have a low blood sugar, an insulin reaction could occur. At the same time, you may have ketones. Always check for ketones if you are vomiting. Vomiting may be due to an infection, a virus, or ketones. Management of vomiting is outlined in Table 5.

- **Insulin:** Keep a bottle of rapid-acting insulin and a syringe available even if you don't usually use them. You may need to give extra insulin during an illness. If using an insulin pump, there may be a problem with catheter occlusion. Be sure the insulin is not outdated.

- **Blood Sugar Levels:** All people with diabetes must have some method of blood sugar monitoring available and be ready to do extra values on sick days (usually every 2-4

TABLE 6:
Sick Day Liquids and Solids

1. **Liquids (in addition to water – particularly if the blood sugar is below 150 mg/dL [8.3 mmol/L]):**
   - Sugar-containing beverages: regular 7-Up, ginger ale, orange, cola, pepsi®, etc.[1]
   - Pedialyte or Infalyte® (especially for younger children)
   - Sports drinks: Gatorade®, POWERADE®, etc. (any flavor)
   - Tea with honey or sugar[1]
   - Fruit flavored drinks: regular Kool-Aid, lemonade, Hi-C® [1], etc.
   - Fruit juice: apple, cranberry, grape, grapefruit, orange, pineapple, etc.
   - JELL-O: regular (for infants, liquid JELL-O warmed in a bottle) or diet[1]
   - Popsicles: regular or diet[1]
   - Broth-type soup: bouillon, chicken noodle soup, Cup-a-Soup®

2. **Solids (when ready) – suggested foods with which to start:**
   - Saltine crackers
   - Banana (or other fruit)
   - Applesauce
   - Bread, toast or tortillas
   - Graham crackers
   - Soup
   - Rice

[1] Sugar-free may be needed depending on blood sugars (e.g., >180 mg/dL [>10.0 mmol/L]). Children under 1 year old should not be given honey.

---

hours). More frequent monitoring of blood sugar and ketones has greatly reduced the need for hospitalizations. Table 4 suggests amounts of water versus sugar fluids to give based on the blood/CGM glucose levels.

- **Extra Snacks:** It is important to take in adequate calories on sick days, or the body will start to break down fat for energy. If this happens, ketones will appear in the urine (see Chapter 15). Sugary soft drinks, popsicles and non-diet JELL-O are suggested to eat if you do not feel like eating food and your blood sugar is below 180 mg/dL (<10.0 mmol/L). Much of eating is psychological, and we often suggest you eat whatever you feel like eating on sick days (also see Table 6).

- **Past Experience:** Base your judgments on past experience. Refer to your record book to see if this illness has occurred before. See what worked in the past, and what didn't.

- **Which Doctor to Call:** Call your family doctor for non-diabetes-related problems such as sore throats, earaches, fever, rashes, etc. (see Table 3). Unless the diabetes specialist also provides general care, only call him/her if the urine ketones are moderate/large or if the blood ketone level is above 1.0 mmol/L. Also call if you need help with an insulin dose, if hypoglycemia is a problem or if you need help with other aspects of diabetes management.

FLUID REPLACEMENT

If you have difficulty eating or keeping food down and the blood/CGM glucose level is below 150 mg/dL (<8.3 mmol/L), take sugar-containing liquids (see Tables 4 and 5). These may include fruit juices, popsicles, slushies, tea with sugar, broth, syrup from canned fruit or even regular pop. Stir the pop to get rid of bubbles and help avoid indigestion. If you are vomiting, take a small amount (juice-glass size or less) of sugar pop. If it stays down 15 minutes, some sugar will be absorbed. If there is no vomiting after ½ hour, increase the amount of fluids. If you have ketones and are not vomiting, keep drinking. Children should receive one ounce of fluid per year of age per hour up to age 16 years. Older teens can consume two cups (16 oz) per hour. The liquids help to avoid dehydration and also to "wash out" the ketones. Specific instructions regarding vomiting are given in Table 5.

A LOW DOSE OF GLUCAGON

Sometimes during illness, the blood sugar can be low (<70 mg/dL [<3.9 mmol/L]), and the person is unable to keep any food down. To elevate the blood sugar level, glucagon can be mixed and given just like insulin. Prepare the glucagon as usual and, using an insulin syringe, measure one unit per year of age. The maximum dose should be no more than 15 units, even for adults.

For example:

- a five-year-old child would get five units of glucagon
- a 10-year-old child would get 10 units of glucagon

If the blood sugar has not risen to at least 90 mg/dL (5.0 mmol/L) in 20-30 minutes, the same dose can be repeated. This treatment has saved many ER visits for our Clinic patients.

FOODS FOR SICK DAYS

Table 6 suggests carbohydrate-containing foods that might be tried during an illness. Eating carbohydrates is important to provide energy and to prevent the body from breaking down fats (and thus making ketones). Drinking liquids is important to prevent dehydration, so liquids are usually tried first. A general rule of thumb is to offer whatever you/your child like(s) best. You may want to have a "sick day kit" on hand which could include items such as sugar-containing 7-UP, sports drinks, regular and diet JELL-O or pudding, apple juice in small cans, regular Kool-Aid mix, Cup-a-Soup, Pedialyte and any other items you would like to have available.

EXERCISE

The person with moderate or large urine ketones or blood ketones above 0.6 mmol/L should not exercise. Fat and muscle can be broken down during exercise, further increasing ketone levels.

CONTACTING YOUR DOCTOR OR NURSE (see Table 1)

Keep a card with your doctor's and nurse's emergency phone numbers in a place where you can easily find it. Also be sure to have the doctor's emergency phone number for nighttime or weekend calls. Take these cards with you if you are going out of town. It is easier to call your own doctor than to go to an emergency room and see a new doctor.

Think ahead! You may want to keep Zofran or Phenergan (Table 5) on hand in case of vomiting. Before you call the doctor or nurse, be sure you have the necessary information (see the list at the beginning of the chapter). **Always check the blood sugar and urine or blood ketones before calling.** Have the number of your pharmacy available in case the doctor needs it. Table 3 tells when to call or get emergency care. Remember to keep sugar pop, popsicles and soups available for illnesses.

CLINIC OR EMERGENCY ROOM VISITS

If you do decide to go to a clinic or emergency room, remember to take your hospital card if you have one, your diabetes records and your insurance information. Take extra clothes in case you must be admitted to the hospital. A relative or friend going with you will need money for food, telephone numbers of people they might need to call, and something to read.

SICK DAY MEDICATIONS

Our general philosophy is that **if you need a medicine for an illness, take it!** The only exception is for people who have complications (eye, kidney, nerve or heart problems) when some medications should be avoided. The diabetes health team will handle the problems related to diabetes. The classic example is asthma. With a severe attack, the person may need medicines which raise the blood sugar. Oral steroids (cortisone) that raise the blood sugar may also be needed. For the short time that these medicines are needed, extra insulin can be taken to help keep the blood/CGM glucose levels in target range. Short-term elevations of blood sugar are not what we worry about in relation to the complications of diabetes.

Over-the-counter medications can be purchased with care. Look at the label to see if sugar is added. Tablets are less likely to have sugar (and alcohol) than are liquids. Again, the small amount of sugar in a medicine taken for a short time is okay. *We do not endorse any products and suggest you discuss these with your primary care physician:*

Generic daytime/nighttime cold capsules are fine to use in children old enough to swallow the capsules. The capsules are alcohol-free and don't have an after-taste as do liquids.

Nasal sprays (Afrin®) can be used for colds and allergies. A nasal spray is less likely to affect the entire body than pills or liquid medicines. If these do not work, or if long-term use is anticipated (as with seasonal allergies), antihistamine tablets or liquids such as Chlor-trimeton® or Triaminic® might be tried next.

Acetaminophen (Tylenol®) can be used to relieve fever if a flu is going through the community. Do not give aspirin to children or adolescents.

Pepto-Bismol®, Kaopectate® or Imodium AD® are fine to use for diarrhea. (Lomotil® should NOT be used in children.)

DI-GEL®, Mylanta®, Gelusil® and Maalox® are all sugar-free antacids.

Cough medications: Use a cold air vaporizer if this relieves the cough. During the day, a cough is often protective, keeping material out of the lungs. Thus, we do not give cough medicines. If the vaporizer does not stop the cough at night, use sugar-free cough medicines with less than 15 percent alcohol. Examples: Colrex Expectorant®, CONTAC Jr.®, Hytuss Tablets®, Queltuss Tablets®, Robitussin CF® liquid, Supercitin®, Tolu-Sed®, Tolu-Sed DM®, Tussar-SF®. Remember, a combined cough and fever means the child should be seen by the primary care physician.

Sore Throats: A throat culture to rule out a streptococcal (strep) infection should be considered, because strep can lead to rheumatic fever or other problems. Saltwater gargles (¼ teaspoon salt in one glass water) may help. Chloraseptic Spray® is sugar-free, as are Cepacol®, Cepastat®, Chloraseptic® mouthwashes or lozenges and N'ICE® lozenges.

FOLLOW THE DIRECTIONS ON THE LABEL FOR ANY MEDICINE YOU USE.

FLU SHOTS

The American Academy of Pediatrics recommends flu shots for all children with diabetes, and we agree. Avoiding an episode of flu may help prevent an episode of ketoacidosis. It is common for the flu (and other illnesses) to raise the HbA1c level by one-half to one point. It is important to get the flu shot early in the fall so it can be working when the flu season begins.

SURGERY MANAGEMENT

Some general guidelines for diabetes management around surgery are outlined in Table 7. The insulin dose may not change if the person is receiving a basal insulin (Lantus [Basaglar]/Levemir/Tresiba or an insulin pump). If NPH is taken in the morning for someone also receiving a basal insulin, the NPH (or boluses of rapid-acting insulin) is often omitted. Any change in insulin dose depends on the person, the type of surgery that is scheduled and the time of day the surgery is to be done. If possible, surgery should be scheduled early in the morning. In general, it is best to call your diabetes care-provider and discuss insulin changes **after** you find out the time of day the procedure is to be done and whether or not food intake will be limited. Sometimes it is also helpful to have the surgeon or anesthesiologist call the diabetes care-provider. This is more likely to be done if the family gives the doctor or dentist a note with the name and phone number of the diabetes specialist. The two of them can then work out the best time for a given person for surgery.

We frequently receive calls from families related to planned dental surgery. Often this can be done under local anesthesia, and sometimes the person can eat regular meals prior to and after the surgery. In this situation it is only necessary to reduce the insulin dose slightly in anticipation of some reduction in food intake due to soreness in the mouth.

If the person is going to have a general anesthetic, eating is usually restricted to avoid vomiting during recovery. Anytime the amount of food intake is to change, the amount of

Check your ketones before calling your doctor when you aren't feeling well.

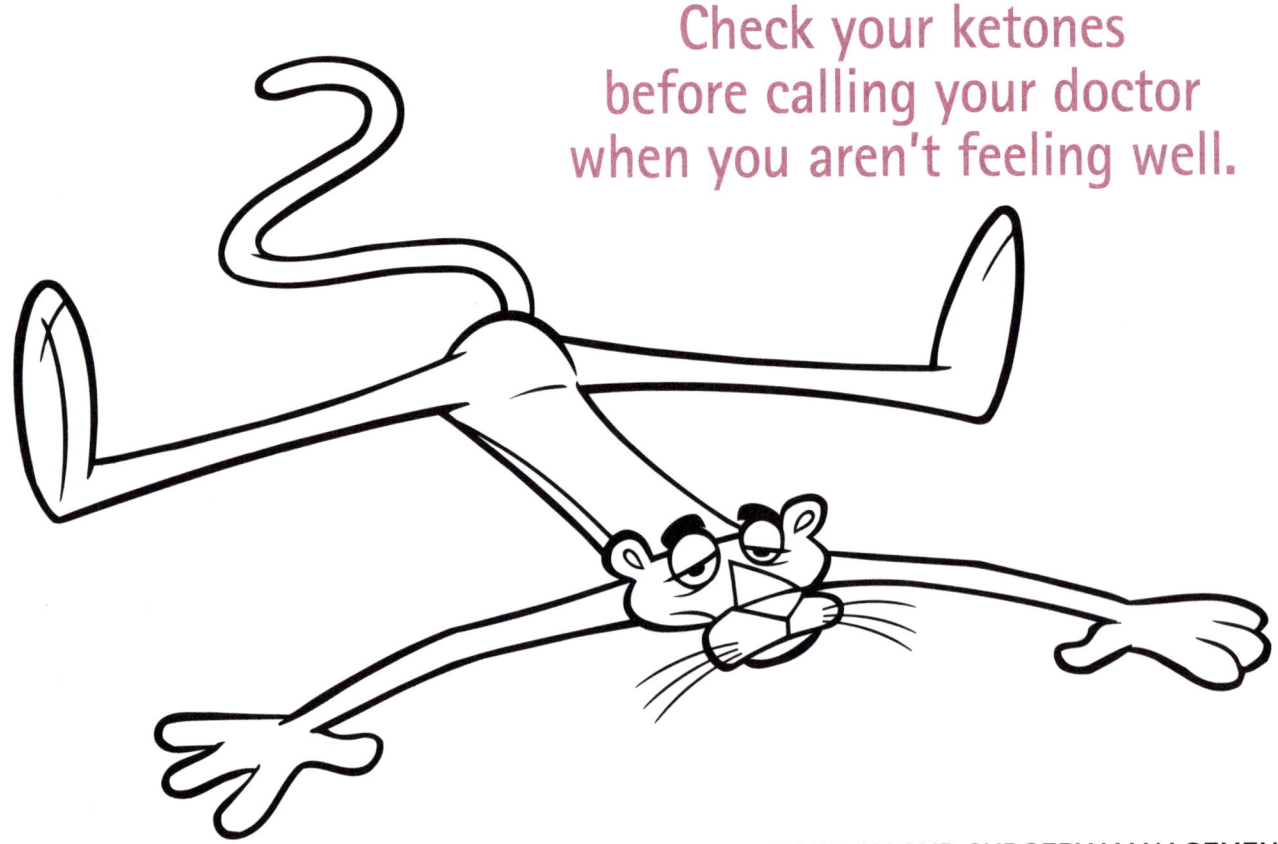

TABLE 7:
Guidelines for Management Around Surgery

- Always contact your diabetes care-provider if surgery is planned – AFTER you find out the time and whether normal food intake will be allowed. You should give the name and phone number of the diabetes care-provider to the person doing the surgery.

- Plan to take your own blood sugar and ketone checking equipment.

- Take your own materials to treat low blood sugar (a source of instant glucose and glucagon).

- Always check the ketones prior to surgery. Then, if they are present at a later time, it will be known that they were negative earlier. If the urine ketones are found to be moderate or large or the blood ketones above 1.0 mmol/L, it may be necessary to cancel the planned procedure. Take the ketone strips with you to the procedure in case vomiting occurs and you need to do a check. It is also wise to check ketones once or twice after the procedure.

- Take your diabetes clinic's phone card so that you may quickly call the diabetes care-provider if needed.

- If on basal insulin therapy (Lantus [Basaglar]/Levemir/Tresiba or a pump), it is best to continue insulin in this way during the surgery. Often no other insulin is needed.

insulin to be given must also be changed. Often the basal insulin (Lantus [Basaglar]/Levemir/Tresiba or pump basal dose) is slightly reduced. The peak-insulins (NPH and rapid-acting insulins) are either reduced or omitted with the reduced food intake. Pumps can be very useful, but require a knowledgeable person to supervise. If the person is going to have a general anesthetic in the hospital, some doctors prefer to give all of the insulin by intravenous infusion.

Any of these methods works. **The important thing is the close monitoring of blood sugars! By doing this, low blood sugars can be avoided. It is also wise to check the urine or blood ketones before and after the procedure.** These may increase with changes in the insulin dose and with the stress of surgery. Be sure to check with your surgeon or anesthesiologist about blood sugar monitoring prior to the procedure. Needless to say, your diabetes care-provider must always be notified if the urine ketones are moderate or large or if the blood ketones are above 1.0 mmol/L following surgery.

Blood/CGM sugar monitoring is usually the responsibility of the parent or the patient when procedures are done in the dentist's or doctor's office. If a meter is used for blood sugar monitoring at home, this should be taken along to the dentist's or doctor's office. If the child is being admitted to the hospital, also take the meter along. If the child is to have a general anesthetic, the blood sugar monitoring is the responsibility of the doctor giving the anesthesia or the doctor doing the surgery. Sometimes the doctor orders dextrose, which is glucose (sugar), to be added to the intravenous fluids if the blood sugar is below a certain level (180 mg/dL or 10.0 mmol/L is a safe level to use).

It is also wise to take along urine or blood ketone checking strips. Many doctors or nurses who do not care for people with diabetes on a regular basis may forget the importance of routinely checking for ketones. Also take your diabetes care-provider's phone numbers with you. If urine ketones are moderate or large, or the blood ketones are above 1.0 mmol/L, you may wish to call your diabetes care-provider.

DEFINITIONS

Anesthetic (anesthesia): A medication (such as ether) used to reduce pain or to allow a person to sleep through an otherwise painful procedure.

Dextrose: The name for glucose (sugar) added to an intravenous (IV) feeding to help avoid low blood sugar.

Suppository: A medication inserted into the rectum (bottom), usually because liquid, food or medicine cannot be kept down (as with vomiting).

QUESTIONS AND ANSWERS FROM NEWSNOTES

Q: In the chapter on "Sick Day Management" in the Pink Panther book, you state four times that ketones must always be checked at least twice daily when someone is ill. Is it necessary to be that repetitive?

a: Forgetting to check ketones with an illness is one of the most common errors families make in managing diabetes. As a result, ketones can build up to high levels in the body, which can then be dangerous (and expensive to treat). There is no charge for a few phone calls to a diabetes care-provider to receive suggestions for supplemental rapid-acting insulin to combat early ketone formation. In contrast, the charge is great for one or two nights in an intensive care unit as a result of large ketones building up in the body. As discussed in Chapter 15, the related risk from ketoacidosis can be avoided if families will just check for ketones immediately (and at least twice daily) when the person with diabetes is ill. The diabetes care-provider must then be called when moderate or large ketones are detected, or the blood ketone level is above 1.0 mmol/L; recheck every 2-3 hours thereafter until the ketones are below these levels.

Q: Should the flu shot be given to children with diabetes?

a: The American Academy of Pediatrics recommends a flu shot for all children with diabetes. Flu is a common cause of ketonuria and of acidosis, so the shot may also help avoid ketoacidosis (and an increase in the HbA1c level). If you do decide to get the flu shot for your child, go to your primary care physician for this purpose. Call first to make sure the doctor's office has the vaccine. If a young child has not previously received the flu vaccine, it may be necessary to get it in two injections, approximately one month apart, and it is best to start during the months of September or October.

Q: Should my child receive the measles and the chicken pox immunizations?

a: Yes. They are recommended by the American Academy of Pediatrics for all children and we support that recommendation. There is an additional factor for children with diabetes who still produce some insulin. Chicken pox may be one of the many infections that stimulate white blood cells in the pancreas to make toxic particles that cause further islet destruction. This is not proven, but we have heard many times of children being diagnosed with diabetes in the month or two after having chicken pox.

The Varivax is a live vaccine. The main side effects are a mild rash (approximately three percent), and/or a temperature elevation (approximately 15 percent) and/or tenderness at the site (approximately 19 percent). Ninety-nine percent of people are protected as a result of the vaccination.

CHAPTER 17
Family and Behavioral Concerns

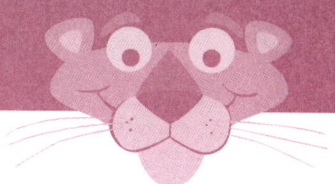

Diabetes affects the entire family. Research has shown that children, adolescents, and even adults do best when there is strong family support and involvement. Immediately after diagnosis there can be a lot of different emotions and frustrations. These typically improve over time, but can resurface throughout an individual's life. Sometimes these feelings persist and affect one's life and diabetes care. This chapter will look into the family life and daily life with diabetes and address behavioral issues that can arise.

DIABETES ONSET STRESS
(See Chapter 10)

The diagnosis of any serious condition, especially in children and teens, is stressful for the whole family (including the extended family). Getting through the initial shock and grief that comes with the diagnosis is difficult. This can be especially hard if families have had previous medical or other serious issues to manage in addition to diabetes.

The crisis of diagnosis can bring up many fears and feelings, and:

✓ an individual can become quite anxious or depressed
✓ children and teens can sense tension between parents and may feel responsible for something they can't help
✓ parents or significant others may feel the strain on the relationship with one another

Parents usually have different coping styles for grief. The period around first realizing that your child or a family member has diabetes can

> **TOPICS:**
> **Psychosocial Adjustment**
>
> **TEACHING OBJECTIVES:**
> The teacher will:
> 1. Describe stresses that a person/family may experience as a result of diabetes.
> 2. Provide healthy coping strategies for individual/family stress.
>
> **LEARNING OBJECTIVES:**
> Learner (parents, child, relative or self) will be able to:
> 1. Identify the stresses experienced by the person/family with diabetes.
> 2. Describe a healthy coping strategy for an identified stress.

be filled with a lot of different feelings, including sadness, anger, and anxiety. Support from friends or other families who are familiar with diabetes can be helpful. These feelings tend to improve over time. If they persist, it is important to communicate with the behavioral health counselor on the diabetes care team.

WORKING AS A FAMILY

It is important for families to share diabetes responsibilities. Parents do the best when they work together and support one another. We encourage **both** parents to share the responsibility for the diabetes care of their child, including blood or continuous glucose monitor (**CGM**) sugar checks, carbohydrate (carb) counting, and insulin injections. Both parents should try to attend clinic visits. Single-parent families may wish to bring a support person.

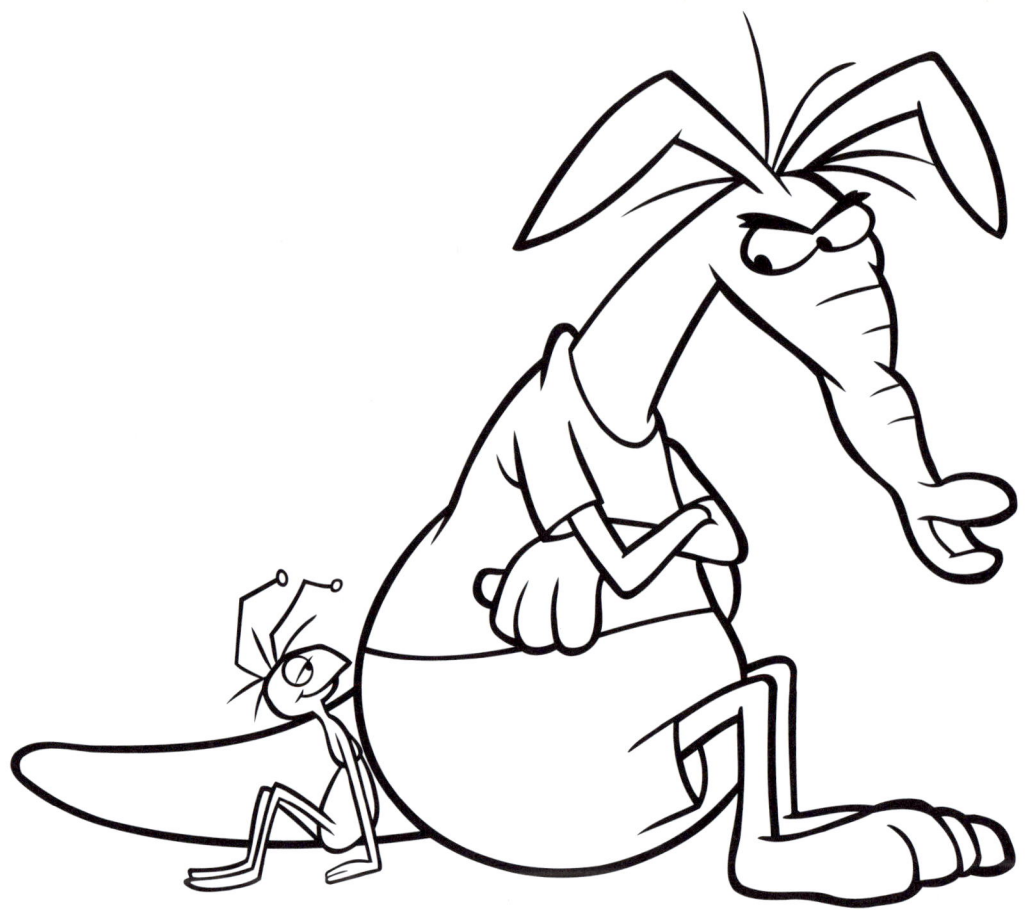

Family support is very important for the person with diabetes.

CONCERNS OF BROTHERS AND SISTERS

When a child first develops diabetes, attention is focused on the new diagnosis. Siblings often feel left out when the child with diabetes needs more attention.

Some common concerns may be:

✔ trouble understanding diabetes

✔ fear that their brother or sister will die

✔ thinking they caused the diabetes by being upset or angry at the child with diabetes

✔ fear that they can catch diabetes and/or that they will also be diagnosed with diabetes

It can be important for the brothers and/or sisters:

✔ to be a part of the initial diabetes education

✔ to visit their sibling in the hospital and come to clinic

✔ to feel comfortable sharing what they think and understand, even if you think everything has been thoroughly explained. For example, *one child used the word "diabetes" very literally. When asked why he was so sad, he said he thought diabetes meant "die of betes."*

✔ to be treated in the same manner as their sibling with diabetes

✔ to have special, dedicated time set aside for each child

Some children with diabetes have the opportunity for special activities, such as diabetes camp. Many brothers and sisters say, "I wish I had diabetes so I could do special things, too." It is important to help siblings understand that these activities provide special supportive care. Make sure the sibling without diabetes gets their special time and activities too.

DAILY LIFE WITH DIABETES

Diabetes care has changed tremendously over the past 20 years. New insulins, insulin pens, blood glucose meters, insulin pumps, CGMs, the artificial pancreas, and flexibility with meal planning and insulin dosing have all made it easier for children and adults to live normal, healthy and active lives with diabetes.

For children, leading a normal life means participating in age-appropriate activities with their family and peers. Diabetes can make fun things like sleepovers and birthday parties a little more stressful. But with some flexibility and creativity, children with diabetes are able to participate in these activities just like their siblings and friends. When in doubt about allowing your child to take part in an activity, ask yourself, "Would I let my child participate if he/she did not have diabetes?" If the answer is "yes," it should not change because of the diabetes. If you are uncertain, contact your diabetes care provider so they can help you create a plan for the activity.

The issue of discipline and diabetes is also an important aspect of leading a normal life. Whether a child has diabetes or not, there will be times when he/she will test limits and act up. Children with diabetes need limits set like any other child. Sometimes it is hard to tell if a child is being difficult because he/she is "acting like a teenager" (or "a toddler") or because their blood sugar is high or low. When in doubt, check the blood/CGM glucose value and then deal appropriately with the behavior.

Care providers, parents and children need to strike a balance between optimal diabetes management and an emotionally healthy lifestyle. It is important for everyone to work as a team to allow children with diabetes to appropriately grow and develop physically and emotionally.

DEALING WITH LIFE STRESSORS

Both positive and negative emotions and stress can have a big effect on diabetes management.

Many different life events can cause stress, such as:

- ✔ family problems
- ✔ arguments with parents or between parents
- ✔ parent separation or divorce
- ✔ death of a relative, friend or pet
- ✔ a move to a new home or school

Other kinds of stressful situations include special events such as:

- ✔ athletic competitions
- ✔ school exams
- ✔ special holidays like birthdays, Christmas, Hanukkah, or Ramadan

Most people will have high blood sugars following stress, although some children can have low blood sugars because of extra activity. It is important to plan ahead and alter the insulin dose or give extra food, as needed. It is also important to monitor blood/CGM glucose levels more frequently to reduce the frequency of low blood sugars at times of increased activity or stress. If the effects of stress do not decrease, the help of a clinical social worker or psychologist should be obtained.

Figure 1 in Chapter 14 shows how the insulin/oral medicine dose, diet, exercise and stress must be in balance for optimal sugar levels. Sometimes, despite our best efforts, blood/CGM glucose levels just don't behave the way we expect! But it helps to keep working at it, and it can keep the person with diabetes much healthier in the long run.

SINGLE-PARENT/ BLENDED FAMILIES

Approximately one-third of children in the U.S. now live in single-parent families. For children who live in two households, it is important to share vital diabetes information between the households. From the first visit, we emphasize that parents in two separate households must communicate about their child's diabetes care.

Information to be shared between households includes:

- ✔ blood/CGM sugar levels
- ✔ recent low blood sugars
- ✔ insulin dosages and recent changes
- ✔ food intake
- ✔ exercise
- ✔ illnesses
- ✔ other events which may affect diabetes management

Communication and cooperation are essential!

Some suggestions for two-household families are:

- ✔ Diabetes supplies should be neatly packed in a carrying case to go with the child between households.
- ✔ Keep a glucagon kit and ketone strips permanently in each household.
- ✔ Keep a **current** log book with insulin doses and important sugar results that go between houses to ensure consistency. Use of computers/cell phones can help with this.
- ✔ remember that the care of the child is the most important thing. Try to put individual differences and conflicts aside and focus on helping the child have a healthy life with diabetes.

PROMOTING A HEALTHY FOOD PLAN
(see Chapters 11 and 12)

When a child is diagnosed with diabetes, one of the first things that parents often wonder about is how their meals will change. Many people still believe sugar causes diabetes. They may think they will need remove all sugar from their child's food. This is not true. A healthy meal plan includes foods from all food groups in appropriate amounts. Eating healthy is important for everyone! With or without diabetes, one should not consume sweets and special treats in excess. Americans already eat more added simple sugars than is recommended, and this contributes to excessive weight gain. Preventing obesity is important for all children, including those with type 1 diabetes, as it can cause insulin resistance (Chapter 4).

It is important that everyone in the family support one another by selecting healthy foods and snacks. Foods in the home should not be restricted from the child with diabetes. If simple carbohydrate foods and drinks are available in the home, they are hard for anyone to resist, including the child with diabetes. It is important to make healthy changes for the whole family and limit the amount of "junk food" available.

For the person with diabetes, the appropriate insulin dose must be given/taken for carbs (including sweets) that are consumed. Diabetes education teaches families about carbs (sugars and starches) and how they affect blood/CGM glucose levels.

SCHOOL OR WORK ATTENDANCE
(see Chapter 25)

People with diabetes typically do not have more school or work absences for illness than people without diabetes. However, they may miss school or work occasionally for routine clinic visits. If a great deal of school/work is being missed for diabetes-related reasons, it is important to review this with the medical team. Working together, the underlying cause can hopefully be identified and addressed.

If a significant amount of school or work has been missed, the following can be helpful:

✔ talking with the school counselor or teacher who can assist in arranging a schedule and homework after a long absence

✔ asking members of the diabetes care team to provide guidance on how to work with the school or office

✔ arranging for a parent or school nurse to talk to the class about diabetes. It allows for the development of peer support and understanding.

BEHAVIORAL AND PSYCHOLOGICAL CHALLENGES IN DIABETES

Behavioral concerns can arise in children or adults with chronic diseases, such as diabetes. These can include anxiety, phobias, depression, and eating disorders, which are discussed in more detail below. Unaddressed behavioral issues can result in poor diabetes management, increased HbA1c levels, and long-term complications. It is important to identify and address concerns with the diabetes care team or a behavioral health counselor. Most clinics have referral lists available.

FEAR OF SHOTS
(see Chapter 9)

Needle anxiety occurs to some degree in almost everyone. Both children and adults have worries about giving and getting shots. In a person with diabetes, it used to be assumed that this anxiety would just go away because they had to have shots every day. We now know that needle anxiety, if strong, doesn't "just go away." But there are ways to reduce this anxiety if it is identified as a problem.

Anxiety about shots is normal. When we fear something, we get tense and tend to hold our breath. Our head becomes filled with thoughts about pain. Parents who have to give shots can be just as anxious as their child. Remember, the syringes used for insulin have much smaller and shorter needles, so shots are much more comfortable these days. With a few easy techniques, shots can be less stressful. Most diabetes educators have parents or significant others practice injections on each other using saline (sterile saltwater). The practice reassures them that giving insulin injections to their child is not as traumatic as they imagine.

Some strategies for needle anxiety include deep breathing and distraction. Before getting a shot, the child can take a couple of deep relaxing breaths ("breathe in through the nose and breathe slowly out through the mouth") and try to imagine they are made of JELL-O. By relaxing the tension, shots can be done more comfortably. Distraction can also help focus the mind away from fear and towards something else. Watching cartoons or listening to some favorite music with headphones can help keep the person from thinking too much about the shot and may aid in relaxation. Parents can be helpful by reassuring the child, and can also use positive rewards (like stickers) when shots go especially well.

Sometimes the needle anxiety persists despite these interventions. Some signs of continued needle anxiety may include:

✔ persistently high HbA1c level

✔ a child wanting to do all their own shots – particularly when they want to do the shots in a room by themselves (some shots will probably be missed)

✔ missed insulin shots

✔ lack of site rotation (hypertrophy or swelling of the injection site)

✔ excuses for wanting to "put off" the shot

The behavioral health counselor on the diabetes care team can be very helpful to children or parents when this problem is identified. They can work with the family to identify techniques specific for the child. As fear of shots decreases, the HbA1c level usually improves.

FEAR OF HYPOGLYCEMIA

Fear of hypoglycemia (very low blood sugars) is seen in individuals with type 1 diabetes as well as in parents of children with type 1 diabetes. Fear of hypoglycemia can include fear of both mild and severe hypoglycemia, including loss of consciousness and seizures. Some anxiety about hypoglycemia is normal and expected.

Signs of significant anxiety about hypoglycemia include:

- ✓ maintaining high blood sugars to avoid hypoglycemia
- ✓ eating large snacks at bedtime despite appropriate bedtime blood/CGM sugar levels
- ✓ waking up multiple times throughout the night to check blood/CGM sugars

Significant anxiety about hypoglycemia can lead to increased HbA1c levels and can affect quality of life of both the child and the parents. Fortunately, with the advances in CGM and in the partial artificial pancreas (see Chapter 30), the fear of hypoglycemia has been greatly reduced. Episodes of hypoglycemia can occur at times, such as with exercise, illness, and when getting an insulin dose that is too high for the amount of carbs eaten. Mild episodes can occur a few times a week even in people with well-managed diabetes. A major goal of diabetes management is to avoid frequent/mild and any severe hypoglycemic episodes. If there is significant anxiety about hypoglycemia, it is important to discuss this with the diabetes care team.

DEPRESSION

Depression is a mood disorder that may be more common in children and adults with diabetes than in the general population.

Symptoms include:

- ✓ change in sleep habits
- ✓ change in appetite or weight
- ✓ feeling guilty
- ✓ decreased energy
- ✓ irritability, sadness, or feeling hopeless
- ✓ decreased concentration, decline in school or work performance
- ✓ lack of pleasure in things previously enjoyed; no longer engaging in social activities

In some people, depression can present as irritability and anger instead of sadness and hopelessness.

Be aware that depression can affect diabetes care in the following ways:

- ✓ high blood/CGM sugar values and high HbA1c level
- ✓ irritability around checking blood/CGM sugars or getting shots
- ✓ not caring about daily diabetes tasks

It is recommended the diabetes care team routinely screen for depression, often using a standard questionnaire. If left untreated, depression can lead to problems in long-term diabetes management. Treatment of depression and other mood disorders through counseling and/or medications (usually antidepressants) can be very effective. If there is any concern about depression, it is important to seek professional help from a behavioral healthcare-provider. Your primary care physician or diabetes care team can provide recommendations and referrals to a behavioral healthcare-provider.

DISORDERED EATING BEHAVIORS/EATING DISORDERS
(see Chapter 20)

Disordered eating behaviors, including insulin omission, and clinical eating disorders are more common in those with diabetes compared to those without diabetes. They can affect management of diabetes, including elevated blood sugars and increased HbA1c levels, leading to diabetic ketoacidosis (DKA) and long-term complications. Two types of clinical eating disorders are:

✔ **Anorexia:** usually involves restricting food intake and, often, engaging in excessive exercise.

✔ **Bulimia:** excessive intake of food followed by self-induced vomiting, use of laxatives and/or excessive exercise.

In those with type 1 diabetes, disordered eating behaviors and eating disorders can be particularly life threatening due to **insulin omission**. Some people *miss shots or under-dose their insulin* to control their weight. Missing insulin doses results in calories consumed going out in the urine instead of being used by the body to make energy. Blood/CGM glucose levels become very high. This can lead to life-threatening DKA in the short term, and chronic complications long-term. Eating disorders can be difficult to treat and require urgent psychological care from a professional with expertise in this area and who understands diabetes.

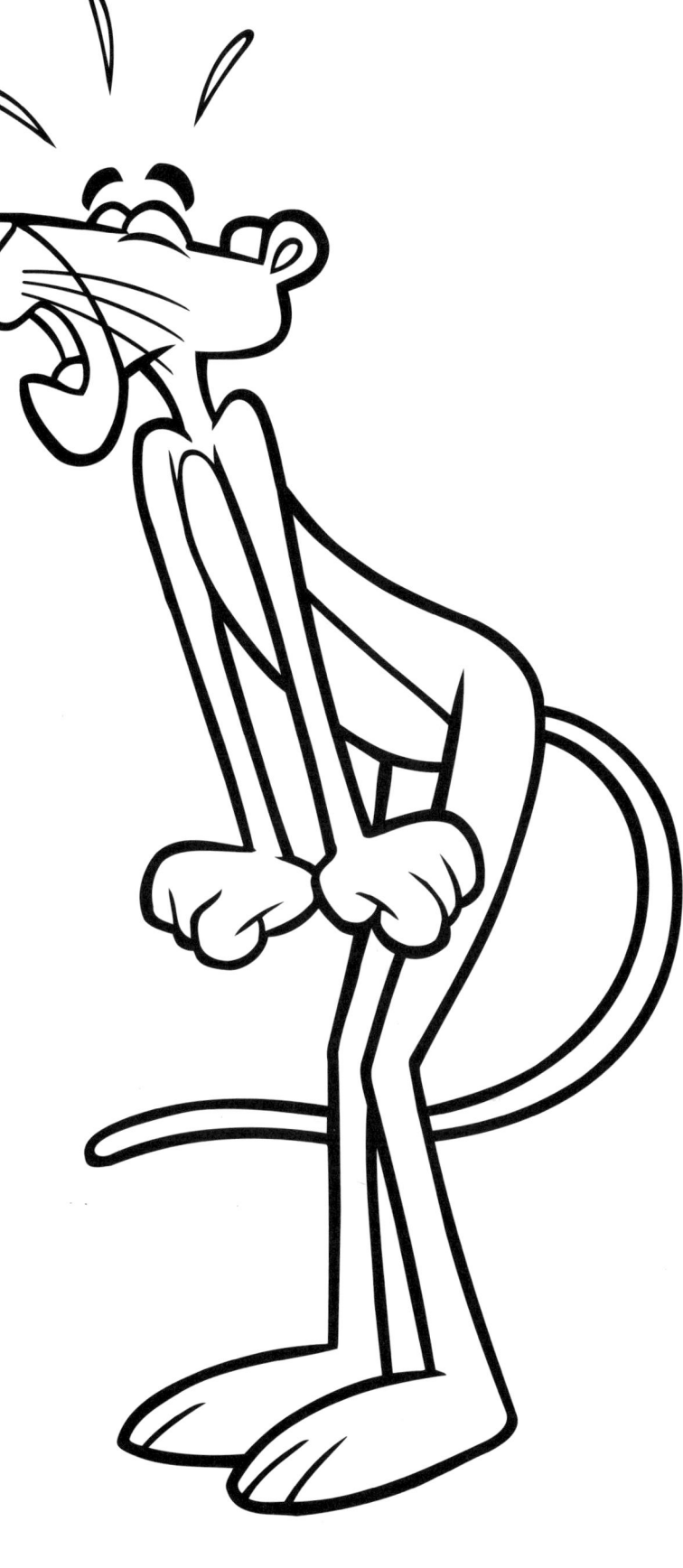

FAMILY AND BEHAVIORAL CONCERNS

DEFINITIONS

Clinical Social Worker: A person licensed at the master's graduate level to provide mental health services to individuals and families.

Psychologist: A person with a doctorate degree trained in diagnosing and treating behavioral health concerns through individual, group, and family therapy.

Psychiatrist: A physician who specializes in diagnosing and treating behavioral health concerns. They can also prescribe medication for treatment of psychiatric disorders.

Stressors: Problems or events that make people feel anxious.

Depression: A mood disorder causing feelings of sadness, hopelessness, and loss of interest.

Eating disorder: Extreme attitudes and behaviors surrounding weight and food issues affecting one's health and quality of life.

QUESTIONS AND ANSWERS FROM NEWSNOTES

What are the occupational restrictions for a person with diabetes?

Parents and young adults often ask this question. Restrictions are based on the idea that all people with diabetes are at a greater risk for hypoglycemia. There are studies that show hypoglycemia does result in an increased risk for accidents.

Our opinion is that restrictions should not be generic and should be individualized. Some people monitor their blood/CGM glucose levels frequently and are careful to eat or make sure they are not low before driving a car or participating in other activities. Others are less careful. Everyone pays the price from the latter group.

Currently, legal restrictions include working in the military, commercial truck driving and flying a passenger plane. Some state and local governments may also deny employment in the police or fire-fighting forces, but this is changing. Most physicians also recommend that people who have frequent low blood sugars do not work at heights, operate heavy equipment or handle toxic substances. Working rotating shifts can also result in more difficulty with blood sugar management. Generally, if the rotations are on a monthly or greater basis, it is possible to alter the insulin dosage to cope. The use of an insulin pump, of basal and rapid-acting insulin, and of a CGM or artificial pancreas can be very effective in providing shift workers the ability to maintain optimal blood sugar levels.

Are psychological problems more or less common in children and adolescents with diabetes compared with people without diabetes?

Psychological problems occur at the same or higher rate in children and adolescents with diabetes compared to those without diabetes. People with chronic diseases tend to have higher rates of psychological problems, which can affect management of their disease. It is not uncommon for those with diabetes to have difficulties and stressors that come and go throughout their life, including feelings of guilt, anger, frustration, sadness, and anxiety. Sometimes these feelings don't go away and start affecting their lives and their diabetes care and need to be addressed by behavioral health counselors. Additional counseling or treatment may be necessary and helpful.

CHAPTER 18

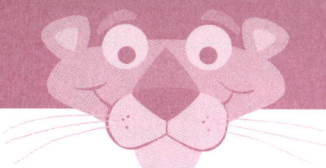

Care of Children at Different Ages

INTRODUCTION

Daily diabetes care has grown more complex in recent years. In addition to the usual family responsibilities, it is common for families to:

✔ take four or more blood sugars per day

✔ give three or more shots or insulin boluses each day

✔ use an insulin pump and/or a continuous glucose monitor (CGM)

✔ balance exercise and blood sugar levels

✔ count carbohydrates or follow other food plans

✔ constantly be on the lookout for high or low blood sugars and ketones

Optimal blood sugar management requires the active involvement of parents for many years. The belief that children should be encouraged to do all their own diabetes care at an early age is misguided. As with all youth, there will be periods of "ups and downs." However, having a supportive (but not overbearing) parent(s) gives the youth the best chance for acceptance of diabetes and its responsibilities. **Diabetes is a family disease.**

Children of different ages are able to do different tasks and to accept different responsibilities. It is important not to expect more from children than they are able to do. If they are unable to do the tasks, they may develop a sense of failure and poor self-esteem, resulting in poor self-care. Family members need to watch for signs that the child needs more

> **TOPICS:**
> **Psychosocial Adjustment**
> **Goal Setting and Problem Solving**
>
> **TEACHING OBJECTIVES:**
> The teacher will:
> 1. Present the importance of long-term family support and involvement in diabetes management.
> 2. Define age-appropriate skills and tasks.
>
> **LEARNING OBJECTIVES:**
> Learner (parents, child, relative or self) will be able to:
> 1. Outline family support roles for diabetes management.
> 2. Identify at least one age-appropriate sign of readiness for learning diabetes skills/tasks.

assistance, especially during times of more frequent high or low blood/CGM glucose levels.

Goals for blood/CGM sugar levels and HbA1c values for children of different ages are discussed in Chapters 7 and 14.

The ability to do certain tasks may vary from day to day, and parents must be available to help as needed. Children should be encouraged to gradually assume care for themselves as they are able. The ability to successfully live independently, both in everyday life and with diabetes care, is the eventual goal for all our children.

A part of the goal of this chapter is to review "normal" child development and how it relates to diabetes care. Although parts of this chapter may not be important for each reader,

TABLE 1:
Age-Related Responsibilities and Traits

	Non-diabetes-related	Diabetes-related
Age below 3 years	• developing gross motor skills • developing speech skills • learning to trust • responding to love	• parents must do all care • acceptance of diabetes care as part of normal life • parents may give shots (pump boluses) after seeing what is eaten • CGM use is common
Age 3-7 years	• imaginative/concrete thinkers • cannot think abstractly • self-centered	• parent does all tasks • gradually learns to cooperate for blood/CGM glucose levels and insulin shots • inconsistent with food choices – may still need to give shots after meals • gradually learns to recognize hypoglycemia • undeveloped concept of time • adult needs to do all insulin pump management
Age 8-12 years	• concrete thinkers • more logical and understanding • more curious • more social • more responsible	• can learn to do own blood sugars (look at CGM values) • at age 10 or 11, can draw up and give shots (boluses) on occasion, although they still need supervision • can make own food choices; can learn initial carb counting • do not appreciate that doing something now (e.g., optimal diabetes control) helps to prevent later problems (e.g., diabetes complications) • can recognize and treat hypoglycemia • by 11 or 12 years, can be responsible for remembering snacks, but may still need assistance of alarm watches or parent reminders • can do own insulin pump boluses (or shots), but needs adult help to remember to give 20 minutes prior to meals
Age 13-18 years	• more independent • behavior varies • body image important • away from home more • more responsible • abstract thinking • able to understand the importance of doing something now to prevent problems in the future	• capable of doing the majority of shots or insulin pump management and blood/CGM glucose measurements, but still needs parental involvement and review to make decisions about dosage and parental reminders regarding premeal insulin • knows which foods to eat; can do carbohydrate counting • gradually recognizes the importance of optimal sugar management to prevent later complications • may be more willing to inject multiple shots (or pump boluses) per day

individual sections may be helpful. It must be remembered that all children develop at different rates (and our own children are always the most advanced). Table 1 summarizes the non-diabetes and the diabetes-related responsibilities and traits for different age groups. Table 2 lists average ages of mastery for various diabetes-related skills. **Age alone, as a guideline, does not tell us when an individual child is ready to assume tasks.** There is no such thing as a "magic age" when the diabetes suddenly becomes the responsibility of the child or teenager. Be patient! Independence takes a long time. The suggestions below may vary for any given child or family. Diabetes is a **"family disease,"** and the family must work together. Family members need to help each other. Sharing tasks will help avoid the diabetes care from becoming the responsibility of just one person.

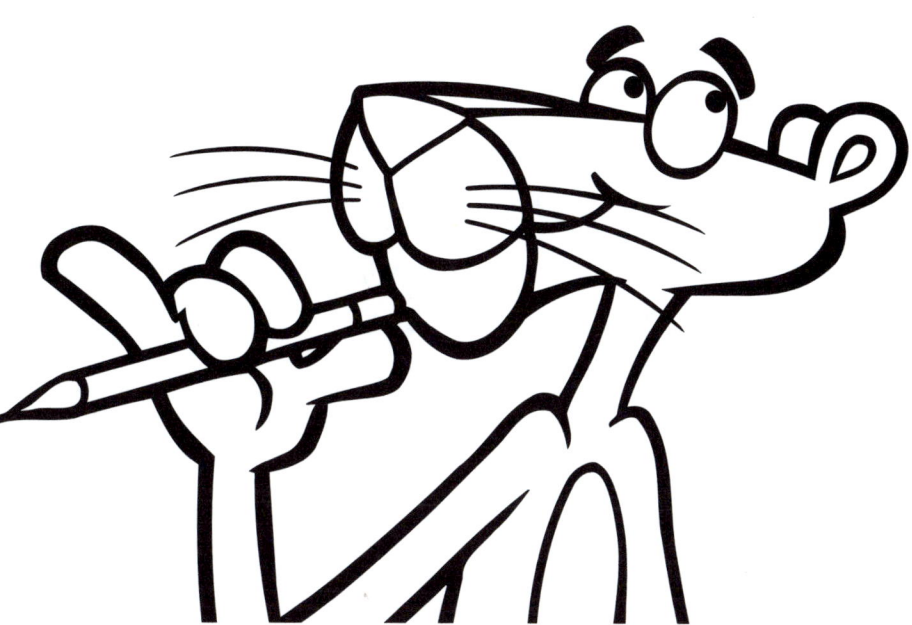

TABLE 2:
Average Ages for Diabetes-Related Skills

Skill	Age of Mastery (in years)	
	Recommended by the American Diabetes Association	Survey of Care Providers
A. Hypoglycemia		
1. Recognizes and reports	8-10	4-9
2. Able to treat	10-12	6-10
3. Anticipates/prevents	14-16	9-13
B. Blood glucose determinations	8-10	7-11
C. Insulin injection		
1. Gives to self (at least sometimes)	—	8-11
2. Draws two insulins	12-14	8-12
3. Able to adjust doses	14-16	12-16
D. Diet		
1. Identifies appropriate pre-exercise snack	10-12	10-13
2. States role of diet in care	14-16	9-15
3. Able to alter food in relation to blood glucose level	14-16	10-15

Abstracted from a survey done by Drs. T. Wysocki, P. Meinhold, D.J. Cox and W.L. Clarke ("Diabetes Care" 11:65-68, 1990).

CARE OF CHILDREN AT DIFFERENT AGES

Child Under 3 Years

Traits and Responsibilities Not Related to Diabetes

This is a time of rapid development of a small, wondrous creature who eats, sleeps, cries, soils diapers and starts to learn about the world.

Motor and brain development are the most rapid of any time in life:

- ✔ sitting (6-8 months)
- ✔ crawling (6-12 months)
- ✔ walking (12-18 months)
- ✔ language development

These developments open up a whole new world.

Accidents are the infant's major danger. *They must be protected from:*

- ✔ stairs where they might fall
- ✔ poisons and medicines they might swallow (from cupboards, garages and purses)
- ✔ auto accidents
- ✔ other dangers (including coffee tables with sharp edges)

All infants with or without diabetes need love. Parents and care-providers need to cuddle and hold infants frequently throughout the day.

This is particularly true after shots and blood sugars, as infants do not understand parents causing pain. Parents must remember that the blood sugars and shots are essential to their infant's life, and they must move beyond feelings of guilt (as discussed in Chapter 10). Much of the fussing around blood/CGM glucose measurements and shots is due to the interruption in the child's activity rather than pain. Infants develop trust during this period and combining the diabetes care with love will help to make it a part of normal life. Young

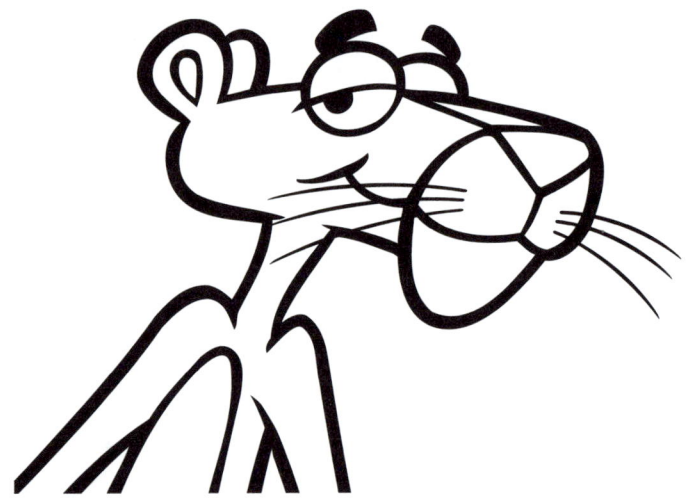

adults often look back with appreciation to their parents for the shots and care they gave them when they were young.

Responsibilities Related to Diabetes

Although babies and toddlers are not able to do any of their own self-care, the following are some special suggestions that may help parents (also see Chapter 19).

- ✔ **Blood/CGM sugar checking:**
  - Toes are used more frequently as a site.
  - The BD Ultrafine™ 33-gauge lancets are smaller and may hurt less. The Accu-Chek FastClix allows dialing a depth from 0.5 to 5.5 and contains six lancets built-in to change daily.

More frequent blood sugar levels or use of a continuous glucose monitor (**CGM**; see Chapter 29), are usually needed. This is because the babies and toddlers cannot tell if their blood sugar levels are low. Over half of infants in this age group in the U.S. (and in our Clinic) now use a CGM.

The parents may learn to recognize a cry, crankiness or body movements that are different than usual and that indicate a need to check a blood sugar level. Teething can be a difficult time when more blood sugars are needed to separate a low blood sugar from normal fussiness. The temptation to let an infant nap longer than usual is offset by the possibility of hypoglycemia.

- ✓ **Blood/CGM glucose levels:**
  - The fasting/pre-meal blood/CGM glucose level to aim for in children under age 6 years is higher (80-180 mg/dL [4.5-10.0 mmol/L]; see Chapter 7), as severe lows may be more dangerous to the infant's rapidly developing brain. We suggest values between 130 and 200 mg/dL (7.2-11.1 mmol/L) at bedtime and during the night. When the family is ready, they may want to consider use of a CGM. There are obvious advantages to being able to look at the CGM glucose values throughout the day.
  - Low glucose levels can be treated with less carbohydrates than for an older child (usually 5-10g due to smaller body size). This amount is found in 1/4 cup of milk, orange or apple juice or 2-3 oz of sugar pop (soda), although the amount needed may vary from infant to infant.
  - Infants who suck on a bottle of milk or juice frequently during the day or night will tend to have higher blood/CGM glucose levels. Overnight sucking on a bottle can also lead to dental decay.

- ✓ **Shots:**
  - Shots are sometimes given while the infant is sleeping (if he/she tends to get very upset). If the child squirms or awakens at the time of the shot, the dad (or mom) should reassure the child. A statement such as, "It is just Daddy (or Mommy) giving you your insulin" may be all that is needed.
  - The bottom (buttock) is used more frequently as a place to give the shot.
  - Insulin pumps are often used in this age group (and in all age groups) with success. Approximately half of diabetic toddlers and preschoolers in the U.S. are now treated with insulin pumps. If the family is ready to consider pump therapy, the option should be discussed with their diabetes care-providers (also see Chapters 19 and 28).
  - Eating is often variable, and parents can wait to give the shot until they see what is eaten. This is easiest to do when the rapid-acting Humalog/NovoLog/Apidra insulin is being used. The dose of insulin can then be reduced if intake is low. HbA1c values will be a bit higher as a result of this practice. However, the safety of avoiding a low blood sugar offsets this concern.
  - The amount of time taken to eat a meal should be the same for all the children, with or without diabetes. Special treatment can result in eating problems. It is important for the parents to stay in control.
  - The amount of rapid-acting insulin is kept low due to body size and due to an increased sensitivity to rapid-acting insulin. With the insulin syringes currently available, it is not usually necessary to dilute insulins. Most parents learn how to judge half-unit dosages using the 0.3 cc (30 unit) insulin syringes. The Precision Sure Dose® 0.3 cc syringes have markings for half-unit measurements (Chapter 9). Similarly, the BD Pen Mini®, the NovoPen Junior, the NovoPen Echo cartridge pen and the Lilly HumaPen LUXURA HD (Chapter 9) can deliver half-unit increments.

It is important for parents of infants with diabetes to incorporate the diabetes into their everyday lives. Children learn through imitation. If parents have adjusted to the diabetes and can view their child with the same positive feelings they had prior to the diagnosis of diabetes, it will help the child to grow up feeling positive and psychologically healthy. A summary of non-diabetes and diabetes traits for each age group is shown in Table 1.

Ages 3-7 Years

(Also see Chapter 19)

Traits and Responsibilities Not Related to Diabetes

✓ *They think concretely.* Concrete thinking means things are either black or white, right or wrong, good or bad. They do not think abstractly. For example, they are unable to realize that "Having a shot of insulin will help me to stay healthy." Instead, a shot may be considered a punishment for doing something wrong. Parents need to repeat over and over that the child hasn't done anything wrong and to try to describe in the child's language why pokes and shots are important.

✓ *They start to see themselves as separate individuals from their parents.* Children gradually become very curious in this period. They often want to know how things work. They can annoy parents with the simple words "how" and "why."

✓ *Children of this age are very self-centered.* They may progress from playing with a toy alone to gradually learning to share a toy or to share the love of their parents. Primary attachments are to parents and family. Interest in other relationships, such as school peers, begins at six to seven years of age.

✓ *Age responsibilities in children 5-7 years old begin to increase dramatically.* They can help pick up their toys, make their bed or put their dirty clothes in the hamper when guided by the parent. They are capable of fixing simple foods, such as cereal or a sandwich, but still do not understand simple dangers such as putting a knife in a toaster or being careful around boiling water. They must have much parental supervision.

✓ *Children 5-7 years old are learning to read, opening a whole new world.* They are discovering many new things, asking lots of questions and practicing new skills. They feel more independent and, in some ways, they are. Usually they are cooperative and love to be helpful. However, they still require a lot of adult supervision.

Responsibilities Related to Diabetes

✓ *The parents must do all diabetes-related tasks.* Fine motor coordination (the coordination of the fingers when handling small items) is not yet fully developed. They cannot do tasks such as accurately drawing insulin into a syringe. This is also true when a child of this age is using an insulin pump. The adult must always be available to do all of the pump management.

✓ *They can gradually learn to cooperate with their parents (e.g., sitting still for blood/CGM glucose activities and insulin shots).* Blood/CGM sugar levels to aim for in children under age six years are listed above and in Chapter 7 (where suggested levels for older-aged children can also be found). CGM use is common in this age group.

✓ *They can help by choosing or cleaning a finger for a blood sugar or by choosing the site for the insulin shot.* Lancets that we prefer for young children's finger pokes are discussed in the "Under Three" section above.

✓ *Children as young as three or four can sometimes recognize low blood sugars.* They can tell parents when they are hungry. Their complaints may be vague or seem strange to us ("Mommy, my tummy tickles," or "Daddy, I don't feel good.") However, these clues can be very helpful to parents. Helping children verbalize the body sensations of low blood sugars is an important task for family members.

✓ *If a shot (e.g., Lantus [Basaglar]/Levemir/Tresiba) is going to be given when the child is asleep, this should be discussed between the child and parents.* Some children will say

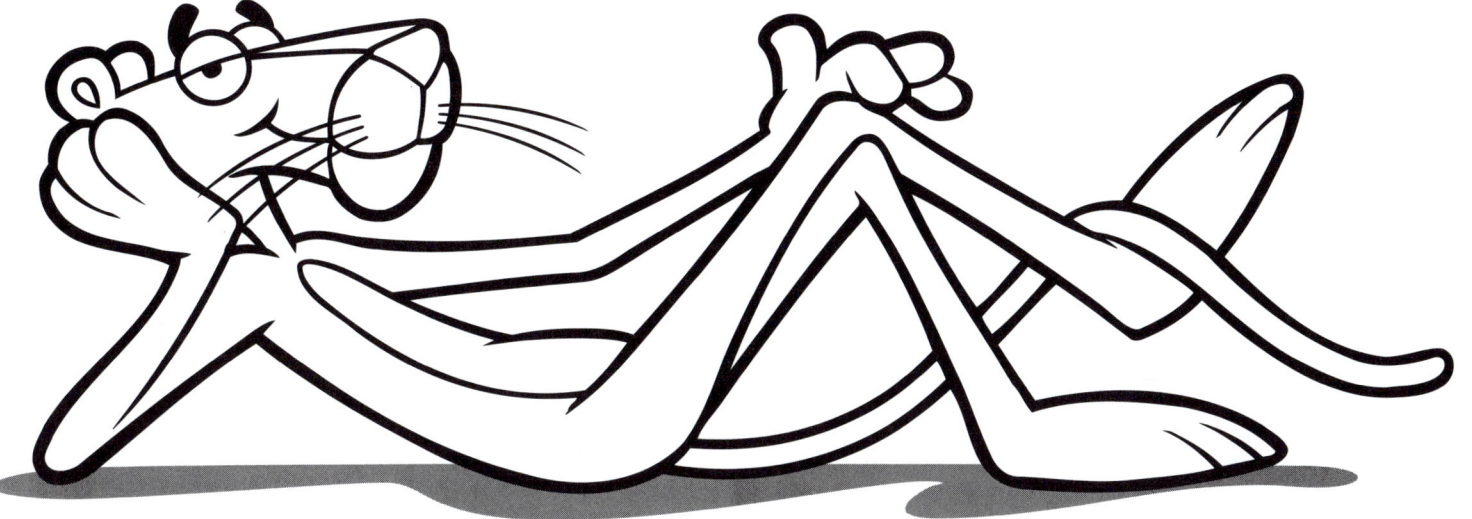

"fine." Others want control and will ask to have the shot given when they are awake.

✔ *By age 5-7 years, recognizing low blood sugars is more completely developed, particularly if the parents have encouraged it.*

✔ *Children of ages 4-7 years may have some concept of which foods they can eat.* They can be taught to ask, "Does it have sugar in it?" or "Do you have a diet pop?" They cannot be expected to always or even very often make the "right" choices over the ones that look or taste good. They will probably choose foods that are similar to what friends or family are eating. They can be expected to have some temper tantrums at being limited in high-sugar food, although healthy family eating habits help this.

There is not much concept of time at this age. An adult will need to make sure that a snack is taken at a specific time. Sometimes a watch that beeps at a set time can be used as a reminder for a snack.

✔ *They usually have no objection to wearing a diabetes ID bracelet or necklace.* It is helpful to get children into the habit of wearing the ID when they are young. This may help them to do this as they get older. Sources of ID bracelets can be found in Chapter 6.

✔ In relation to insulin pumps, parents (adults) are "in charge" of the pump to make certain insulin boluses are consistently given.

✔ Pumps provide more flexibility with insulin doses (by 0.025-unit increments). Multiple doses can be easier with a pump than with shots (see Chapter 28).

It is important for parents of children in this age group (as in all age groups) to keep a positive attitude. Remember the blood/CGM glucose data and insulin shots help to keep the child healthy. Playing games around diabetes chores and gradually getting the child to help (even in little ways) may be beneficial. One fun game is to use quarters or stickers to reward the child for guessing what the blood sugar number will be. Whoever is closest "wins." It will help the child to learn to tell when they are high or low. Hugs and kisses will reassure the child that the parents' love continues. To be able to keep a positive attitude, parents need their own support for their worries and hard work. Friends, family, diabetes support groups or other sources of support can be extremely helpful.

CARE OF CHILDREN AT DIFFERENT AGES

Ages 8-12 Years

Traits and Responsibilities Not Related to Diabetes

✓ *Children of this age continue to think in concrete ways.* They can gradually think more objectively and understand another person's point of view.

✓ *Fairness and meeting their needs are very important.*

✓ *Children at these ages are more social, and peers begin to play a more important role in their lives.* They usually begin to spend nights at friends' houses. They have more peer activities than do younger children. Becoming involved in some team sports can help them to stay involved as they get older (and athletic activity is helpful for diabetes management). This is a great age to do classroom education about diabetes. The more peers understand, the more likely they will be supportive. Peer support is important, especially later during adolescence.

✓ *Children can be helpful by learning to take on increased responsibilities.* They may help with doing dishes, feeding pets, cleaning their own room and other rooms or taking out the garbage. Special rewards, such as stars on a calendar, may be helpful in encouraging certain activities.

✓ *They are capable of more complex food preparation and can better understand safety and danger issues such as using a hot stove.*

Responsibilities Related to Diabetes

✓ *Some children begin to do their own blood sugars at ages 8-10.* CGM use is common.

✓ *At about this age some children wish to begin to give some of their own insulin shots.* The ability to accurately draw up the insulin is a bit slower in developing, but it is usually present at 10 or 11 years of age. The coordination needed between seeing something and using the fingers to successfully do the job (eye-hand coordination, fine motor skills) develops during this age. Use of an insulin pen may help with accuracy. They may learn to give insulin boluses if using an insulin pump. This is an exciting time to watch a child develop. Adult supervision is essential for all of these important tasks.

The child can get "burned out" if:

✓ they begin any of these tasks at too young an age

✓ they have too much responsibility without the parent being available to take over when needed

They will be more likely to rebel later, during the teen years, by missing shots or not checking blood/CGM glucose levels. In addition, they may have difficulty requesting their parents' help when needed if they are expected to perform self-care tasks alone. **Parents must stay involved in diabetes management with this age group!**

✓ *Children of this age sometimes feel that "life isn't fair,"* particularly as it pertains to diabetes. It is helpful to just listen to them if they express such feelings.

✓ *Children may be able to give their own shots when staying at a friend's house.* As children are usually very active when staying at a friend's, we often suggest reducing or omitting the dose of rapid-acting insulin and reducing the dose of the evening long-acting insulin by 10-20 percent. The parent can draw up the shot ahead of time and put it in a small box, toothbrush holder or other container and leave it at the friend's home. They may ask the friend's parent to supervise the shot (or pump bolus). It is important to remember to roll a syringe containing NPH insulin between the hands to re-mix it prior to giving the shot.

It is also essential that the friend's parents be informed about hypoglycemia. The handouts in the school or child-sitters sections (Chapters 25 and 26) may be helpful.

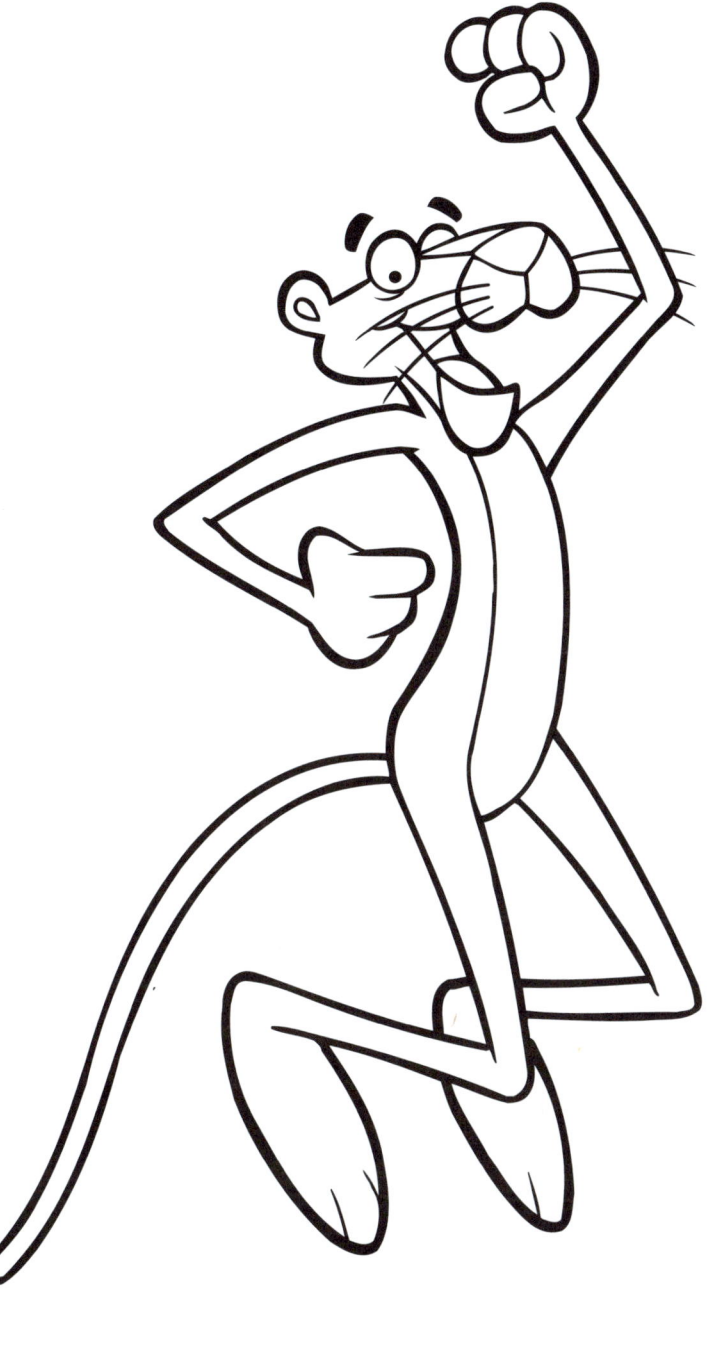

✔ *Children of this age can eat lunch at school and make choices to avoid high sugar foods.* Some will begin to learn to count carbohydrates.

✔ *They can gradually learn to recognize and treat their own hypoglycemic reactions.*

✔ *They are also more aware of time and can learn to be responsible for eating a snack at a set time.*

✔ *Insulin pumps and CGMs are often considered by the family in this age group.* It is important for the family to meet with all diabetes care team members before transitioning to a pump (Chapter 28). This helps to determine who is truly ready to start using the pump. Children of this age can start to assume some pump-related activities/responsibilities.

✔ *Sports can be very important at this age.* A child who learns to enjoy athletics is starting a healthy pattern for his/her life as well as for managing diabetes. Parents of the child in this age range must be patient in teaching the child about diabetes and how to do diabetes-related tasks. **The parents must still be very involved in supervision of the diabetes care.** They must also be secure enough to let the child begin to assume some responsibilities on his/her road to becoming an independent person. Diabetes camp, group ski trips, hikes or other events allow the children to receive invaluable support from each other and to realize that they are not the only person in the world with diabetes.

Chapters 13 and 28 discuss changes in insulin dosages for safely managing possible low blood sugars in relation to exercise.

CARE OF CHILDREN AT DIFFERENT AGES

Ages 13-18 Years

(Also see Chapter 20)

Traits and Responsibilities Not Related to Diabetes

✓ *Teens gradually develop independence and a sense of their own identity.* As noted in Chapter 20, "Special Challenges of the Teen Years," this age group varies greatly between wanting independence versus needing supervision and guidance. Some rebellious behavior may be demonstrated toward parents as teens grow into separate individuals.

✓ *Skills increase greatly in this age group.* Automobiles can be driven legally, and power lawn mowers can (hopefully) be used. Teenagers may take jobs to earn their own money. Activities, in general, are greatly increased.

✓ *Body image becomes a major concern.* Teenagers worry about how others view them. The slightest pimple may become a catastrophe. Early in this period, friends of the same sex are very important, whereas later, interest in the opposite sex usually begins.

✓ *More time is spent with friends.*

✓ *The older teen is away from the home more and stays out later with friends.*

✓ *Experimentation with alcohol or illegal drugs at some point may occur.*

Responsibilities Related to Diabetes

✓ *Teens gradually take over more of their diabetes care.* Parents still need to be available to assist with friendly reminders and with giving a shot from time to time. They may need to take over the diabetes care for a period of time if the youth seems "burned out." Teens generally do better if they get extra help, particularly with insulin dosage. A decrease in the number of blood sugar checks per day is a major reason for the HbA1c value increase in teenagers. Use of a CGM can be very helpful.

As noted in Chapter 20, **A SUPPORTIVE ADULT CAN BE AN ASSET FOR A PERSON WITH DIABETES, REGARDLESS OF AGE.** Even parents of older teens still need to help with making sure adequate diabetes supplies are available (and paying for them) and making sure that clinic appointments are made and kept every three months. Parents should come to the clinic, although the staff may request to see a teen individually to discuss issues that may be difficult to talk about with parents present.

✓ *Many teens dislike the chore of writing blood sugar results in a logbook or emailing results to the care-providers.* If the parents agree to do this (with the teenager's OK), it is a way for the parents to keep tabs on the diabetes. Having values written down or downloaded (and faxed or emailed to the diabetes care-provider if needed) is important in looking at trends and knowing when changes in insulin dosages need to be made. If using a CGM, the family should do a weekly download of the data and discuss the results and any insulin dose changes. Results can also be sent to the care-providers if the family has questions.

✓ *Experimentation with alcohol may upset the diabetes management (see Chapter 11) and can cause severe hypoglycemia.*

✓ *Experimentation with illegal drugs upsets schedules and diabetes as well. The use of drugs can result in:*

- impaired judgment
- increased appetite and higher blood sugars
- loss of incentive for optimal diabetes management
- eating meals irregularly

✔ *Peer support can help the continuation of:*
   - an exercise regimen
   - a healthy diet
   - a consistent lifestyle
   - not using tobacco products (an added risk for diabetic complications). Most people who are going to use tobacco will begin prior to age 20 years. Usually, if the peer group does not smoke or chew, the youth will make a similar choice. Identification with peers is so important in this age group that their support (or lack of it) may greatly affect the teen's diabetes management.

✔ *A belief in God and church, synagogue or mosque activities may help guide the teen.*

✔ *Continued involvement with parents can provide stability, limits, love and support.*

✔ *Grandparents and other relatives can be a tremendous help at any age (see Chapter 26).*

✔ *There is often a feeling of invincibility or "it can't happen to me." Regular clinic visits at this age may help the teen realize that diabetes care and responsibility are important. Teens with diabetes are faced with more difficult tasks and more serious life issues than their peers. Teens with diabetes often seem to mature earlier than teens without diabetes. They learn at an earlier age when they have to be serious in life and when they can have fun.*

✔ *Transition to college or to an adult care-provider are discussed in Chapter 20.*

✔ *Insulin pump use is often considered in this age group (Chapter 28), if not begun earlier.* **Transition to a pump is more successful if**

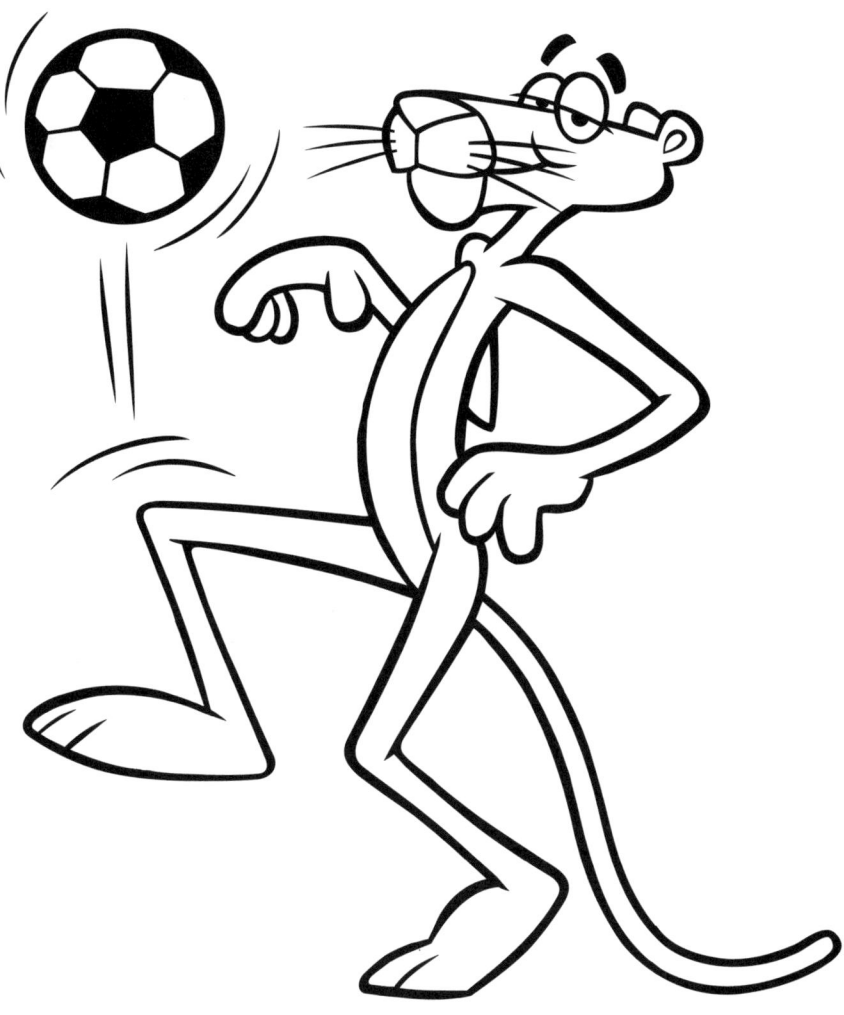

this is the teen's choice. If the parents "push" for an insulin pump, but the teen is not ready, there is a lower chance for success. It is important to have the help of the entire diabetes care team when making this decision. Readiness for the pump can be assessed together. This age group is often quicker than parents in learning the use of the pump (a mini-computer). Glucose levels will improve ONLY if meal and snack boluses are remembered. This activity can often require adult help.

The parents' role for the teenager is to be available to help when either forward or backward steps toward adult maturity are taken. Providing support, stability, limits and love are essential at this difficult age (as at all ages).

Age alone should not be the primary factor in deciding that a person should assume responsibility for diabetes self-management. Parents who offer continued assistance and who share the responsibilities with the teen will generally have a teen with better diabetes management.

The average ages for mastering tasks as recommended by the American Diabetes Association and by a survey of care-providers are shown in Table 2.

DEFINITIONS

Fine motor control: The ability to carefully move the fingers with precision (e.g., drawing insulin to an exact line on a syringe). This ability usually develops around age 10 or 11.

Hand-eye coordination: The ability to use the hands to finely adjust what is seen with the eyes. This ability usually develops around the age of 10.

Self-esteem: How a person feels about himself/herself.

QUESTIONS AND ANSWERS FROM NEWSNOTES

Q It seems like every time our eight-year-old son stays at his friend's house, or has his friend stay overnight at our house, he has low blood sugar the next morning. Should we be making changes?

A "Overnights" are an important social and developmental step in our society. It is important that a bedtime snack is also available. Remember the "pizza factor," that pizza tends to keep a blood sugar up better than most other foods. If there is a frozen pizza in the freezer, it may be a good night to eat it. It is also wise to awaken the child at a reasonable time in the morning and to get a glass of juice or milk down sooner rather than later.

Do remember that if the child is able to do a shot but is not yet old enough to draw it up, the morning insulins can be pre-drawn. The syringe(s) can be put into a little box or toothbrush holder. If NPH is part of the morning insulin, the syringe containing the NPH (± rapid-acting insulin) can be rolled between the child's hands for mixing. Think about reducing the dose again for the morning shot if it is likely that the two friends will be playing together much of the next day.

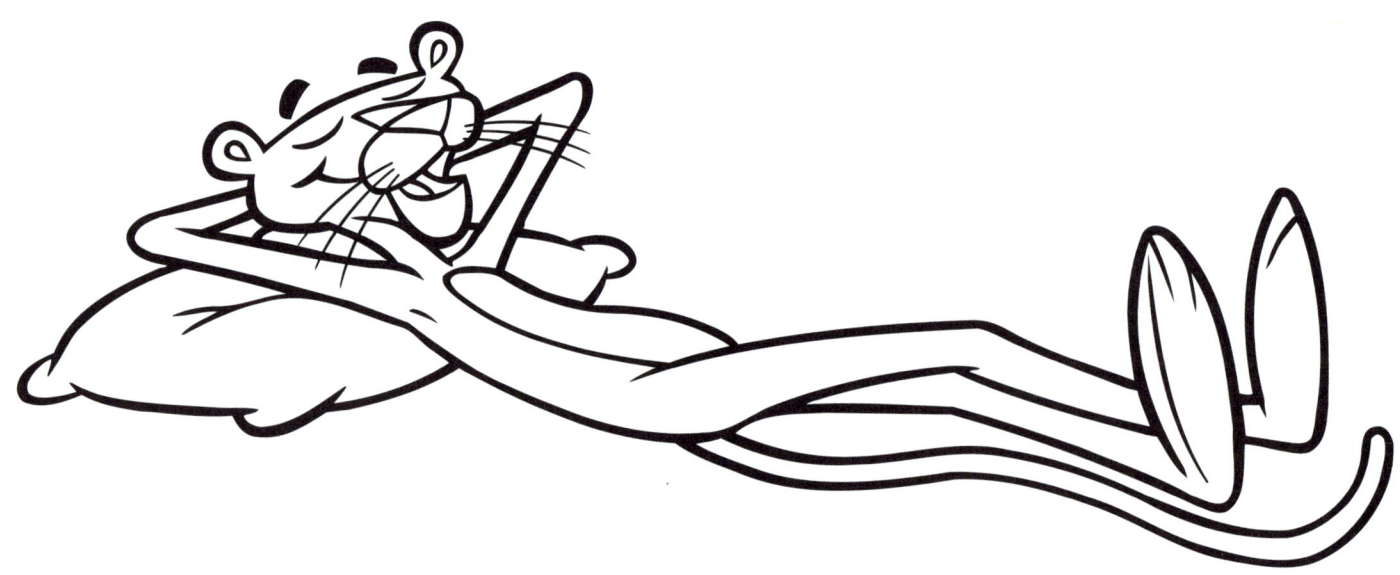

CHAPTER 19

Diabetes Management in the Toddler/Preschooler

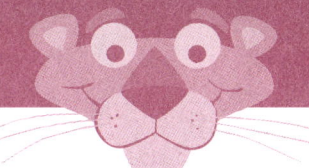

Preschool children (age six and under) make up about 10 per cent of all children and adolescents with type 1 diabetes. It has been clearly shown that diabetes is NOT due to infant immunizations, and these are important for all children. Consuming cow's milk protein in infancy has also been ruled out as a factor. The causes of diabetes are discussed in Chapter 3.

As with all age groups, family education about the many aspects of diabetes covered in this book is essential. Diabetes education for preschools/schools (Chapter 25) and for other care-providers (Chapter 26) is also essential.

Chapter 18, Responsibilities of Children at Different Ages, has special sections dealing with "Children Under Three Years" and "Ages Three to Seven Years." Chapter 18 deals with typical traits for these age groups that are not diabetes-related, as well as traits that are related to diabetes. For this age group, all diabetes responsibilities fall on the parents or other caregivers.

The focus of this chapter is on helping the parents to incorporate blood sugar and/or continuous glucose monitoring, insulin administration (by shots or insulin pump), and other diabetes care as part of the child's normal life. The four- and five-year-old child can gradually learn to cooperate with diabetes-related tasks, even though they cannot yet reliably do the tasks. They may also begin to recognize low blood sugars and to tell the parent/care-provider when those occur. A healthy lifestyle, including exercise (Chapter 13) and nutritional management (Chapter 12), are as important for this age group as for older children.

TOPICS:
Psychosocial Adjustment
Goal Setting
** and Problem Solving**
Medications (Insulin)

TEACHING OBJECTIVES:
The teacher will:
1. Present the importance of long-term family support and involvement in the diabetes management.
2. Discuss options for insulin therapy, pump and continuous glucose monitor (CGM) use in the toddler/preschooler.

LEARNING OBJECTIVES:
Learner (parents, child, relative or self) will be able to:
1. Outline family support roles for diabetes management.
2. Identify what is most important in the treatment of a toddler or preschooler and what this might involve.
3. Identify the best option for insulin therapy for the child, and possible advantages of insulin pump therapy.
4. Identify advantages of use of a CGM.

The major focus of the present chapter will be to discuss insulin management in the preschooler. Parents often ask if there is anything they can do to keep their infant's pancreas working longer. This includes questions about achieving lower sugar levels or about using dietary supplements. Unfortunately, there are no dietary supplements that have been proven to help. Similarly, a recent study showed that even starting an insulin pump and continuous glucose monitor (CGM) at the time of diagnosis did not preserve insulin production for this age group. What then is the goal of insulin therapy for the preschooler?

THE NUMBER ONE GOAL FOR THE TREATMENT OF THE PRESCHOOLER IS SAFETY. **This includes minimizing severe hypoglycemia and hyperglycemia (with or without ketones).** Other goals include incorporating diabetes care into the daily routine as early as possible. There is no one magic formula for safety or convenience. What works best for one family may not be the answer for another family.

BLOOD SUGAR AND HbA1c LEVELS (See Chapters 7 and 14)

We generally recommend a goal for blood/CGM sugars in this age group of 70 to 180 mg/dL (3.9-10 mmol/L). It is often wise to have 8 to 12 blood sugar checks per day in young children. This is due to their inability to recognize hypoglycemia. If the child enters a "honeymoon" period (Chapter 2), it is common to see frequent values down to 70 mg/dL (3.9 mmol/L). This is the lower level of normal for all people and is not a concern, even though the recommended lower levels in the Table are higher. In 2015, the American Diabetes Association (ADA) changed their recommendations for blood sugar levels and advised the same goals for children of all ages (see Table). For children who are not having excessive hypoglycemia, and particularly when a CGM and insulin pump are used, the ADA recommendations are appropriate.

It is now recommended that children of all ages have HbA1c values below 7.5% (<58 mmol/mol). This goal has an aim of decreasing the number of high blood sugars and episodes of acidosis (Chapter 15). There is now evidence that high blood sugars and episodes of ketoacidosis may have adverse effects on the developing brain (as with low blood sugar).

Achieving even lower HbA1c values in this age group may be possible, especially in the honeymoon period, but must be balanced with the primary goal of safety (see Table).

CONTINUOUS GLUCOSE MONITORING
(**CGM**; See Chapter 28)

As with insulin pumps, CGMs can be discussed with the diabetes care team **when the family is ready.** The CGM may provide convenience in not having to do so many finger, toe, or heel pokes for blood sugar levels. Alarms for high and low sugar levels may be helpful. With consistent use of an insulin pump and a CGM, HbA1c levels and safety are usually both enhanced. Computer connections are available for parents' bedrooms, and alarms are helpful. In addition, apps are now available to continuously monitor the child's glucose values from a distance. The Dexcom SHARE™ allows parents or caregivers to remotely receive notifications about glucose levels and trends on their Apple iPhone® or iPod® Touch (see Chapter 29). The Guardian™ Connect CGM will also transmit CGM glucose values to an iPhone® or Android® phone.

The major drawback is once again body "real estate." The diabetes nurse-educator can help to determine if adequate fat is available for both an insulin pump and a CGM. Chapter 29 discusses CGMs in detail and the Pump/CGM book (see above) provides further information.

INSULIN THERAPY
(See Chapter 8)

A. Basal Insulin

First, when possible, "basal-bolus" insulin therapy should be used. Previous research has shown that low blood sugars in preschoolers are less likely to occur using a basal insulin (e.g., Lantus [Basaglar], Levemir, Tresiba, or an insulin pump) in comparison to NPH insulin.

TABLE:
ADA Blood Glucose and HbA1c Recommendations for All Children

Before Meals	Bedtime/Overnight	A1C	Rationale
90-130 mg/dL (5.0-7.2 mmol/L)	90-150 mg/dL (5.0-8.3 mmol/L)	<7.5% (<58 mmol/mol)	A lower goal (<7.0% or 53 mmol/mol) is reasonable if it can be achieved without excessive hypoglycemia.

Key concepts in setting glycemic goals:
- Goals should be individualized, and lower goals may be reasonable based on benefit-risk assessment.
- Blood glucose goals should be modified in children with frequent hypoglycemia.
- Post-meal blood/CGM glucose values should also be checked routinely. When possible, CGM use is valuable.
- It should be realized that the ADA recommendations for blood/CGM sugar levels in this age group are different from the values that we suggest (Chapters 7 and 14).

The evening NPH insulin peaks during the night, increasing the risk of nighttime lows. Since the brain is still increasing in cell numbers during the first four years after birth, low blood sugars may be detrimental. We usually suggest giving the basal insulin in the morning in this age group. Then, if the insulin does not last for 24 hours, the insulin activity falls off during the early hours of the next morning, reducing the likelihood of early morning lows. Some families give it in the buttocks before the child awakens.

B. Bolus Insulin (Humalog, NovoLog, Apidra)

The rapid-acting insulin for meals is sometimes divided if eating is inconsistent, giving part of the dose before the meal and the remainder during or after the meal. This is easiest to do when using an insulin pump (see below). It is risky if a shot/bolus has been given and the child does not eat. Giving the shot/bolus after the meal results in higher blood/CGM sugar values after meals (in contrast to giving it 20 minutes before meals as in older age groups, see Chapter 9), but results in increased safety. The dose, or part of the dose, can be chosen after seeing what the child eats. This is a compromise to avoid hypoglycemia and can be changed when the child starts to eat consistently. If using an artificial pancreas, there will be an increase in insulin as a result of the meal blood sugar rise, and the usual meal bolus will need to be reduced. If a very young infant is nursing, start with a low dose (one-half or one unit) and gradually work up if the blood/CGM sugars at any time after meals are above 180 mg/dL (>10.0 mmol/L). Weighing the infant before and after nursing is tedious and usually not necessary.

Smaller (3ml) vials of Humalog can be ordered from pharmacies. The NDC number (to tell the pharmacist) is 002-7510-17. There is also a 3ml NovoLog FlexPen® and the NovoPen® Junior which give 0.5-unit doses. Hopefully, the co-pay will also be less with lower amounts of insulin.

INSULIN PUMPS

Although insulin pumps (Chapter 28) and CGMs (Chapter 29) are discussed elsewhere, their use in this age group is especially important. Many physicians consider their use, when available, as the preferred method of treatment for young children.

The first question often asked by parents is, "Is pump therapy safe in this age group?" The answer is, "Absolutely, **YES.**" In fact, this age group often has the best results with pump therapy. One of the reasons for this is that day-to-day glucose levels are more variable in this age group, and can be more easily modified when using a pump.

The second question often asked is "When should my infant be placed on an insulin pump?" The answer is simple: **"When the parents are ready."** We do not usually start insulin pumps at the time of diagnosis in this age group, as we feel the parents already have enough to handle, and they need to become comfortable with injections. If the family is ready, an insulin pump can be discussed with the diabetes care team members at the one-week visit or anytime thereafter. Families often worry about other care-providers being able to manage the pump. Data from Yale University shows they do just as well as the parents. There can be some initial stress for the parents with pump initiation, but this usually subsides in a few weeks.

Another reason for considering a pump is for the convenience of both the infant and the parents. Multiple small insulin boluses (for corrections or for food - see Chapter 28) can be given. This often results in eight to 12 boluses per day, which would be difficult if giving shots. For example, a small correction bolus, plus insulin for food most certain to be eaten, can be given before the meal. Then, additional insulin can be given as more carbs are eaten. This can more safely match insulin dosing to the child's needs.

The total units of basal insulin given in a 24-hour period (after the honeymoon) is usually lower in preschoolers (e.g., 0.6 units/kg body weight or 0.27 units/pound body weight) compared to older children. In contrast, teenagers usually need approximately 0.9 units/kg (0.41 units/pound) body weight as basal insulin. In older youth, basal insulin usually provides about half of the total daily dose and bolus insulin the other half.

Preschoolers, however, often need 60 to 80 percent of their daily insulin dose as bolus doses. As discussed in Chapter 28, the use of temporary basal rates (for low or high blood sugar levels) can be very helpful in management. The toddler who has an active play day often does best with a 50 percent basal insulin reduction during play and another 20 percent reduction from 9 p.m. to 3 a.m. (just like older children). This approach can help to reduce the likelihood of delayed hypoglycemia during the night (see Chapter 6).

Two studies have not found significant differences in HbA1c values as a result of insulin pump use in young infants. However, this may vary between families. The major reasons for pump use in this age group are safety and convenience.

Parents sometimes wonder if adequate "real estate" is available on their infant to place a pump. Fortunately, even infants have adequate fat in the buttocks, and the upper buttocks (seat) is where the pump catheter is usually inserted. The pump trainer will assist with suggesting sites and methods for cleanliness. Chapter 28 discusses pumps in greater detail, and a pump/CGM/artificial pancreas book is also available (see order form in the back of this book).

PSYCHOLOGICAL ASPECTS

A. Preschoolers:

Allowing an older preschooler to pick the next infusion site position can make the task easier to accomplish. A reward system (e.g., stickers) for each site change can also be helpful. Pump cases with belts or fanny packs often work better than clipping them on the child's clothing. Picking out his or her own pump case can also encourage the child to feel some ownership of their diabetes, and some children even give their pump a name. During site changes, a child may choose to use numbing cream such as EMLA or LMX to minimize pain, but this can be left to the child to decide.

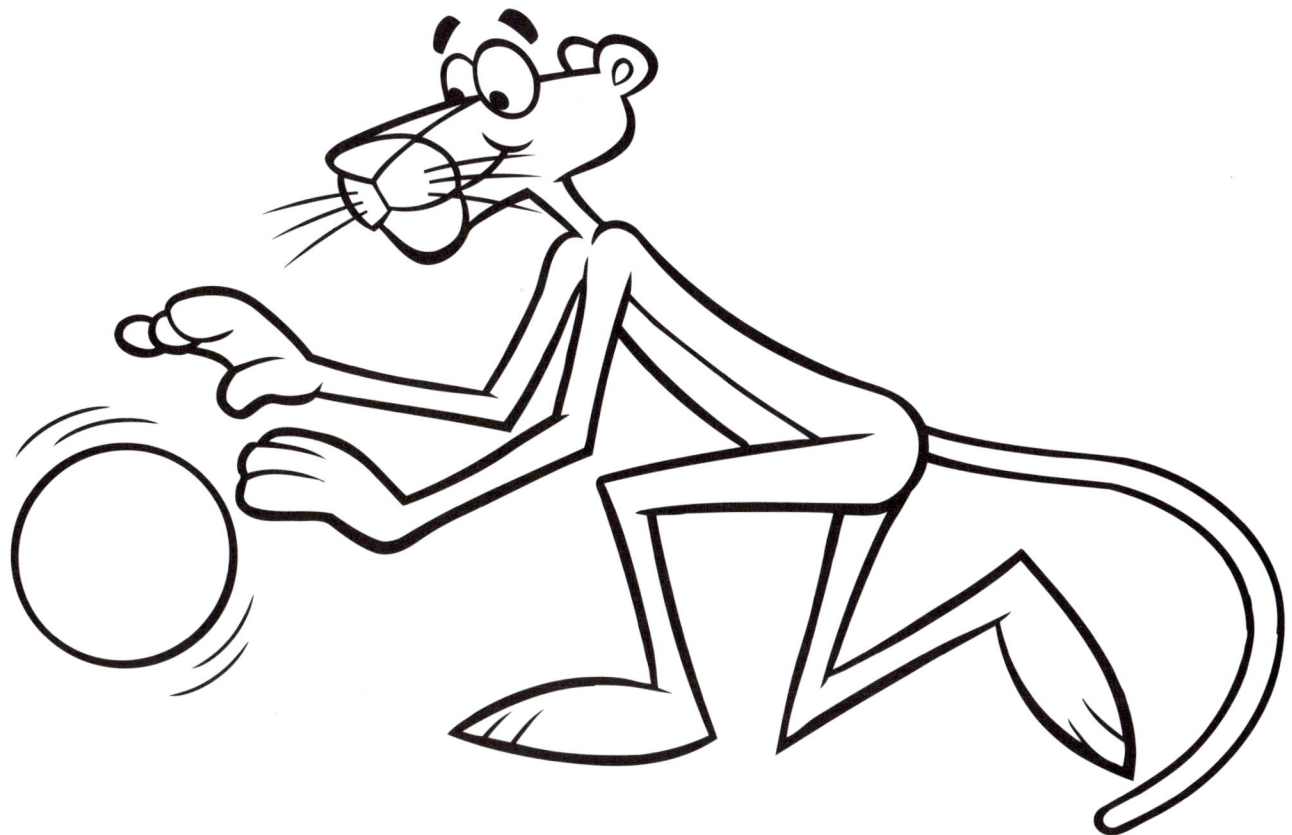

B. Parents:

Some studies (not all) have reported an improved quality of life for the parents of preschoolers using insulin pumps and CGMs. Some observers note that the management of diabetes with a pump is associated with higher degrees of stress (particularly in the early period of pump use). The use of CGM (see below) may reduce the number of blood sugar checks done per day and usually helps with hypoglycemia fears. It can be very comforting for parents to receive their child's CGM glucose levels "via the cloud" when they are apart from each other. Nearly all families of preschool-aged children have chosen to continue pump therapy after participating in research studies.

Parents express that diabetes management style can make a difference. A positive, non-judgmental attitude will likely have a positive influence on the way a young child views and manages his/her type 1 diabetes as he/she gets older. Parents should be encouraged to adopt a "matter-of-fact" approach to the routines (injections/pump site changes, finger pricks, and meal times), treating numbers as just numbers/data points, and not apologizing for aspects of care such as finger pricks, site changes, and injections that cannot be avoided. (From: Hitchcock, Jeff; Dooley, Greg; et. al.: Managing Diabetes in Preschool Children, Pediatric Diabetes, 2017.)

NEONATAL DIABETES

A final reminder—all children diagnosed under the age of six months should be tested for genetic alterations that cause diabetes. They may have a genetic defect that allows treatment with an oral medicine rather than insulin. This genetic defect is rarely found to be the cause of diabetes in anyone diagnosed after age six months.

DEFINITIONS

Neonatal Diabetes: An inherited genetic alteration usually resulting in the onset of diabetes in the first six months after birth. It has many differences from the usual type 1 diabetes and may even be able to be treated with oral medicines.

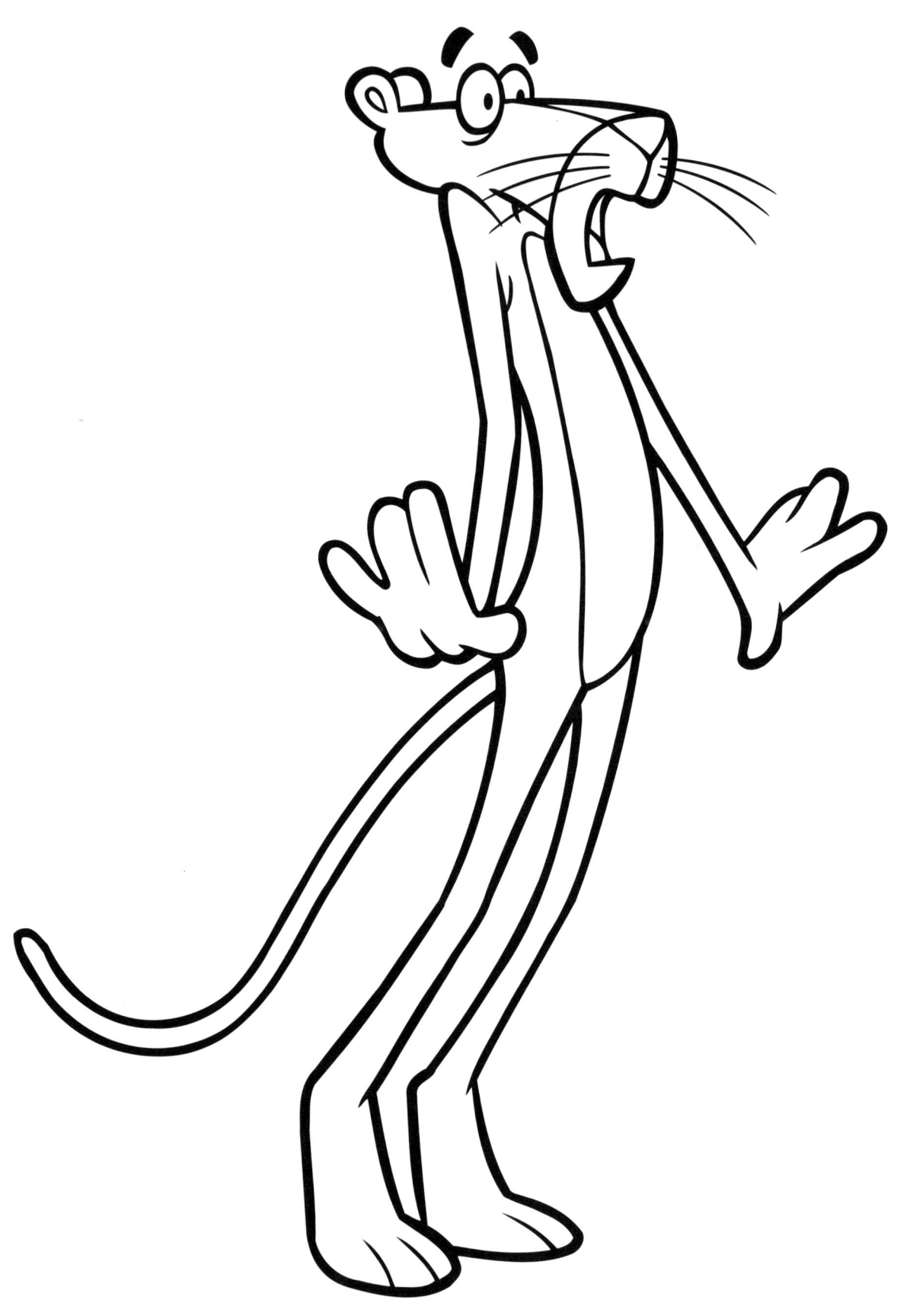

CHAPTER 20

Challenges of the Teen Years

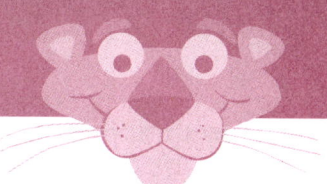

Shideh Majidi, MD
H. Peter Chase, MD
Brigitte I. Frohnert, MD, PhD

- Also see Chapter 18
- This chapter will follow the outline given in Table 1:

A. STRUGGLE FOR INDEPENDENCE

Parents often despair at the thought of their "angelic" child becoming an adolescent. The teen years have been defined as the period in life when one varies between wanting to be a child and wanting to be an adult. These feelings vary from hour-to-hour, day-to-day, week-to-week and year-to-year. The "child" part of the adolescent still wants to be completely dependent on parents and other adults. The emerging "adult" wants to be an entirely independent person. There are many shades between these two extremes that may linger for some time. Parents must realize that this developing person does not always react or reason as an adult. The part of the brain responsible for problem solving, judgement, planning, organization, controlling emotions, impulse control and reasoning continues to develop until the age of 25. Daily life has become more complicated, and the task of independence is not easy. In the past, we believed that children with diabetes should assume their own management at a certain age, and that they would suddenly become independent. **We now know that independence is not age specific and is a**

TOPICS:
**Psychosocial Adjustment
Goal Setting and Problem Solving
Pregnancy**

TEACHING OBJECTIVES:
The teacher will:
1. Discuss how teenagers typically assume responsibility for diabetes care and the role of their family.
2. Discuss special challenges of teen years, including tobacco use, alcohol, substance abuse, sex, identity issues and lifestyle.

LEARNING OBJECTIVES:
Learner (parents, child, relative or self) will be able to:
1. Support teenagers with diabetes to assume independent care for their diabetes.
2. Develop action plan with diabetes provider(s) to minimize health risks.

TABLE 1: Special Challenges for the Teenager

A. Struggle for independence
B. Growth and body changes
C. Identity
D. Peer relationships, alcohol, drugs, tobacco
E. Sexuality
F. Consistency (exercise, eating, emotions and lifestyle)
G. Driving
H. College
I. Emotional changes
J. Transition to an adult diabetes clinic

gradual process. We think of diabetes as a family condition. Daily diabetes care has become far more complicated in recent years. It requires a great deal of parent-child partnership to achieve optimal blood sugar control and healthy independence.

The "child vs. adult" struggle can greatly influence diabetes management during the adolescent years. A teenager may want entire responsibility for the diabetes management at one time – faithfully following blood/CGM glucose levels, exercising, watching food and "treat" intake and taking the responsibility for the injections/boluses, (or oral medicines for type 2). Yet, at another time, blood/CGM glucose values will not be checked unless the parent is there to help, injections/boluses or oral medicines may be forgotten, or "treats" may be consumed in large quantities. Exercise, which is critical for persons with type 1 or type 2 diabetes, may be ignored. Parents can lessen the effects of this variable attitude toward the diabetes care by remaining involved and offering to share these responsibilities with their teenager. Offering to exercise with the teen makes it more fun and challenging for everyone. **We believe that a supportive adult who provides continued and open communication with their child is one key to diabetes care during the adolescent years. Family conflict can occur, but implementing methods of open communication as early as possible can decrease and minimize conflict significantly.**

Parental partnership (involvement) with the teen can be accomplished in a variety of ways:

✔ drawing up and/or giving injections

✔ keeping a logbook or using downloads to record blood/CGM sugars and noting trends and problems

✔ helping to fax/email blood/CGM glucose values to the diabetes care team (fax sheets are found in Chapter 7)

✔ helping with weekend dosing when teens may want to sleep in and could use some assistance

These not only help the teenager, but also help keep the parent "in the loop" and aware of what is going on with management.

Diabetes care is usually NOT the top priority for a teenager. Their main interests may be their peers, schoolwork, sports, a car, a job, etc. (in varying orders of importance for different teens). The parents may need to help in keeping a focus on the care necessary for optimal diabetes management.

If the teenager's actions (or lack of them) result in possible serious dangers to his/her health, then the parents have no choice but to step back in and take over the majority of care for a time. This is particularly true when insulin shots/boluses or oral medicines (with type 2 diabetes) are being missed. Once things are back on course and the teen feels ready to take on more again, responsibility can be shifted. This back-and-forth in degree of care provided by the parent or adolescent is a natural part of the transition to independent care. Remember to take things one step at a time. Just because a young person has had diabetes for many years, that does not mean he or she has assumed ownership of the care. Occasionally, professional counseling is necessary.

The majority of teenagers gradually assume adult independence without too much difficulty. In contrast to the parents' worst fears, they do grow up! In fact, the teenager with diabetes may assume adult responsibilities earlier than other teenagers.

Achieving independence step by step:

The task of how to help children grow to be independent young adults is a challenge for most families. Diabetes complicates that task somewhat. It is normal for parents of children with diabetes to feel anxious about normal separations such as overnights, camp and school trips. Parents worry about injections, low blood/CGM glucose values and whether the schedule and snacks will be remembered. With preparation and supervision, these separation experiences are an important part of growing up and eventually becoming independent. These experiences are also usually a lot of fun for kids. It is best to start with brief periods of separation, like staying at a relative's or friend's house overnight.

- **Overnights**

Staying at a friend's home, even for one night, can be a big step, as can a visit to relatives. This often begins prior to the teen years. We generally suggest a small reduction in insulin dosage (rapid- and long-acting insulins) for overnights at home or away, since young people are usually up later at overnights and tend to burn more energy. This way, the parents do not need to worry quite as much about low blood sugars!

- **Summer Camps**

Follow these short visits with longer stays at a diabetes camp or other summer camps (often beginning prior to the teen years). Youth learn that they CAN survive without parents and parents learn that their children CAN survive without them! (Re-education for both is important.)

- **School and Athletic Trips**

Eventually teens will want to participate in longer school excursions and/or sports trips. With some insulin adjustments and education of staff, these should be a safe and important part of independence and life experience.

- **Clinic Visits**

Teenagers can begin seeing diabetes care team members by themselves at diabetes clinic visits. Parents are still needed at these visits to review plans and problems with their teens and the diabetes care team. Some clinics have teen-group clinics, which can be very helpful in sharing feelings and experiences. As noted in Chapter 18, better diabetes management usually results if parents stay involved in offering continued assistance and sharing responsibilities with the teenager.

B. GROWTH AND BODY CHANGES

The adolescent growth spurt and the development of adult sexual characteristics result in many changes, probably more than occur at any other single time in life.

- **Growth Hormone**

The gain in height seen during puberty is a result of increased hormone levels (growth hormone, testosterone and estrogen). Growth

Julie's Challenge:

Julie is a 16-year-old girl who has had diabetes for seven years. She and her family have always prided themselves on Julie's diabetes control. Julie is a talented dancer and hopes to become a professional dancer someday. She dances on Mondays, Wednesdays and Fridays at 5:30 p.m. At a clinic appointment, it is discovered that her blood sugars have been consistently high with her HbA1c unexpectedly being over 10 percent (>86 mmol/mol). In talking with Julie, she admits to missing evening injections sometimes when she goes to dance class. She says she just doesn't have time to get her homework done, check her blood/CGM sugar value, get her injection done and still get something to eat before leaving for dance class.

PLAN: Julie's parents volunteered to help with the blood/CGM sugar check and injection on those nights and to make some dinner for her. Julie was relieved to have her parents take over some of the diabetes care, but admitted it was hard to ask for help after being responsible for her own diabetes care for several years.

NOTE: Another possibility is the missed shots were done on purpose in order to lose weight for dancing. If so, this is more serious. More discussion on this topic can be found later in this chapter under the topic "Emotional Changes," and in Chapter 17 under "Eating Disorders."

hormone partially blocks insulin activity. Insulin requirements increase dramatically and are usually the highest per pound of body weight that they will ever be. The insulin requirement usually decreases when growth is completed. If blood sugar levels are maintained during puberty, full growth is usually reached. Research from our Center has shown that better growth (to full adult potential) is more likely with optimal sugar levels.

- **Sex Hormones**

Female sexual development includes breast and pubic hair development and the onset of menstrual cycles. These pubertal changes may be slightly delayed in girls with diabetes. Blood/CGM glucose values may increase during menstruation. Many girls will increase their Lantus (Basaglar)/Levemir/Tresiba or pump basal insulin and/or their rapid-acting insulin during this time. Some girls who use an insulin pump will switch to a different basal rate setting to provide more insulin during menses.

Males have enlargement of the testes and penis, and facial and other body hair begins to grow. When body odors become noticeable, for males or females, the use of deodorants is desirable. Acne or pimples ("zits") may develop in either sex, making skin care important. Antibiotics, such as Minocycline or Doxycycline, or other treatments are fine to use if acne becomes a problem. Some athletes may be tempted to try steroid drugs to try to make their muscles larger. Use of these drugs can prevent full height attainment and lead to increased blood cholesterol levels and risk for heart attacks later in life. They also may cause aggressive behavior, resulting in problems getting along with others. The drugs reduce insulin sensitivity and cause increased blood/CGM sugar levels. Non-prescribed steroid drugs should not be used.

- **Thyroid Hormone**

The thyroid gland (in the neck) must function properly during this time, or growth will not progress normally. As part of the regular diabetes check-up visits, the diabetes care-provider will monitor the size and function of the teen's thyroid gland. About half of teenagers with diabetes get some thyroid gland enlargement, although in most cases no treatment is necessary. This is an "autoimmune" disorder, as is diabetes, and is discussed in Chapter 24.

- **Body Image**

Teenagers are often very concerned about "body image" (self-consciousness). Diabetes does not usually result in visible body alterations. Having diabetes may make teens feel different from their peers. Wearing an insulin pump (see Chapter 28) or a continuous glucose monitor (CGM) is often a visible and a constant reminder of having diabetes. This is a reason why an insulin pump or CGM should not be "pushed" on a person until they are ready. The refusal to wear an identification (ID) bracelet or necklace, to wear an insulin pump or CGM or to refrain from eating high-carb foods may relate to not wanting to feel different from peers. Some teens hide their pump or CGM under baggy clothes. They may choose not to give an insulin bolus or not to look at their CGM if eating with friends. As they gain confidence and maturity, they will bolus when needed without regard to their peers. Often, peers can be a helpful, supportive part of a teen's diabetes care.

C. IDENTITY

- **Who Am I?**

Teens are searching for the answer to the question, "Who am I?" It is important to emphasize the positives about who they are at this stage of their lives (e.g., someone who loves a sport, music, mechanics, school plays or other interests) and who only secondarily has diabetes. Reinforcement should be given when a positive attitude toward living with diabetes is demonstrated. Compliments are important. For example, "Good job on managing your blood/CGM glucose measurements even with the stress of finals" (even though the stress and not exercising may have resulted in high values). A sincere offer to record results or give injections during busy times can be helpful for both the teen and the parent.

As later adolescence is reached (often ages 16 to 21 years), a firmer identity with a sense of their future becomes apparent. They are better able to delay gratification and to reason through problems. Practical, realistic goals can start to be set. Reacceptance of parental advice and values often occurs.

- **Risk-taking**

The "in-the-middle" age range of adolescence (approximately ages 14-17 years) is usually the most difficult time. The teen often sees himself/herself as "invincible." Risk-taking and experimentation tend to occur more frequently.

Some of the experimentation may include:

✔ bright hair colors or styles
✔ unusual clothing
✔ piercings
✔ a tattoo(s)

Some diabetes-related risk behaviors are:

✔ "I don't need to wear my diabetes ID; I've got an ID card in my wallet."
✔ "I'm not going to carry sugar; I can get something at my friend's house if I need it."
✔ making poor food choices without taking stteps to maintain sugar control
✔ not checking blood/CGM glucose levels (particularly prior to driving; see section G below)
✔ missing shots/boluses

Regular or more frequent clinic visits and measuring HbA1c levels at this time may help the teen. The HbA1c level is often a measure of how the teen is coping with life, as well as of the sugar management. Parents need to let the teen know that they trust their child to act maturely. Patience on the part of the care-providers and from the parents is a real virtue.

D. PEER RELATIONSHIPS

Peer relationships are very important to teenagers, often more so than relationships with parents. Early in adolescence, close friends are usually of the same sex. In later adolescence this often changes or is "added to" by members of the opposite sex. Being like their peers is very important. Having diabetes and "being different" can be a challenge. Some teenagers are comfortable monitoring blood/CGM glucose levels or giving themselves injections in front of their friends. Others will absolutely refuse to let anyone other than their closest friend know that they have diabetes. The willingness or refusal to wear an ID, as well as doing diabetes tasks in front of friends, may reflect the teen's own degree of acceptance of diabetes.

Much of a teen's identity relates to conforming to their peer group. Peer groups can be important in helping the teen make decisions about the use of drugs, alcohol or tobacco. If the peer group rejects or accepts these, the teen with diabetes may do likewise.

Effects of the use of these substances on diabetes are listed below:

✔ **Tobacco use** (smoking or chewing) affects blood vessels in anyone. Tobacco use by a person with diabetes is particularly harmful as it increases the risk of diabetes complications later in life.

✔ As in all people, **chewing tobacco** can lead to dental problems and cancer of the mouth.

✔ **Smoking cigarettes** is associated with an increased likelihood of lung cancer and heart disease in all people.

✔ **Alcohol consumption** can result in delayed severe insulin reactions and impaired judgment related to diabetes care. (This is discussed in more detail at the end of Chapter 11.)

✔ **Drugs** that alter awareness of time have their greatest effects on diabetes by interfering with consistency in eating and insulin injections. Alterations of judgment can also be very dangerous.

✔ **Chronic drug use (including marijuana)** may result in an "I don't care" attitude toward diabetes management with poor health outcomes.

Warning signs which should alert investigation of behaviors:

✔ withdrawal from the usual routines
✔ change in sleeping pattern (sleeping more/less)
✔ changes in friends
✔ not communicating with family members
✔ mood changes and irritability

Participation in an activity group for teenagers with diabetes can be helpful. We also encourage participation in our group clinics, which includes meeting with other teens who have diabetes. It may help the teenagers share their feelings with others who also have diabetes. They soon realize that others have many of the same feelings that they do, and they are quite normal in spite of having diabetes!

Teens in an area without such groups might find a useful resource on-line, such as www.childrenwithdiabetes.com/fsn (the 'fsn' is for Family Support Network), for information and support.

Research has shown that the teen with diabetes who involves his/her peers by sharing knowledge about diabetes is more likely to have better diabetes management. We encourage teens to bring a friend to the clinic visit to continue to learn how to support a person with diabetes.

E. SEXUALITY

- Teenagers with diabetes run the same risk as non-diabetic teens of contracting diseases such as AIDS, herpes, chlamydia and other sexually transmitted diseases (STDs). It is very important to talk with the healthcare-provider about prevention, protection and contraception to reduce the risk of an unplanned pregnancy or STD.

- PREGNANCY in a woman with diabetes (also see Chapter 30) carries added risks for the baby and the mother.

- Attaining a HbA1c level close to the non-diabetic level PRIOR to becoming pregnant will reduce the risk for miscarriage or birth defects in the baby. Advanced planning for pregnancy is essential for a person with diabetes.

- Research has shown that there is no increased risk for teenage girls with diabetes to use contraception compared with non-diabetic teenage girls.

- The only sure way to absolutely prevent a sexually transmitted disease or pregnancy is to abstain from sex. If the teen chooses to have sex, a condom should always be used. This will help to prevent sexually transmitted diseases, although there is no guarantee for absolute protection.

- **If a male or female believes they cannot cause pregnancy or become pregnant due to diabetes, they are absolutely wrong. People with diabetes can cause a pregnancy or become pregnant just like anyone else.**

- The stress of the teen years may be heightened by conflicts about emerging sexuality, and sensitivity to this is important.

F. CONSISTENCY (EXERCISE, EATING, EMOTIONS AND LIFESTYLE)

The word CONSISTENCY is in capital letters throughout Chapter 12, "Food Management and Diabetes." If everything could be the same every day, diabetes management would be much easier. Unfortunately, there is no such thing as consistency in many teenagers' lives.

Bedtime may be at 10:00 p.m. on school nights but then at midnight or later on Friday and Saturday nights. Many teens like to sleep late on weekends. If the teen is on Lantus (Basaglar)/Levemir/Tresiba insulin or on the pump, this may work well, though we would continue to urge glucose monitoring in the morning to make sure the blood/CGM glucose level is not low. Teens who are still on NPH dosing will need to take their insulin on schedule. We suggest an absolute limit of 9:00 a.m. as the time when the NPH insulin must be taken with at least a small snack. The teenager can then go back to sleep for an hour.

Consistent exercise is often a challenge. Seasonal sports, such as football or soccer, call for heavy exercise for a few months, but may be followed by weeks or months of little activity. Erratic exercise will cause blood/CGM glucose levels to vary. The insulin dose and eating plan may need frequent adjustments for changes in activity level. It is wise to have a "back-up" activity such as biking, walking, jogging or aerobics so that there is some exercise every day. Daily exercise is also very effective in controlling weight. Some teens who use an insulin pump use one set of basals for exercise days and another set for days without exercise.

G. DRIVING

Perhaps no new function in this age group requires more responsibility than the driving of a car. The teen's own life, as well as the lives of friends or total strangers, may be in the balance. **It is essential to check a blood/CGM glucose level before driving.** This is particularly true after a sports activity or exercising. It has been shown that driving with a low blood sugar results in greater impairment than driving when drunk. **FRIENDS DO NOT LET A FRIEND DRIVE WHEN LOW!**

If a person does feel low while driving, it is essential to pull over and have a snack. They should never assume they can "make it" home or to the nearest convenience store. The person

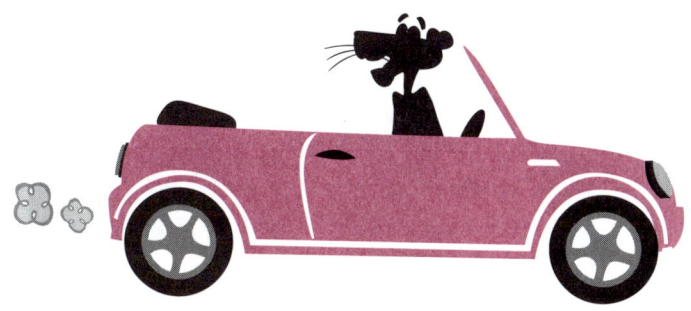

should not resume driving until a repeat blood sugar is shown to be back up. Snacks (a small can of juice, granola bar, etc.) should be kept in the glove compartment. Teens need to be extra careful not to drive with a low blood sugar.

As for all drivers, do not drive if impaired by alcohol or drugs!

H. COLLEGE

Starting college is a challenge for anyone. It is even more so for the person with diabetes. Our Center has offered a "Beyond High School" workshop for the past thirty years. Students who have completed one or more years of college are the most helpful in preparing the pre-college students at the seminar. Getting all the needed diabetes supplies together in addition to the usual packing for college is an extra chore.

Other important issues to remember or consider are:

✔ If the college student is to live in a dorm, getting the (meningococcal) meningitis vaccine is important and should be discussed with your primary care physician.

✔ The flu shot is also advised.

✔ Hepatitis shots should be current.

✔ It is important to take emergency phone numbers. Because of health privacy laws, a release for parents to be contacted during illness should be signed and filed with the student health service.

✔ A copy of this book (or the *First Book*) may be helpful with questions about sick days or other diabetes-related problems.

- ✔ This book, or the condensed *First Book* version, may also be helpful in educating a roommate about diabetes, and especially about hypoglycemia.
- ✔ A plan for how to discuss the diabetes with new roommates/friends must be made.
- ✔ A roommate and/or dorm counselor must be able to recognize and treat low blood sugars.
- ✔ Be aware of the usual high calorie/high-fat cafeteria food. Selecting alternatives may help prevent weight gain (often referred to as the "freshman 15").
- ✔ Doing more frequent blood/CGM glucose checks will help to make the transition safer.
- ✔ Some teens start using an insulin pump and/or a CGM, or the artificial pancreas (see Chapters 28, 29 and 30) the summer prior to college. These devices can provide extra information and safety.
- ✔ University peer-led groups, such as the College Diabetes Network (collegediabetesnetwork.org) can provide students with counselling, support, and knowledge of special accommodations.

I. EMOTIONAL CHANGES

Much of the above sections of this chapter are about the usual changes in adolescence. However, a few other areas still need to be considered. Rapid mood swings are more common during adolescence. Mood swings may change the blood adrenaline level, affecting blood sugars. Adrenaline (epinephrine) causes the blood/CGM glucose levels to rise. In general, normal adolescent mood changes should not affect overall diabetes control significantly. Adolescence is frequently an age when other behavioral conditions may emerge. Anxiety and mood disorders, such as clinical depression, are common even though they are often unrecognized conditions. Research has shown depression is more common in teens with diabetes than in other teens. The ADA recommends that all teens with diabetes be screened annually for depression. If your teenager shows unusual changes which concern you, please talk with your healthcare team. (Also see Chapter 17 for discussions of depression and eating disorders.)

Such changes to watch for include:

- ✔ frequent irritability or anger
- ✔ a drop in grades or school performance
- ✔ loss of interest in activities that were previously enjoyable
- ✔ suspected substance abuse
- ✔ changes in sleep habits (unable to go to sleep or sleeping all the time), loss of appetite
- ✔ "hanging out" with a different group of friends or dropping friends altogether

The above changes may be symptomatic of an underlying mood disorder.

Teenagers' eating habits may be affected by their emotions. Teenagers are notorious for rather unusual eating habits, and this poses a challenge for teens with diabetes who might not want to see themselves as "different."

Some teenagers develop mild to severe eating disorders (also see Chapter 17):

- ✔ Anorexia: limiting or avoiding eating
- ✔ Bulimia: binging on food and self-induced vomiting and/or use of laxatives. With diabetes, skipping insulin shots is a dangerous way to control weight.

Parents should be concerned about possible eating disorders. For example, if their teen overeats or doesn't exercise and still doesn't gain weight, there may be a cause. Weight loss without dieting or exercise should also alert the parents to possible missed insulin injections or boluses. If the HbA1c level is above 9% (>75 mmol/mol), then insulin is usually being missed (for any reason). Teens tell us that their main reason for missing shots or boluses is just "forgetting."

Stress is a normal part of life (e.g., arguments with friends, worrying about grades or concern about making a team). Learning to deal with stress is an important part of growing up.

It should be apparent that the saying "DIABETES IS A COMPROMISE" fits particularly well with the teenage years. Consistency in areas that would benefit diabetes control sometimes needs to be compromised in helping a teenager to develop normally.

J. TRANSITION TO AN ADULT DIABETES CLINIC

There has been much written in recent years about the importance of transitioning patients, usually between the ages of 18 and 22 years, from a pediatric to an adult diabetes care-provider. The transition from pediatric to adult care is not determined by age, but rather is marked by the adolescents' behavior, such as seeing clinicians without their parents and taking on greater responsibility for diabetes self-management. The ADA recommends beginning to prepare at least a year in advance of the transfer from pediatric to adult care, with a gradual transition of self-care responsibilities such as scheduling appointments, glucose monitoring, and insulin administration. The pediatric team should provide the adult care clinicians with a report of the patient's glycemic control, self-care proficiency, and a complications history. Ideally, a patient liaison could help the adolescent or young adult with a smooth transition and provide him or her with patient resources.

The Barbara Davis Center is fortunate in that the Young Adult Clinic is just down the hallway from the Pediatric Clinic. The transition process should be discussed over several visits. We often walk down with the patient/family to introduce them to adult providers and to make certain that the initial appointment is made. It is essential that the parents and clinic staff ascertain that follow-up actually occurs when the transition time arrives. It may be more important that the patient continues to be seen every three months than whether it is at a pediatric or an adult clinic.

The transition from pediatric to adult care is particularly necessary from the medical standpoint because most adult diabetes clinics have the ability to follow parameters not evaluated in a pediatric clinic (Doppler blood flow, EKGs, etc.). Many studies have shown that there is a subset of young adults at high risk for severe hypoglycemia, diabetic ketoacidosis, and the eye and kidney complications of diabetes. Needless to say, focused and timely transition is essential.

More information is available at: http://ndep.nih.gov/transitions/index.aspx

SUMMARY

The teen years can be stressful for everyone. However, they can also be the happiest years of an individual's life. The teen with diabetes has extra stress, but with a supportive family, these can be managed. Diabetes is a partnership between the parents and the teenager. It is often important for parents to be patient and to remember that they, too, were once teenagers. Parents must find ways to stay involved in the diabetes management, but not to be overbearing. They must be available to help and to be supportive but still let the teenager gain independence. The positive news is they do grow up!

DEFINITIONS

ADA: American Diabetes Association

Adolescence: The term given to the teenage years.

Adrenaline (epinephrine): The stress hormone made in the adrenal gland in the abdomen. It causes blood sugars to rise.

Estrogen: Female hormone made in the ovary (located in the abdomen) that causes female body changes.

Growth hormone: A hormone made in the pituitary gland at the base of the brain that is important for growth. It blocks the insulin activity.

Peers: One's group of friends.

Self-consciousness (body image): Concern about how one appears to others.

Sexually transmitted diseases (STDs): Diseases contracted through sexual contact, such as herpes, chlamydia, gonorrhea (clap) or syphilis.

Testosterone: A male hormone made in the testes that causes male body changes.

QUESTIONS AND ANSWERS FROM NEWSNOTES

Q At the last clinic visit, we expected a great HbA1c because my daughter's blood sugar record looked decent. We were shocked to find out that she had not been checking blood sugars and was falsifying her results! Her HbA1c was the highest ever. What should we do?

A Blood sugar checks can be difficult for some youth, particularly when they see high blood sugars. Unfortunately, they can feel discouraged or worry that they will be criticized for their high blood sugars ("what did you eat?"). When youth stop checking blood sugars or falsify numbers, it is important that we find out why they were doing so. Sometimes they worry about disappointing their parents; sometimes high values make them feel like a failure; and sometimes they want to avoid lectures from well-intentioned adults. There are many reasons why they do this. If we understand, we are in a better position to help them. Talk with them about how blood sugars are not "good or bad" but helpful information to guide dosing. They may need more involvement by parents for a while to support their efforts to check their blood sugar.

Q Is it true that growth is reduced by poor sugar control?

A Research using longitudinal HbA1c values showed that optimal growth was not reached if long-term HbA1c values were elevated. In addition to the growth rate of the person with diabetes, the final adult height was compared to that of siblings, as well as the expected adult height based on the parents' heights. All were reduced in people with chronically increased HbA1c values. In contrast, growth was not altered in people who kept their HbA1c values in the desired range.

Q Our teenage son has had an elevated HbA1c value (approximately 9% [75 mmol/mol]) over the past year. His physician and his mother and I have warned him about kidney failure and vision problems, but it doesn't seem to faze him. He currently receives Humalog and NPH insulin before breakfast and dinner. What would you suggest?

A First, it has long been known that scare tactics do not work with teenagers. This is particularly true in the mid-teen period (14-17 years) when they are "invincible," which may in itself lead to risky behavior. If you want your son to change, you and his healthcare-provider might start with "planting seeds." Second, our Clinic recommends basal-bolus insulin therapy (see Chapter 8). The use of Lantus (Basaglar)/Levemir/Tresiba rather than of NPH in the evening might be helpful. Likewise, use of an insulin pump and/or a CGM could be beneficial. It might be suggested that extra shots each day of Humalog/NovoLog/Apidra, possibly using an insulin pen, would help at lunch or with snacks. Continue to offer education, but without the scare tactics. Any positive change should be praised and encouraged.

CHAPTER 21

Outpatient Management, Education, Support Groups and Standards of Care

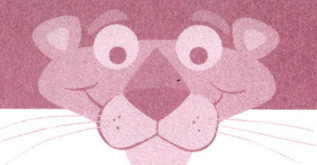

INTRODUCTION

The majority of new-onset treatment is now usually done in an outpatient setting. Outpatient care is less traumatic for the person with diabetes and the family. It also saves money compared with the cost of hospital treatment. In addition, it is now relatively rare to hospitalize people with known diabetes in the U.S. to "assess how they are doing." It is possible to have diabetes for decades and never have a diabetes-related hospitalization.

This is a result of many factors, some of which are:

✓ age-appropriate education
✓ family support
✓ regular clinic visits (every three months, or every two months for very young children)
✓ close communication with the diabetes healthcare-providers
✓ Adhering to the diabetes standards of care

TELEPHONE/EMAIL MANAGEMENT

Much of diabetes management can be done over the telephone, by fax or by email. Some glucose meters and continuous glucose monitor (CGM) systems have downloads allowing email transmission. The extra equipment needed can be obtained from the meter or CGM company (see website or call phone number on back of device).

> **TOPICS:**
> **Goal Setting and Problem Solving**
> **Monitoring (clinic visits and laboratory values)**
>
> **TEACHING OBJECTIVES:**
> The teacher will:
> 1. Indicate the importance and frequency of clinic visits as related to positive diabetes outcomes.
> 2. Present the minimum standards of care for diabetes management.
>
> **LEARNING OBJECTIVES:**
> Learner (parents, child, relative or self) will be able to:
> 1. State the anticipated clinic visit schedule, relate its importance as well as necessary items to bring (meter, written materials [especially Pink Panther book], labs, etc.).
> 2. List three expected tasks in diabetes management.

The diabetes care team should be called (or emailed):

✓ if at least half of the blood/CGM glucose values are not in the desired range for age (see Chapter 7) and help is needed
✓ excessive time is spent above or below range (see Chapter 14) and help is needed
✓ prior to the next regularly scheduled injection if a severe hypoglycemic reaction has occurred

- ✓ if more than two mild reactions occurred within a short time (e.g., one week)
- ✓ anytime the urine ketones are moderate or large or blood ketones are above 1.0 mmol/L
- ✓ prior to any planned surgery

People with diabetes should have checkups with the health team about every three months. This is the recommendation of the ADA Standards of Care. Some of these Standards of Care are included in this chapter.

FAX AND EMAIL MESSAGES

Most families have access to a fax machine or email. Blood sugar record sheets can be found in Chapter 7. Meter, insulin pump and CGM downloads can now usually be sent by email.

If the family is using an insulin pump or a continuous glucose monitor (CGM), there are also ways to make the data available to the diabetes care-provider. The diabetes nurse-educator or the company (number on back of device) may be able to help. It is usually necessary to call or email the provider to let them know the pump or CGM data has been downloaded. The alternative is to take the CGM into the diabetes clinic and ask to have it downloaded. The data can then be given to the diabetes care-provider.

We ask that records be faxed or emailed anytime the family feels they need some help. We prefer faxes or emails to phone calls to report blood/CGM sugar values. The fax or email saves time and confusion when trying to listen and write down values while on the phone.

If the parents do not have access to a fax machine or email, most schools (and especially the school nurse) will provide a way to transmit the blood/CGM sugar results.

When families fax/email the records, please remember to:

- ✓ include the insulin dosages
- ✓ record the time of any symptomatic low blood sugars (even if it was not possible to do a blood sugar) and include any information relating to why lows occurred
- ✓ include the sender's fax/email and phone number and when that person can best be reached
- ✓ include the family's plan on what adjustments to make. (We want families to be active in the decision-making process.)

The forms from Chapter 7 can be downloaded to use when emailing records. It is only when records are kept that trends can be seen. Faxing/emailing the healthcare-provider when values are out of the target range is very helpful. Adjustments can then be made immediately. This prevents delaying changes until the next clinic appointment.

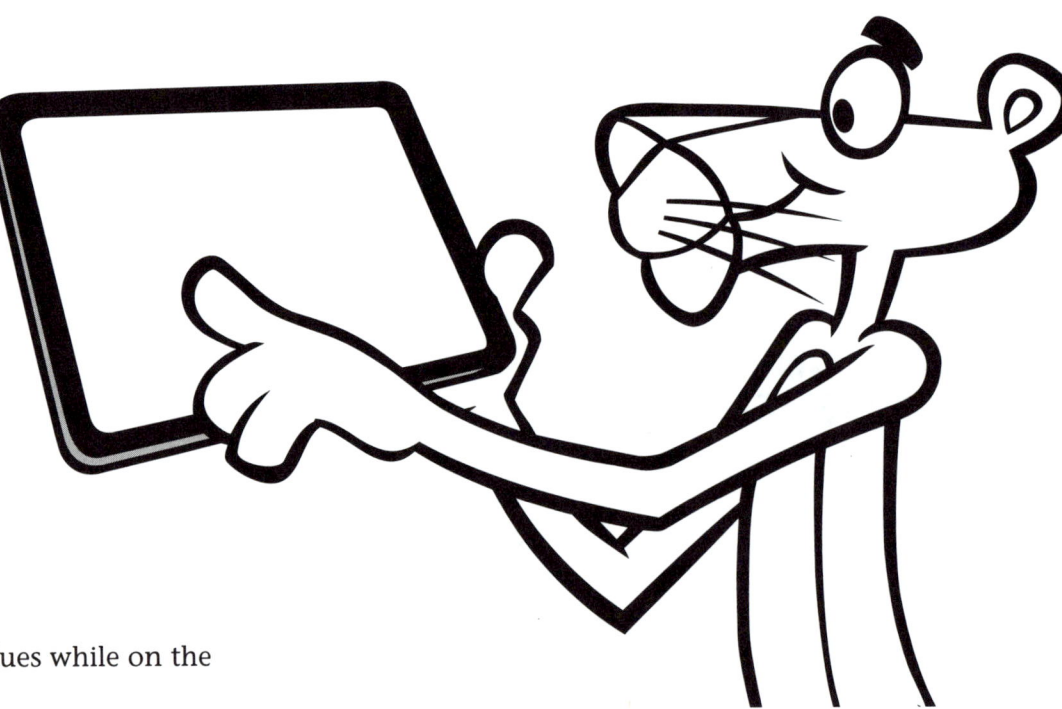

CLINIC VISITS

When someone is attending our clinic for the first time, the visit usually takes a half to a whole day. Later visits will be shorter. Snacks should be brought to the appointment. Blood sugar records, meters and CGM devices must **ALWAYS** be brought along for the clinic visit. All meters that we recommend have memories to store the last 100 to 250 blood sugar values and the ability to download the data upon arrival in the clinic. It is important to analyze this data at the time of the clinic visit.

Having a clinic visit every three months allows:

- ✔ a review of high and low blood/CGM glucose values and "Time in Range"
- ✔ changes in insulin dosage
- ✔ the HbA1c to be done (Chapter 14)
- ✔ growth to be followed
- ✔ a check for any problems
- ✔ continued education and introduction of new information/devices

In the clinic, the following people may help:

The Clinic Nurse or Medical Assistant will:

- measure height and weight
- check the blood pressure
- check a blood sugar
- measure the hemoglobin A1c (HbA1c)
- check for urine ketones and protein
- download blood glucose meters, CGMs and pumps

The Diabetes Nurse Educator will:

- continue the diabetes education
- introduce any new information and/or new devices available
- check prescription needs
- review diabetes management
- do the school health plan (if needed)

The Doctor, Physician's Assistant (P.A.) or Nurse Practitioner will:

- check to see how the person/family is doing with diabetes care goals
- review the blood/CGM glucose values and the HbA1c result
- change insulin or oral medication doses if needed
- evaluate the pump download, if using an insulin pump
- do a partial physical examination (including checking growth, thyroid size, injection sites and any signs of diabetes complications)
- coordinate the recommendations of all team members

The Dietitian will:

- review food intake and make suggestions for changes if needed
- provide nutrition education and information about snacks and other food needs

The Social Worker or Psychologist will:

- assess personal, family, school or other problems
- provide resource options for the individual or family
- monitor current family issues and their effect on diabetes management

It is also helpful to bring this educational book so that it can be used to review knowledge about diabetes.

CLINIC VISITS BY TELEMEDICINE

Clinic visits by telemedicine are now available in some areas. These should be alternated with regular clinic visits so physical exam changes can be checked. The family may want to discuss the mechanism for using telemedicine during a routine clinic visit. It may become essential during pandemics (e.g., COVID-19) or other crises.

SUPPORT GROUPS AND CONTINUING EDUCATION

Some families gain extra support from meeting with other families who also have a family member with diabetes. *This meeting can happen at:*

✔ the time of the clinic visits (e.g., group-clinics arranged by age)

✔ special group meetings

✔ special events: sports, picnics or Halloween parties

Additional education courses are important for families who do not live near a specialized diabetes clinic. These courses are important for people who were diagnosed at a young age and have now reached an age when they are able to understand material they could not understand earlier.

Some of the additional education courses offered at our Center are:

✔ **Transition to Work- and College-Bound Workshop:** Offered as people become independent from their parents. A boost in knowledge at this time can be helpful in limiting later problems.

✔ **Grandparent's Workshop:** A one-day course. It is important that children with diabetes have the same relationships with grandparents as do other children (see Chapter 26). This likely involves staying with the grandparents. The workshop may also be useful for aunts and uncles, babysitters or others who are close to the child.

✔ **Insulin Pump or CGM classes** for those starting to use a pump (Chapter 28) or a CGM (Chapter 29)

✔ **Carb Counting Classes:** These may be helpful as a review, when families start an insulin pump, or for newly diagnosed families.

WEBSITES

There are many excellent websites for people and families with diabetes. Some that we recommend are:

1. www.childrenwithdiabetes.com
2. www.childrensdiabetesfoundation.org
3. www.barbaradaviscenter.org
4. www.jdrf.org
5. www.diabetes.org
6. collegediabetesnetwork.org – The College Diabetes Network is also available online (no cost) for helping students with diabetes "to thrive in all of their personal, healthcare, and scholastic accomplishments."

STANDARDS OF MEDICAL CARE

Standards of medical care for people with type 1 and type 2 diabetes have been published by the American Diabetes Association (ADA) and by ISPAD. The standards are both for care-providers and for people with diabetes.

The ADA standards can be found in: *Diabetes Care*, January, Supplement 1 every year.

Knowing these standards will allow people with diabetes to:

✔ assess the quality of medical care they receive

✔ determine their role in their medical treatment

✔ compare their treatment outcomes to standard goals

✔ The person and/or family must assume some of the responsibility for meeting the standards of care outlined below.

For example:

✔ If the family member with diabetes has reached age 10 or puberty, and has had diabetes for at least five years, annual eye and kidney evaluations are needed. The family must set up the eye evaluation with an eye doctor covered by their HMO.

✔ They need to help the family member do two timed overnight or first morning urine collections, or the spot screen in clinic, for the measurement of microalbumin leakage by the kidneys (directions at end of Chapter 23).

Some of the recommended **ADA's Standards of Care**, with a few modifications, are outlined below:

- Insulin-treated people should have clinic visits at least every three months.

- An HbA1c level should be done at least every three months. This is done in our clinic using the DCA Vantage Analyzer. The method is very accurate, and the result is available in six minutes. It is important for the care-provider to have the result during the clinic visit so that changes can be made if needed.

- All people with diabetes must be taught how to do blood glucose values.

- A comprehensive physical examination, including sexual maturation in adolescents, should be done annually by either the diabetes or primary care physician.

- Parts of the physical exam affected by diabetes (e.g., height, weight, blood pressure, eyes, thyroid, liver size, deep tendon reflexes, injection sites, feet, etc.) should be checked every three months.

- People ≥10 years of age or at puberty should have a dilated eye examination by an eye doctor within 5 years after the onset of diabetes. Screening for diabetic eye disease is NOT necessary before 10 years of age.

- Laboratory measurements for microalbuminuria (Chapter 23) should be done annually after age 10 or in post pubertal people who have had diabetes for at least five years. People with type 2 diabetes should be checked at diagnosis and then annually.

- The occurrence of severe hypoglycemic episodes (episodes requiring the help of others when not usually required, seizures or loss of consciousness) is serious and requires the help of a diabetes specialist in reducing the likelihood of further episodes.

- The stress of illness frequently affects sugar levels and necessitates more frequent monitoring of blood sugar and urine or blood ketones by the family. Medical help must be constantly available when moderate or large urine ketones or blood ketones above 1.0 mmol/L are detected.

- In type 1 diabetes, a lipid profile including cholesterol, triglyceride, LDL- and HDL-cholesterol should be performed by age 12, and then yearly (see Chapters 11 and 23). In type 2 diabetes, lipids should be checked at diagnosis and then yearly.

- High blood pressure (hypertension) and borderline elevations in blood pressure contribute to the development and progression of the chronic complications of diabetes. Elevations in blood pressure must be treated aggressively to achieve and maintain blood pressure in the normal range.

For people with known diabetic complications:

✔ Known diabetic eye disease requires care by an ophthalmologist (eye doctor) experienced in the management of people with diabetes.

✔ The person with abnormal kidney function requires heightened attention, reduction of other risk factors (e.g., hypertension and tobacco use) and possible consultation with a specialist in diabetic kidney disease.

✔ People with cardiovascular risk factors, who have usually had type 1 or type 2 diabetes for many years, should be carefully monitored. Evidence of cardiovascular disease (such as angina, decreased pulses and ECG abnormalities) requires efforts aimed at correction of contributing risk factors (e.g., obesity, use of tobacco, hypertension, sedentary lifestyle, hyperlipidemia and poorly regulated diabetes), in addition to specific treatment of the cardiovascular problem.

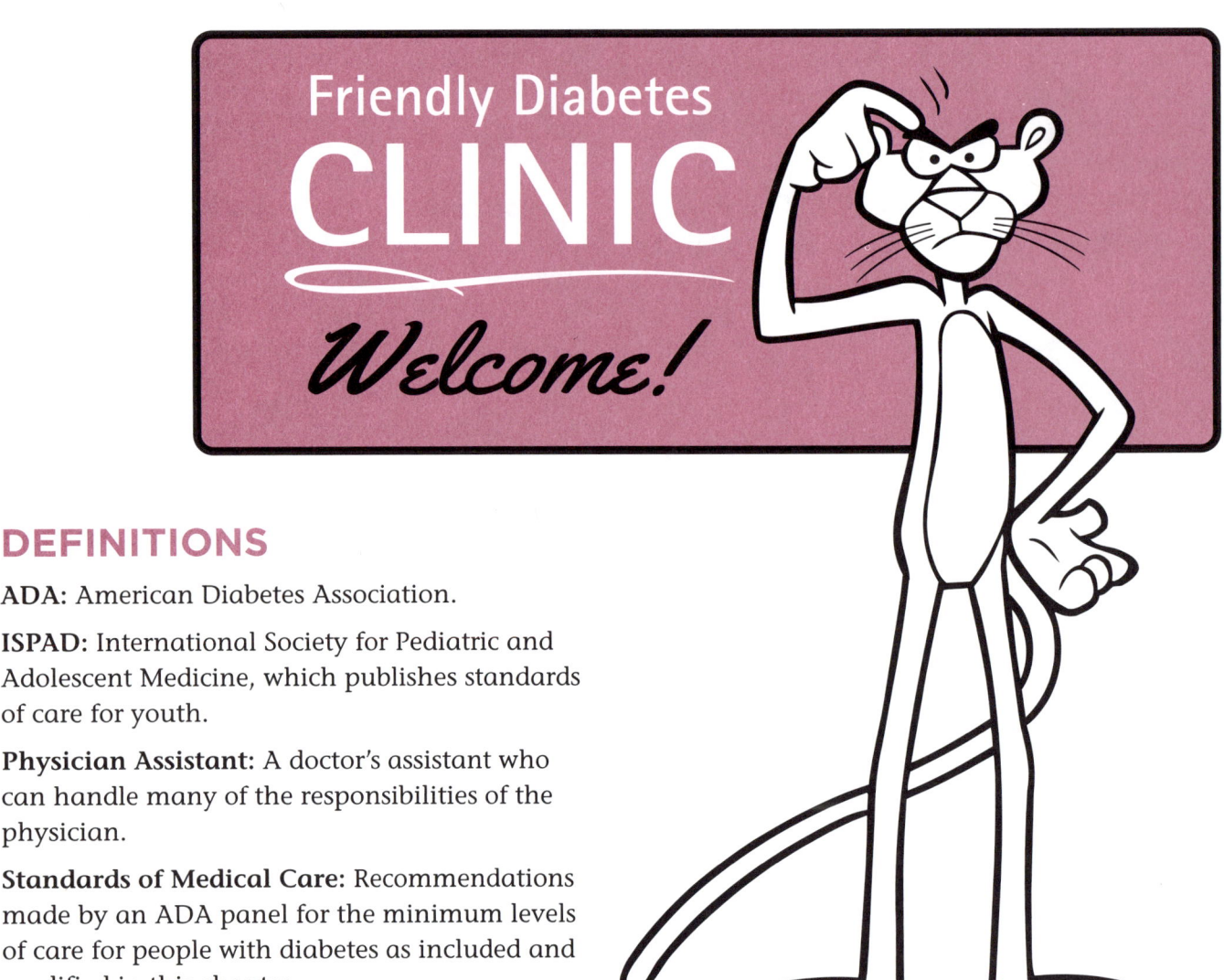

DEFINITIONS

ADA: American Diabetes Association.

ISPAD: International Society for Pediatric and Adolescent Medicine, which publishes standards of care for youth.

Physician Assistant: A doctor's assistant who can handle many of the responsibilities of the physician.

Standards of Medical Care: Recommendations made by an ADA panel for the minimum levels of care for people with diabetes as included and modified in this chapter.

QUESTIONS AND ANSWERS FROM NEWSNOTES

Q Why are regular clinic appointments necessary and how often should these be scheduled?

a Clinic appointments should be scheduled approximately every three months. This is the recommended interval in the ADA "Standards of Medical Care." The reasons for this are primarily preventive, since this is where the emphasis in healthcare now lies. In the early 1900s, the emphasis in healthcare was on the treatment of acute problems. Medicine has now switched to a more preventive-based healthcare, particularly relating to chronic diseases.

For people with diabetes, the visits every three months allow continued education and increased motivation for doing day-to-day monitoring of the diabetes. Also, the HbA1c level provides an estimate of blood/CGM glucose levels over the past three months, and of the time blood/CGM sugars are "in range." If regular visits do not occur, diabetes monitoring and knowledge become lax.

In summary, the best management occurs with the family and diabetes-team working together. Although every three months seems to be an average best time to return to the clinic, there are obviously some situations where more frequent visits are important.

CHAPTER 22

Adjusting the Insulin Dosage and "Thinking" Scales

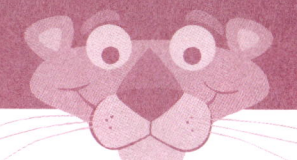

BLOOD/CGM GLUCOSE GOALS AND SUGGESTED RANGES

It is our goal to have blood/CGM glucose levels in the ranges shown in Table 1 (also see Chapters 7 and 14). Values are given in mg/dL and in mmol/L (in parentheses). A person who has difficulty recognizing low blood sugars or who has severe insulin reactions may need to keep the blood/CGM glucose at a slightly higher level. Families and the diabetes care-provider should discuss the desired range. This range should be written down for future reference. It is important to remember that this is a target goal.

TABLE 1: Blood/CGM Glucose Goals (suggested ranges)

Age	Before Meals/Fasting	Bedtime/Overnight
Under 6 years	80-180 (4.5-10)	130-200 (7.2-11.1)
6-17 years	70-150 (3.9-8.3)	90-150* (5.0-8.3)
Adult (18 and older)	70-130 (3.9-7.2)	90-150* (5.0-8.3)

* After heavy exercise a goal of 130-150 (7.2-8.3) might be a safer level.

These values differ from the 2015 ADA recommendations stating that the values for all ages of youth should be between 90-130 mg/dL (5.0-7.2 mmol/L) before meals and 90-150 mg/dL (5.0-8.3 mmol/L) at bedtime/overnight.

TOPICS:
Medications (Insulin Adjustments)
Monitoring

TEACHING OBJECTIVES:
The teacher will:
1. Discuss when and how to adjust insulin doses.
2. Integrate factors that influence insulin dose into a "thinking" scale.
3. Demonstrate the application of dose adjustments to blood sugar trends.

LEARNING OBJECTIVES:
Learner (parents, child, relative or self) will be able to:
1. Describe when and how to increase or decrease insulin doses.
2. Explain insulin adjustments using blood/CGM glucose records.
3. List two factors that affect blood sugars and describe the appropriate insulin adjustments.

Aim for 70 percent of glucose values to be in the desired range. Not all blood/CGM glucose values will be in the target range. If more than half of the values are in range and the HbA1c is still high, additional blood/CGM sugar levels at other times of the day should be evaluated. Chapters 7 and 14 give suggestions for other times – including two hours after meals. The ADA recommends that all values following meals be below 180 mg/dL (10.0 mmol/L).

After six to 12 months of dealing with diabetes, many families and older teens begin making some of their own insulin adjustments. The longer people have diabetes, the more comfortable they become making adjustments.

FIGURE 1:
The Four Time Periods of Insulin Activity

Period 1: a.m.	Humalog/NovoLog Apidra/Regular	Works primarily from breakfast (B) to lunch (L)
Period 2: a.m.	a.m. NPH	Works primarily from lunch to dinner (D)
Period 3: p.m.	Humalog/NovoLog Apidra/Regular	Works primarily from dinner to bedtime (BT)
Period 4: p.m.	NPH (evening) Lantus (Basaglar) (Basaglar)/Levemir/Tresiba; anytime)	Works primarily from bedtime to the following morning (NPH) or all day

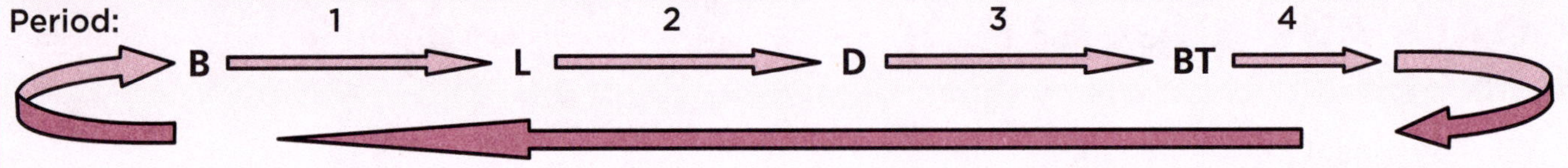

Period: B → 1 → L → 2 → D → 3 → BT → 4

This can be discussed with the diabetes care-provider at a clinic visit. We encourage patients and families to be actively involved in making insulin dose adjustments. When blood/CGM sugar logs are faxed/emailed, we ask that families include their plan on how they would adjust the insulin dose. Guidelines for insulin adjustments can then be discussed with the care team.

ADJUSTING THE INSULIN DOSAGE

The first step in learning to adjust insulin is to know the times of action of the insulins used. Refer to the figures in Chapter 8 and Figure 1 in this chapter to review the times of action of various insulins.

The three rapid-acting insulins are Humalog, NovoLog, and Apidra. All of these have similar activity (Chapter 8). They can be used interchangeably.

Changes in insulin dosage will be considered under five categories:

A. Reducing the Insulin Dose
B. Increasing the Insulin Dose
C. Insulin Adjustments for Basal-Bolus Insulin Therapy
D. Insulin Adjustments for Correction/Sensitivity Factor
E. "Thinking" Scales

A. REDUCING THE INSULIN DOSE TO AVOID LOW BLOOD SUGARS:
(Figure 1 and Table 2)

Reducing a specific insulin dose should be done if:

✓ Frequent (>2 per week) blood/CGM glucose values occur below 60 mg/dL (<3.3 mmol/L), which we consider is the level of true hypoglycemia, or below 70 mg/dL (<3.9 mmol/L) in a preschooler.

✓ Many of the blood/CGM sugar values in a day are below the desired lower limit. The insulin doses should be reduced with the next injection. How much the insulin is reduced depends on the age and size of the person and the dose being given.

We do not always know why blood/CGM glucose values will suddenly be low for a day or longer in a person who has had stable levels. Most often this is due to increased physical activity, eating less food or opening new bottles of insulin. If you use NPH insulin, we do know it has to be carefully mixed and may still have variable absorption from day to day.

When are the low values occurring?

- If the reactions are during the night or in the early morning hours, the Lantus (Basaglar)/Levemir/Tresiba (given at any time of the day) or evening NPH can be reduced by one or two units.
- If the values are still low the next day, reduce the insulin again.
- If the low values occur before lunch or dinner, the morning NPH or the breakfast or lunch rapid-acting insulin can be reduced by one or two units.

Think about what time of the day the reactions are occurring and which insulin is having its main action at that time of day. Reduce the insulin that is working at that time by one or two units.

Remember that the rapid-acting insulins (Humalog, NovoLog, Apidra) have their peak activity 90 minutes after the injection or pump bolus). Thus, when considering a time for a high or a low glucose value, it is important to consider the rapid-acting insulin dose having its peak effect starting 90 minutes after the injection.

Sometimes the values are high the day after the insulin dose is reduced. This is because the insulin-balancing hormones may require a day or two to adjust. It is important to be patient when a dose is reduced, and **DO NOT GO BACK UP ON THE DOSE** just because blood/CGM glucose values are a bit higher. Wait a few days to let the balancing hormones decline before deciding to go back up on the dose. Remember that even though we suggest waiting a few days to make further changes if the blood/CGM glucose level is high, this is NOT necessary if it is low. **It is important to make a further reduction the next day if values are still low.**

Thinking ahead to help avoid lows (reactions)

Although discussed in more detail in Chapter 6, families need to **"think ahead"** to help avoid lows. Reduce the insulin dosage during days of high excitement and activity or when eating less. **When children stay overnight at a friend's house (or have a friend spend the night)** there is often an increase in activity and less sleep. More energy is expended, and it is wise to reduce the p.m. insulin dose and/or the Lantus (Basaglar)/Levemir/Tresiba dose or the pump basal rate. Some people use the temporary basal rate on their pump on a daily basis to increase or reduce insulin (Chapter 28).

The following can all lead to low blood sugars:

- ✓ school trips and field days
- ✓ family picnics and playing with cousins
- ✓ long hikes or bike trips
- ✓ spending the night with a friend
- ✓ vacations to places like Disneyland® or the beach
- ✓ deciding to begin a diet
- ✓ when school is out and the weather is nice, children will play outside after dinner. The evening rapid-acting insulin almost always has to be reduced.
- ✓ getting cold when playing outside in cold weather (not wearing enough warm clothing)
- ✓ starting sports or a new exercise program

Temporary reductions in dosage of insulins acting at the time of activity or excitement can help to avoid problems. It is better, when possible, to reduce an insulin dose rather than having to eat extra snacks. Frequent snacking can lead to excess weight gain. If there are questions about reducing the insulin dosage, call the diabetes care-provider during office phone hours. (Save home calls and pager calls for emergencies.) **Remember it is generally best to err on the safe side.** Alterations in the insulin dose for sick day and surgery management are discussed in Chapter 16, "Sick Day and Surgery Management."

TABLE 2:
Insulin Dosing Algorithms for LOW BLOOD/CGM SUGAR (B.S.) in mg/dL (mmol/L)

	Birth - 5 years	6 - 17 years	18 years and older
Target glucose levels	80-180 (4.5-10.0)*	70-150 (3.9-8.3)*	70-130 (3.9-7.2)*
Morning (a.m.) B.S.	B.S. <80 (4.5) ↓ dinner or bedtime N or Basal insulin by ¼ to ½ unit.**	B.S. <70 (3.9) ↓ dinner or bedtime N or Basal insulin by ½-1 unit.**	B.S. <70 (3.9) ↓ dinner or bedtime N or Basal insulin by 1-2 units.**
Noon B.S.	B.S. <80 (4.5) ↓ a.m. RAI or R ↓ N by ½ unit if given in a.m.	B.S. <70 (3.9) ↓ a.m. RAI or R by ½-1 unit ↓ N by 1 unit if given in the a.m.	B.S. <70 (3.9) ↓ a.m. RAI or R by 1-2 units ↓ N by 1-2 units if given in the a.m.
Afternoon (dinner) B.S.	B.S. <80 (4.5) ↓ a.m. N or noon RAI or R by ¼ to ½ unit.	B.S. <70 (3.9) ↓ a.m. N or noon RAI or R by ½-1 unit.	B.S. <70 (3.9) ↓ a.m. N or noon RAI or R by 1-2 units.
Bedtime B.S. (higher goals)	B.S. <130 (7.2) ↓ dinner RAI or R by ¼ to ½ unit.	B.S. <90 (5.0) ↓ dinner RAI or R by ½-1 unit.	B.S. <90 (5.0) ↓ dinner RAI or R by 1-2 units.

↓ = lower, decrease; < = less than; N = NPH;
RAI = Rapid-acting insulin (Humalog, NovoLog or Apidra); R = Regular insulin
*Values in parentheses represent mmol/L.
**Decrease Lantus (Basaglar), Levemir or Tresiba (given at any time of day).

Continuous Glucose Monitors
(**CGM**; Chapter 29)

Many people now use CGMs, which can help with making insulin adjustments (particularly with weekly downloads to see patterns). Goals for percent of times within, above and below range are presented in Chapters 14 and 29. The trend graphs and direction-arrows may help with immediate changes in insulin dosage. The artificial pancreas (Chapter 30), using the threshold and predicted low glucose suspend features, provides safely in avoiding lows.

Responding to severe insulin reactions (also see Chapter 6)

If a severe insulin reaction occurs, it is important to call the diabetes healthcare-provider before giving the next scheduled insulin shot. The stores of balancing hormones (e.g., adrenaline) are reduced with a severe reaction and there is a greater risk for more reactions. The insulin dose should be reduced temporarily (often for 2-3 days). It is important to decrease the risk of a severe reaction from occurring again. Sometimes it is helpful to schedule a clinic appointment to discuss this.

TABLE 3:
Insulin Dosing Algorithms for HIGH BLOOD/CGM SUGAR (B.S.) in mg/dL (mmol/L)

	Birth - 5 years	6 - 17 years	18 years and older
Target glucose levels	80-180 (4.5-10.0)*	70-150 (3.9-8.3)*	70-130 (3.9-7.2)*
Morning (a.m.) B.S.	B.S. >180 (10.0) ↑ dinner or bedtime basal insulin** by ¼ to ½ unit.	B.S. >150 (8.3) ↑ dinner or bedtime basal insulin** by ½-1 unit.	B.S. >130 (7.2) ↑ dinner or bedtime N or basal insulin** by 1-2 units.
Noon B.S.	B.S. >180 (10.0) ↑ a.m. RAI or R by ¼ to ½ unit.	B.S. >150 (8.3) ↑ a.m. RAI or R by ½-1 unit	B.S. >130 (7.2) ↑ a.m. RAI or R by 1-2 units
Afternoon (dinner) B.S.	B.S. >180 (10.0) ↑ a.m. N or noon RAI or R by ¼ to ½ unit.	B.S. >150 (8.3) ↑ a.m. N or noon RAI or R by ½-1 unit.	B.S. >130 (7.2) ↑ a.m. N or noon RAI or R by 1-2 units.
Bedtime B.S. (higher goals	B.S. >200 (11.1) ↑ dinner RAI or R by ¼ to ½ unit.	B.S. >150 (8.3) ↑ dinner RAI or R by ½-1 unit.	B.S. >150 (8.3) ↑ dinner RAI or R by 1-2 units.

↑ = raise, increase; > = greater than; N = NPH;
RAI = Rapid-acting insulin (Humalog, NovoLog or Apidra); R = Regular insulin
*Values in parentheses represent mmol/L.
**Increase Lantus (Basaglar)/Levemir/Tresiba or p.m. NPH.

B. INCREASING THE INSULIN DOSE TO TREAT HIGH BLOOD SUGARS:
(Figure 1 and Table 3)

Understanding why more insulin is required

An insulin dose may need to be increased:

✔ if the blood/CGM glucose levels have been above the desired range for three or four days in a row and there is not an obvious illness or stress that will soon go away

✔ when children grow, their insulin needs generally increase by one unit for every two pounds (or 1kg) gained. Also, when growth hormone levels increase, insulin activity is decreased.

✔ because in most people with diabetes, their own pancreas gradually makes less insulin

✔ in the winter when many people exercise less and their insulin needs increase

✔ during times of high stress or during menses (menstrual period)

✔ if HbA1c values are high (reflecting blood/CGM glucose levels over the past three months)

✔ during an illness, there may be a temporary need for more insulin (especially if ketones are present); see Chapter 16.

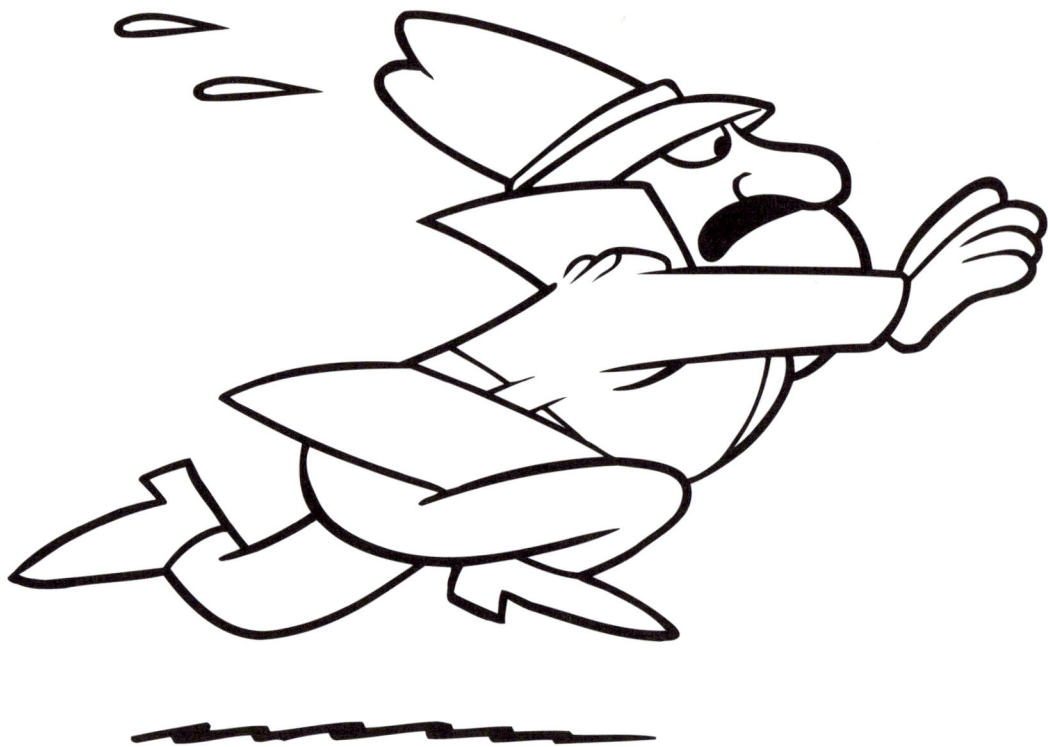

Resistance to increasing the insulin dose

Some people resist increasing the insulin dose. When blood/CGM glucose levels have been running high, the person's body becomes accustomed to higher levels. They may feel uncomfortable with glucose levels in the target range. This unpleasant feeling lasts for a short period and will gradually disappear. Also, the most frequent fear of people with diabetes (and their family members) is of low blood sugars. This is particularly true if severe reactions have occurred. People may resist (sometimes subconsciously) increasing the dose and lowering the blood/CGM glucose levels. An increase in the dose may mean a loss of further insulin production in the eyes of some families. This can seem like a time of additional loss.

Knowing which insulin to increase

It is essential to know the times of action of the insulins and the desired ranges for the blood/CGM glucose levels. The insulins working during the four time periods are shown in Figure 1. *When the blood/CGM glucose levels are above the desired range for three to seven days with no obvious cause, the insulin acting in that time period should be increased. Thus:*

✔ if the sugars are high before lunch, increase the morning rapid-acting (Humalog/NovoLog/Apidra) or Regular insulin

✔ if the sugars are high before dinner, increase the morning NPH or the rapid-acting insulin or Regular insulin at lunch. Also, remember that rapid-acting insulin is needed for afternoon snacks!

✔ if the sugars are high before the bedtime snack, increase the dinner rapid-acting or Regular insulin

✔ if the sugars are high before breakfast, increase the dinner (or bedtime) NPH or the Lantus (Basaglar)/Levemir/Tresiba insulin

The increases are usually by a half unit for a preschooler or by a unit for an older child or adult. The blood/CGM glucose levels will tend to run lower on the first day of increased insulin.

The dose may need to be increased again as the balancing hormones adjust. Extra blood/CGM glucose checks on the first day of an increased dose are often wise. If the blood/CGM glucose levels are still above the desired range

TABLE 4:
Algorithm for Adjusting Basal-Bolus Insulin*

1. Basal Insulin Dose (Lantus [Basaglar], Levemir or Tresiba):
When using only a basal insulin (no NPH), determine the dose based on the pre-breakfast blood sugar

If morning blood/CGM sugar value is:

- 60-80 mg/dL (3.3-4.5 mmol/L) = decrease the basal insulin dose by one-half to one unit
- <60 mg/dL (<3.3 mmol/L) = decrease the basal insulin dose by one or two units

} Daily changes can be made

- 180-240 mg/dL (10.0-13.3 mmol/L) = increase the basal insulin dose by one or two units
- >240 mg/dL (>13.3 mmol/L) = increase the basal insulin dose by one or two units

} Wait 2-3 days between changes

2. If using an a.m. NPH dose:
(if afternoon or dinner blood sugar goal = 70-180 mg/dL [3.9-10.0 mmol/L])*

If afternoon blood/CGM sugar value is:

- 60-70 mg/dL (3.3-3.9 mmol/L) = decrease a.m. NPH dose by one-half to one unit
- <60 mg/dL (<3.3 mmol/L) = decrease a.m. NPH dose by one or two units

} Daily changes can be made

- 180-240 mg/dL (10.0-13.3 mmol/L) = increase a.m. NPH dose by one-half to one unit
- >240 mg/dL (>13.3 mmol/L) = increase a.m. NPH dose by one or two units

} Wait 2-3 days between changes

3. Humalog, NovoLog or Apidra (H/NL/AP)
(two hours after a meal blood/CGM sugar goal = 70-180 mg/dL [3.9-10.0 mmol/L])*

If blood/CGM sugar value two hours after the meal is:

- 60-80 mg/dL (3.3-4.5 mmol/L) = decrease the H/NL/AP dose prior to the meal by at least one unit**
- <60 mg/dL (<3.3 mmol/L) = decrease the H/NL/AP dose prior to the meal by at least two units**

} Daily changes can be made

- 180-240 mg/dL (10.0-13.3 mmol/L) = increase the H/NL/AP dose prior to the meal by one-half to one unit
- >240 mg/dL (>13.3 mmol/L) = increase the H/NL/AP dose prior to the meal by one or two units

} Wait 2-3 days between changes

*For ages 6-17 years, the healthcare-provider may wish the blood/CGM sugar goal to be 70-150 mg/dL (3.9-8.3 mmol/L) rather than 70-180 mg/dL (3.9-10.0 mmol/L). For 18 years and older, a goal may be 70-130 mg/dL (3.9-7.2 mmol/L). Older ages will likely need double the suggested insulin dose changes.

**If carb counting, it may be helpful to talk with the dietitian to change the I/C ratio.

Call your healthcare-provider if you need help.

after three to seven days, repeat the increase again. **Continue this program until at least half of the blood/CGM glucose levels at the time of day being worked on are in the desired range.** A general rule is to increase the dosage slowly. If you are not sure whether to make further increases in the insulin dose, fax or email the values. Most glucose meters will display a 7, 14 and 30-day average. These averages can be used to know if you are making progress with adjustments. See Chapter 14 on how average blood glucose levels relate to HbA1c. You can also call to discuss changes with your diabetes care-provider. Faxing or emailing the blood/CGM glucose values allows the diabetes care-provider time to review and think about recommendations. Some families use their phone to take pictures of blood/CGM sugar values and then email or text message the information. Sample fax sheets are included in Chapter 7. This reporting should be done during office phone hours. Save home calls and pager calls for emergencies.

C. INSULIN ADJUSTMENTS FOR BASAL-BOLUS INSULIN THERAPY (Table 4)

In Chapter 8 you can find:

✔ The most common ways we currently use the basal insulins, Lantus (Basaglar), Levemir and Tresiba.

✔ A method to determine the starting dose of basal insulin

✔ An example for the basal insulin given at dinner or in the evening. The dose of Lantus (Basaglar)/Levemir/Tresiba is increased or decreased until most of the morning blood/CGM glucose levels are in the desired ranges (see above).

Most people will adjust up or down by one or two units of Lantus (Basaglar)/Levemir/Tresiba insulin (or one-half unit for toddlers) every two or three days until morning values are in the ranges listed above.

If NPH is given at breakfast, the amount of NPH is adjusted up or down until the blood/CGM glucose levels at dinnertime are mostly within the ranges listed above. If given at night (preferably bedtime), the dosage is adjusted up or down based on the morning blood sugar levels. Table 4 provides an algorithm that may be helpful in adjusting insulin dosages.

The H/NL/AP dosages for meals are best adjusted by measuring blood/CGM glucose levels two hours after the meal. The ADA recommends that all blood/CGM glucose levels after a meal be under 180 mg/dL (<10.0 mmol/L). Others routinely aim for a glucose level below 140 mg/dL (7.8 mmol/L) two hours after meals. These levels are easier to attain if the pre-meal insulin can be taken 20 minutes prior to the meal. If the values are not in the desired range two hours after eating, the Insulin-to-Carbohydrate (I/C) ratio may need to be changed. If the blood/CGM glucose levels are high, more insulin for carbohydrate in the I/C ratio will need to be given. An example would be to change from 1:15 (1 unit/15g carbohydrate) to 1:10 (1 unit/10g carbohydrate). If the blood/CGM glucose level is below the lower limit, less insulin is needed. An example would be to change from a ratio of 1:15 (1 unit/15g carbohydrate) to 1:20 (1 unit/20g carbohydrate; with pumps smaller changes can be made). Call your healthcare-provider if you need help.

Snacks are usually not necessary with Lantus (Basaglar)/Levemir/Tresiba insulin. However, if there has been exercise that day, and the blood/CGM glucose is below 130 mg/dL (7.2 mmol/L) at bedtime, it is usually wise to have a bedtime snack. When the glucose is above this level and the person is having a bedtime snack, H/NL/AP may be necessary.

Special care is needed if switching to or from Tresiba insulin, as it lasts longer than Lantus (Basaglar) or Levemir (or NPH) insulin. Contact with the diabetes care-provider is important.

TABLE 5:
Example of Insulin Adjustments

| Blood Sugar | | Correction Factor* | Carb Choices** | Total units |
mg/dL	mmol/L	Units of Insulin	(15g carb)	of Insulin
150	8.3	0	1	1
200	11.1	1	2	3
250	13.9	2	3	5
300	16.7	3	4	7
350	19.4	4	5	9

*Assuming a correction factor of one unit of rapid-acting insulin per 50 mg (2.8 mmol/L) above 150 mg/dL (8.3 mmol/L).

**One carb choice = 15g carbohydrate. In this example, one unit of insulin is given for each 15g carb choice.

D. INSULIN ADJUSTMENTS FOR CORRECTION/SENSITIVITY FACTOR
(Table 5)

When choosing a dose of rapid-acting insulin at meals/snacks, it is important to think about both the blood/CGM glucose level and the food to be eaten. Many families and careproviders choose a **correction factor** which can be added to the food insulin dose to cover high blood/CGM glucose levels. The **correction factor** refers to the units of insulin needed to correct a blood sugar to a given level. The goal is to return the blood sugar level into the desired range in approximately two hours. If the blood sugar remains high after two hours, an additional correction insulin dose can be given. A correction factor is generally used when Humalog/NovoLog/Apidra has not been given within the previous two hours. A common correction dose is one unit of rapid-acting insulin per 50 mg/dL (2.8 mmol/L) of glucose above 100 mg/dL (5.5 mmol/L). Corrections may aim for 130 mg/dL (7.2 mmol/L) or 150 mg/dL (8.3 mmol/L) during the night. However, every person is different. If the correction insulin dose is correct, an elevated blood sugar value should be back in range after two hours. Pumps with bolus calculators make the calculation easier. A preschooler may do better with one unit per 100 mg/dL (5.5 mmol/L) above 150 (8.3 mmol/L) or 200 mg/dL (11.1 mmol/L). The person or family will need to find out what works. It is a helpful way to get the blood/CGM glucose levels back on track.

If food is to be eaten at the time of doing the correction (e.g., time for lunch or afternoon snack), the insulin to cover the food should be added to the correction dose. For example, in Table 5, if a person planned to eat 45g of carbohydrate and their blood sugar level was 150 mg/dL (8.3 mmol/L) and their I/C ratio (Chapter 12) was 1:15, the dose of rapid-acting insulin would be three units. If their blood/CGM glucose level was 250 mg/dL (13.9 mmol/L), the correction factor would be two units (if their correction was one unit of rapid-acting insulin per 50 mg/dL [2.8 mmol/L] for glucose levels above 150 mg/dL [8.3 mmol/L]). The total dose to be taken would be five units (three units plus two units). If no food were to be eaten, then the dose to be taken would just be the two-unit correction factor.

If the correction dose is to be given after an exercise-induced high sugar, it should be reduced by half. (Delayed hypoglycemia may

TABLE 6:
Suggested "Thinking" Scale for Humalog/NovoLog/Apidra (H/NL/AP) or Regular (R) Insulin Dosage

Blood CGM Sugar Level	Morning H/NL/AP/R		Afternoon H/NL/AP/R		Dinner H/NL/AP/R	
	Active (or not eating much)	Not Active (eating normally)	Active (or not eating much)	Not Active (eating normally)	Active (or not eating much)	Not Active (eating normally)
_____ =	_____	_____	_____	_____	_____	_____
_____ =	_____	_____	_____	_____	_____	_____
_____ =	_____	_____	_____	_____	_____	_____
_____ =	_____	_____	_____	_____	_____	_____
_____ =	_____	_____	_____	_____	_____	_____
_____ =	_____	_____	_____	_____	_____	_____

NOTE: This table does not apply to sick day management (see Chapter 16). Call your diabetes care-provider AFTER CHECKING THE BLOOD/CGM SUGAR AND KETONES if you have questions. Scales may also be used for rapid-acting insulin dosages given at other times during the day. Copy this table as often as you wish.

follow as adrenaline levels decrease and sugar goes back into muscle – see Chapter 13.) Also, if a correction is to be done at bedtime, many people use half of the usual dose. Avoiding lows during the night is important.

Correction insulin doses are also discussed in Chapter 28 on insulin pumps. Insulin-to-carbohydrate (I/C) ratios are also discussed in Chapter 12 on food management.

E. "THINKING" SCALES (REPLACING THE TERM "SLIDING" SCALES)

The term "sliding" scale is often used for the system of giving rapid-acting (or Regular) insulin at meals based on the blood sugar value. We prefer to use the term "thinking" scales. They give the person or family ranges of H/NL/AP and/or Regular insulin to "think about." **The blood sugar level SHOULD NEVER be the only factor considered. Food intake and both recent and expected exercise also need to be considered with every shot.** An example would be a five-year-old going out to play with friends after dinner in the summer. If the blood/CGM sugar was 100 mg/dL (5.5 mmol/L) before dinner, it might be wise to reduce the evening dose of rapid-acting insulin. This would also apply if Mom (or Dad) was making tuna noodle casserole for dinner, and they knew that the five-year-old disliked tuna noodle casserole. **"Sliding" scales that do not account for food and exercise can be dangerous. In contrast, "thinking" scales in which insulin is adjusted based on multiple factors are helpful.** Thinking scales for different aged children are often based on whether they are still quite sensitive to rapid-acting insulin or not as sensitive. Possible scales should be discussed with your diabetes care-provider.

Many families adjust Humalog/NovoLog/Apidra and/or Regular (not NPH) insulin dosages with every injection. *They use a thinking scale in which the amount of rapid-acting insulin given is based on:*

1. the blood/CGM glucose level
2. the expected food intake
3. both recent and expected exercise
4. the CGM trend graph and the rate of glucose change (arrows)
5. other factors (e.g., illness, stress, menses)

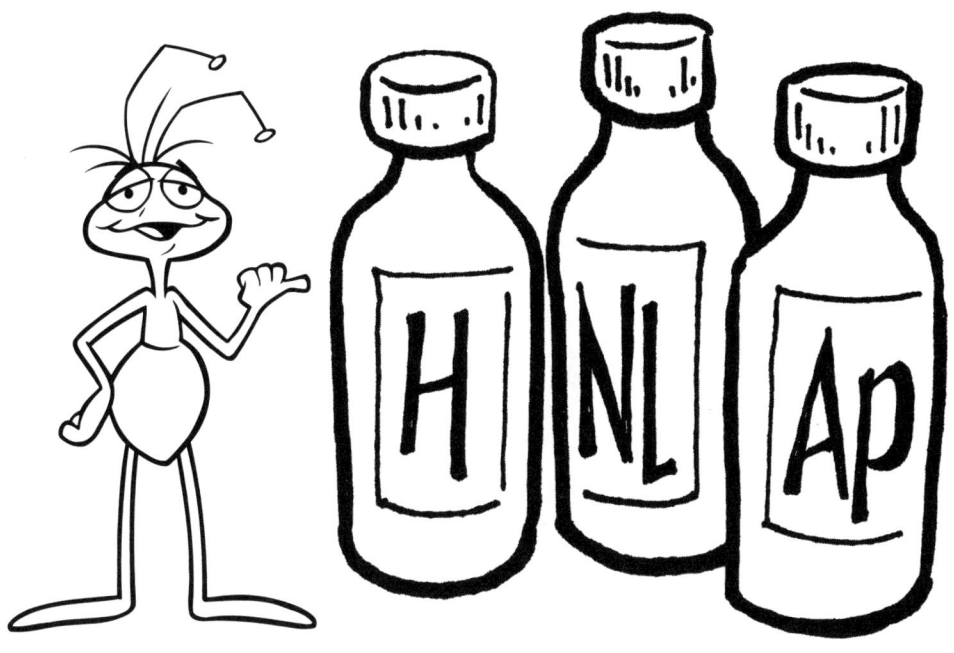

The insulin scale can be written down in Table 6. If the blood/CGM sugar is low, the amount is decreased. In contrast, the dose is increased for higher blood/CGM glucose levels or if less exercise is expected or if a large meal is to be eaten. Smaller children generally have lower dosages than larger children. Children in the first year after diagnosis (who make more of their own insulin) are usually more sensitive to rapid-acting insulins and will have lower dosages.

The blood/CGM glucose level must always be measured if the thinking scale is to be used. Sometimes one scale is used for the morning and a different scale for the evening. As indicated in Table 6, it may even be necessary to use one scale for an active day and a different scale for a quiet day.

It is important to remember that thinking scales are not "written in stone." A scale that works fine for a few months may have to be altered if the blood/CGM glucose levels are not in the desired range. Always bring the scale along to clinic visits so the dose can be reviewed with the diabetes care-provider. Also, write down the dose of insulin given in each shot on the blood sugar record sheet (see Chapter 7). This makes it possible for you and the diabetes care-provider to more easily review dosages and how the scales being used are working.

While "thinking" scales are an improvement on "sliding" scales, a disadvantage of "thinking" scales is that it can be challenging to determine how to make changes. Using "rules" for carbohydrate counting and for correction factors is preferred.

SUMMARY

In summary, it is important for families to consistently look at blood/CGM sugar levels. The HbA1c value may be up to one point lower in families who review values and look at patterns. They then make insulin adjustments to attain or maintain optimal blood sugar values. It is most frustrating when high blood/CGM glucose values are obtained week after week and no adjustments have been made. If a family is uncertain whether changes in insulin need to be made, fax, email or mail the blood/CGM sugar values and insulin dosages to the diabetes care-provider to get help. Remember to bring your meter and log book to the clinic visit.

DEFINITIONS

Correction factor: Use of a set amount of insulin to correct the blood sugar into the desired range. An example is giving one unit of Humalog/NovoLog/Apidra insulin for every 50 mg/dL (2.8 mmol/L) above 150 mg/dL (8.3 mmol/L) blood sugar level.

Sliding scale: Altering the insulin dose based on the blood/CGM sugar levels only.

Thinking scale: Altering the insulin dose considering factors in addition to blood/CGM sugar levels. The other factors might include food amount and type, exercise, stress, illness and menses.

QUESTIONS AND ANSWERS FROM NEWSNOTES

Q: What is meant by "sliding" scales for insulin adjustments, and who should use them?

a: "Sliding" scales generally refer to giving different dosages of Humalog/NovoLog/Apidra or Regular insulin depending on the level of blood/CGM sugar. They should not be used for NPH or Lantus (Basaglar)/Levemir/Tresiba. We prefer the term **"thinking"** scale to emphasize that the blood/CGM glucose level, food intake and exercise must all be considered before each insulin dose is chosen. On some occasions, illness, stress and menses must also be considered. Although thinking scales can be helpful for some people, most now use carb counting and correction factors to calculate the insulin dosage.

Q: Do the needs for insulin change with the seasons?

a: The short answer is "yes." To illustrate this, think of summer camp. Nearly every person going to camp has their routine dose of insulin substantially reduced because of all the extra activity. To a lesser degree this happens in spring – over a week or two the snow suddenly disappears, the sunshine appears, and children are out playing, bicycling, etc. With the increased activity, low blood/CGM glucose levels are more likely. Snacks may have to be adjusted and/or insulin doses may need to be lowered.

In contrast, the opposite happens with going back to school in the fall, especially for those going to new schools. This may be a time of extra stress as well as reduced activity. Activity is decreased with the evening homework. Blood/CGM glucose levels may go up and insulin doses may need to be raised.

CHAPTER 23

Long-Term Complications of Diabetes

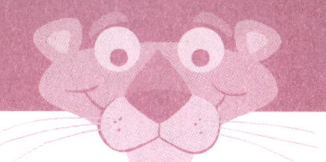

INTRODUCTION

In addition to the acute complications of diabetes, hypoglycemia and acidosis, there are also problems known as "long-term" complications. Generally, the long-term complications occur in people who have had diabetes and high blood sugar levels for many years. Maintaining a healthy weight with exercise and a healthy diet is important for good health.

About this chapter:

✓ Many families may prefer to read this chapter when they are ready to deal with the subject.

✓ Adults and teenagers may be able to understand the material better than pre-teens.

✓ It is important to know that good diabetes care reduces the risk of future complications.

✓ Many new and difficult words are used in this chapter. They are introduced and defined in the back. If your diabetes care-provider uses them, you will have a place to find their meaning.

The four most common parts of the body to be affected by high sugar levels are:

1. Eyes (retinopathy)
2. Kidneys (nephropathy)
3. Nerves (neuropathy)
4. Heart and blood vessels (cardiovascular)

TOPICS:
Prevent, Detect and Treat Chronic Complications Through Risk Reduction
Monitoring (Complications and Associated Diseases)

TEACHING OBJECTIVES:
The teacher will:
1. Discuss the relationship of glucose levels and other risk factors on diabetes complications (eye, kidney, nerve and heart).
2. Summarize the methods to monitor eye and kidney complications.

LEARNING OBJECTIVES:
Learner (parents, child, relative or self) will be able to:
1. Describe the relationship between glucose levels and complications.
2. Describe the effect of smoking on diabetes complications.
3. Identify routine methods used to monitor the eyes and kidneys.

Three other areas that can be affected by high sugar levels are:

5. Joints (finger curvatures)
6. Birth defects in infants born to mothers with high HbA1c levels
7. Foot problems

THE DCCT

The Diabetes Control and Complications Trial (DCCT) has been mentioned previously in this book (Chapter 14). The results of this study became available in 1993 and proved without question that **eye, kidney and nerve problems of type 1 diabetes were decreased in people ages 13-39 years whose blood sugars were kept closer to normal. They also reported that lower HbA1c levels resulted in a 57 percent reduction in nonfatal heart attacks, strokes and coronary vascular disease.**

For people with type 2 diabetes, studies in the U.K. and Japan showed the risks for eye, kidney and nerve complication were reduced as a result of better diabetes management.

Some important factors that affect the complications:

- ✔ **optimal blood sugar levels:** Although this is one important factor in relation to these complications, **IT IS NOT THE ONLY FACTOR**
- ✔ **high blood pressure and abnormal blood lipids** are important in relation to eye, kidney and heart complications
- ✔ **tobacco use** adds to the risk for kidney, eye and heart damage
- ✔ **increased blood clotting** is also a possible risk factor
- ✔ **other unknown factors, including genetics**

Some facts about the occurrence of complications:

- ✔ Most of the long-term complications do not occur in young children.
- ✔ The years of greatest risk for complications seem to start after puberty. Research has shown that in people with diabetes, the small blood vessels showed no changes before puberty, whether optimal sugar management was present or not.
- ✔ After puberty, the blood vessels usually remain healthy in people with low HbA1c values, but changes are more likely to appear in people with chronic high HbA1c values.
- ✔ Around the time of puberty, levels of growth hormone, sex hormones and other hormones increase greatly. These hormones cause increased blood sugar levels.
- ✔ The risk of complications after puberty may increase because of the changes in hormone levels, because of high sugar levels caused by the changes in hormone levels, or possibly due to both.

We are continuing to learn more about how the high blood/CGM glucose levels cause the complications.

Sugar does attach:

- ✔ to the protein (hemoglobin) in the red blood cells to form hemoglobin A1c or HbA1c (see Chapter 14)
- ✔ to the skin proteins in people who have curvatures of several fingers (see "Finger Curvatures" in this chapter)
- ✔ to other proteins in the blood vessels and other parts of the body when the blood sugar levels are very high

Once the sugar attaches to a body protein, the protein may not work as well as when sugar is not attached.

Although not yet proven, there is some evidence that wide fluctuations in blood/CGM glucose levels may also add to the risk for complications. Until people began to use continuous glucose monitors (CGM), it was not realized how much glucose levels fluctuated. These fluctuations usually decrease in people who consistently wear a CGM.

Even though the vascular complications are not usually seen before puberty, it is important to work for optimal blood/CGM glucose levels in the pre-pubertal years. There are some side effects of high blood/CGM glucose levels that can occur at any time (see Chapter 14). Also, the habits for the future are formed when the person is young.

COMPLICATIONS IN PEOPLE WITH DIABETES

Complications related, at least in part, to high blood sugar levels:

1. EYE PROBLEMS

Cataracts

Cataracts are small thickenings in the lens (which is located at the front of the eye; see picture in this chapter).

- The damage to the lens is believed to be caused by sorbitol, a compound made in the lens from glucose.
- Sorbitol damage occurs when blood glucose (sugar) levels have been very high in the body for a long time.
- Sorbitol in foods is changed by the body (liver) and does not cause this damage.
- Damage to the lens can happen at any age.
- Rarely, cataracts can be present at the onset of diabetes if sugar levels have been high for a long time before insulin is started.
- They may show some improvement with optimal sugar levels.
- These lens changes are not the same as the more severe retinal complications in the back of the eye that are discussed next.
- The eye doctor (ophthalmologist or optometrist) will do a detailed exam for cataracts in the yearly eye exam, starting around the time of puberty.
- If cataracts interfere with vision, they can be removed surgically by the eye doctor.

Retinal Changes or Retinopathy

The word retinopathy refers to changes of the retina, which is the layer of tissue at the back of the eye (see picture of the eye). This part of the eye has many small blood vessels similar to those found in the kidney.

A. *Retinopathy facts:*

Retinopathy is a change in the small blood vessels found in the back of the eye (retina), which occurs mainly after puberty. The DCCT showed that in people without eye changes from diabetes, lower blood sugars delayed development of retinopathy by 76 percent. The DCCT also showed that, in people with known early eye changes from diabetes, intensive therapy slowed the progression of retinopathy

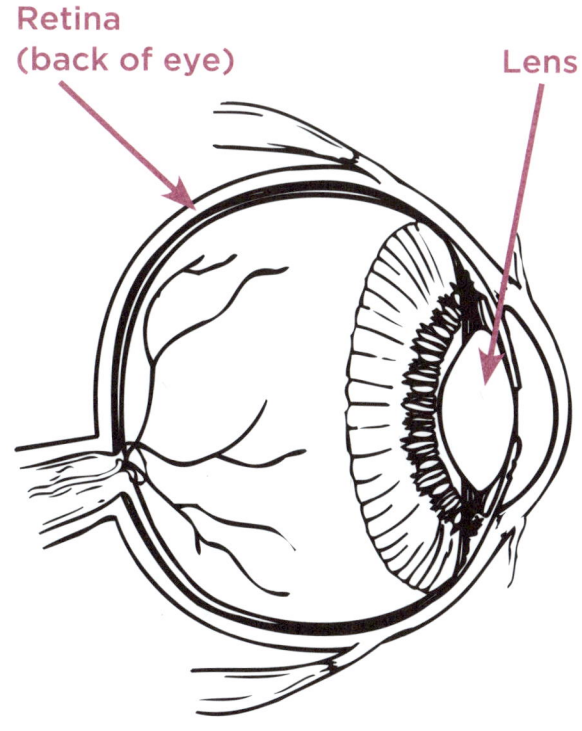

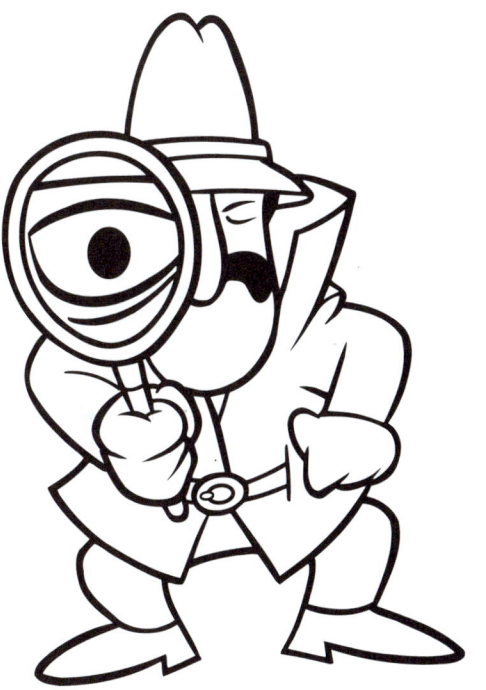

by 54 percent and reduced the incidence of severe retinopathy by 47 percent.

▼ increased blood pressure also results in a greater risk for retinal changes

▼ tobacco use makes these changes progress more rapidly

We do not understand all of the causes of the eye changes from diabetes. There is a small group of people for whom the presence or absence of eye changes does not seem be associated with sugar levels.

B. *Diabetes*:

✔ Early detection is very important and is one clear argument for having diabetes check-ups every three months.

✔ The diabetes care-provider doing the physical exam should be able to detect eye changes and make appropriate referrals to an eye doctor (ophthalmologist) who specializes in diabetic changes (retinal specialist).

✔ **The ADA recommends annual screening for people who have had type 1 diabetes for five or more years, starting at age 10 years or at puberty, whichever is first. How long someone has had type 2 diabetes before diagnosis is often not known. For this reason, people with type 2 diabetes should see the eye doctor soon after diagnosis (if ≥10 years old).**

✔ Thereafter, if there are no diabetic eye changes, or if the changes are minor, yearly visits to the diabetes eye specialist are adequate.

✔ Minor eye changes include a ballooning of the small retinal blood vessels; these changes are reversible and are called **"microaneurysms."** Some people can have these minor changes for many years and not develop more severe eye disease. Careful blood sugar management is particularly important when any changes are detected. If more severe eye changes occur, then more frequent visits to the diabetes eye specialist are needed.

C. *More severe eye disease:*

"Pre-proliferative" and "proliferative" retinopathy:

• Usually involves formation of new (proliferative) and fragile retinal blood vessels, which are at a greater risk for breaking (hemorrhaging).

• The more severe changes are referred for **laser treatment**. This involves the use of a very bright light. It was begun in the 1970s as a way to save vision in people with diabetes who have severe eye changes.

• Laser treatment destroys the fragile (proliferative) new blood vessels and has been very effective in reducing the loss of vision.

• The most important factor is to have close follow-up once the more severe changes appear. Laser treatment can then be done at the proper time.

• The biggest danger is a hemorrhage. It could damage the retina or send blood into the vitreous fluid between the lens and retina (vitreous hemorrhage) or cause the retina to separate from the other layers in the back of the eye (retinal detachment).

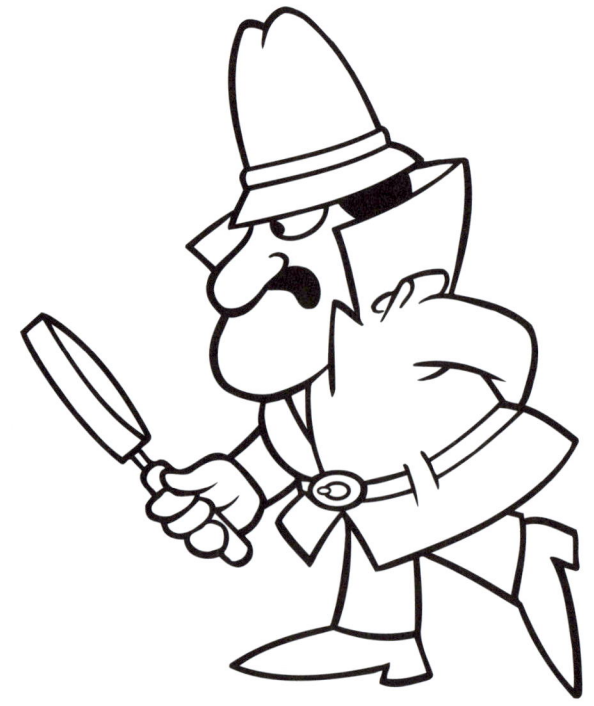

LONG-TERM COMPLICATIONS OF DIABETES

2. KIDNEY DISEASE OR DIABETIC NEPHROPATHY

A. *The job of the kidneys in the body:*

✔ They normally filter wastes and water from our blood and make urine (Chapter 2).

✔ When blood/CGM glucose levels are high, sugar is passed into the urine. When this happens, the pressures are higher in the kidney filtering system (the glomerulus), and changes in the small blood vessels of the kidney can occur. This increased pressure causes damage to the filtering system so that some proteins start leaking through the filter and appear in the urine.

B. *Kidney disease, or nephropathy, is more likely to occur in people:*

✔ after puberty
✔ who have had diabetes for a long time
✔ with high HbA1c values
✔ with elevated blood pressure
✔ who smoke or chew tobacco

Outcomes for kidney disease have improved in diabetes in the past few decades. However, it still occurs in 20 to 40 percent of people with diabetes.

C. *Signs of kidney disease may include:*

▼ increased blood pressure
▼ ankle swelling, also known as edema (due to fluid collection)
▼ excessive urine protein spillage
▼ elevation of the waste materials in the blood (increased blood creatinine and urea nitrogen or BUN)

D. *The Microalbumin level:*

• detects diabetic kidney damage at an early stage when it might still be reversible
• is often initially done on a random spot or first morning void urine sample for albumin-to-creatinine ratio (ACR). A normal value is considered to be less than 30 micrograms of albumin per mg of creatinine
• should be measured annually for people who have had type 1 diabetes for five or more years, starting at age 10 years or puberty, whichever is first
• should be done soon after diagnosis for people with type 2 diabetes
• should then be done once yearly so that the interval is not missed when the early damage is still reversible
• if the screening sample is elevated, further evaluation is best done by collecting the overnight urine sample (see directions at the end of this chapter)

If there is an increased level of microalbumin in the overnight urine on two separate evaluations:

▼ A "borderline microalbumin level" for timed overnight urine collections is a value between 7.6 µg/minute and 20 µg/minute. This "borderline" range represents a time period when optimal sugar and/or blood pressure levels may help to lower the value or keep it from going higher.

▼ Medications should not usually be given for a "borderline" level, as it is possible to return the value to normal by lowering the HbA1c or blood pressure.

▼ If the urine microalbumin value is between 20 and 200 µg/minute, it is called **"microalbuminuria"** and is reversible with lowering of blood/CGM glucose values, of blood pressure, and/or with medications (e.g., ACE-inhibitor, see Part E). There can be spontaneous regression from microalbuminuria to normal, and two (of three) samples above 20 µg/min are required prior to diagnosis.

▼ The term "persistent albuminuria" has been used to indicate albumin spillage in a 24-hour urine at levels of 30-299 mg or at a level above 300 mg per 24 hours. Normal 24-hour albumin excretion is below 30 mg per 24 hours.

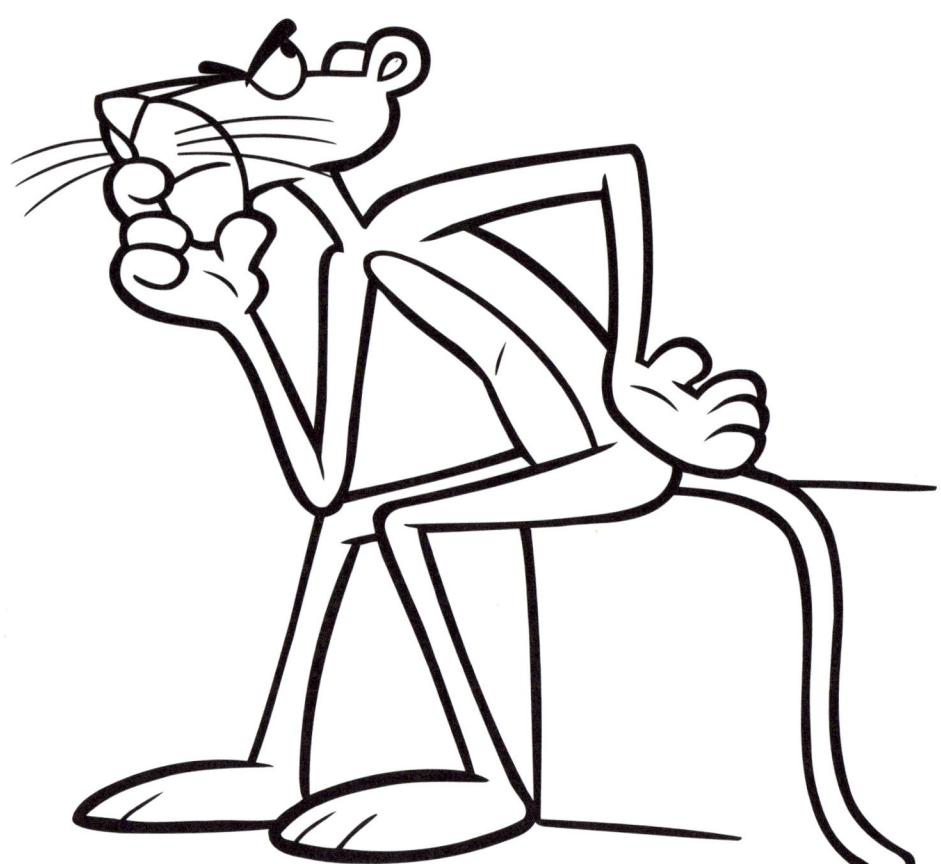

- ▼ Smoking cigarettes and chewing tobacco lead to a greater risk for kidney damage and must be avoided by people with diabetes.

- ▼ The DCCT showed that improved glucose management reduced the occurrence of microalbuminuria by 39 percent. Gross kidney damage (nephropathy or albuminuria) was reduced by 54 percent. It must once again be remembered that high glucose levels are NOT the only cause of diabetic kidney damage.

- ▼ The DCCT/EDIC study showed that after 18 years, the Intensive Treatment group had 17.5 percent of subjects with persistent albuminuria (4 percent >300mg/24hrs) compared to 28 percent (7.4 percent >300mg/24hrs) for the Conventional Treatment group.

E. ***The past three decades have brought significant advances in attempting to prevent, detect and treat diabetic kidney damage.***

- ✔ It is up to the family and the physician to make sure that the urine collections to detect kidney changes are done at the recommended times.

- ✔ If the microalbumin levels are not done, the "window" during which changes may be reversible could be missed.

- ✔ If the microalbumin levels on the overnight or 24-hour urines are high, medicines may be effective in reversing or slowing the kidney damage.

- • The usual medicine that is tried first is an **ACE-inhibitor** (ACE = **A**ngiotensin-**C**onverting **E**nzyme). This medication reduces formation of angiotensin II, which is a very potent constrictor of blood vessels. The result is less pressure buildup in the kidneys. There are several varieties of ACE-inhibitors, all of which are probably effective if given in adequate dosage. Another similar class of medications is called **ARBs** (or **A**ngiotensin **R**eceptor **B**lockers).

- • Early kidney damage is detectable, and methods to reverse or slow down kidney damage are available. This has now resulted in a decline in the incidence of kidney failure from diabetes.

3. NEUROPATHY (NERVE DAMAGE)

Diabetic neuropathy, or "damage to the nerves," is a condition seen after puberty, usually in people who have had very high sugar levels for a long time. Neuropathy screening is done as part of the physical exam.

About neuropathy:

- ✓ It is a complex condition that we still do not completely understand.
- ✓ The DCCT found that the incidence of neuropathy was 60 percent less in the group with the lower HbA1c levels.
- ✓ As with cataracts, neuropathy is believed to be related, at least in part, to increased sorbitol levels deposited in the nerves. The sorbitol is made from sugar.
- ✓ There is also a decrease in another compound (myoinositol) which is important for the nerves.
- ✓ Some people with type 2 diabetes have neuropathy when they are diagnosed with diabetes.

The neuropathy usually makes itself known with:

- ▼ numbness, tingling, sharp pains in the lower legs or feet
- ▼ changes in other parts of the body: e.g., the rate at which food moves through the intestines may change (gastroparesis)

Much research is being done to find new and better medications for the treatment of neuropathy.

4. CORONARY (HEART) AND OTHER LARGER BLOOD VESSELS (Cardiovascular; see Table)

The "larger" blood vessels are in contrast to the very small (sometimes microscopic) ones found in our eyes and kidneys. The larger ones include the heart blood vessels that provide blood (and thus nutrition and oxygen) to the heart. When a heart blood vessel is blocked, a "heart attack" can result. Approximately 50 percent of deaths for older people with diabetes are due to heart attacks. Heart attacks have many causes, some of which are outlined in the table.

- ▼ Until a few years ago, diets that contained 40 percent of calories from fat were routinely recommended. Most dietitians now recommend that no more than 30 percent of calories be from fat sources. High fat intake is known to raise blood cholesterol levels (see Chapters 11 and 12).
- ▼ Heredity and chronic high HbA1c levels also can be causes of high cholesterol levels.

Recommendations:

- Blood cholesterol and LDL-cholesterol levels should be checked at puberty and then

TABLE:
Heart and Blood Vessel (Cardiovascular) Risk Factors

Risk Factors	Aim to Reduce Risk
high glucose (sugar) levels	HbA1c in recommended range for age
blood pressure	below 130/80 or 90th percentile for age
tobacco use	don't use
elevated total cholesterol	below 200 mg/dL (5.2 mmol/L)
elevated LDL cholesterol	below 100 mg/dL (2.6 mmol/L)
elevated (fasting) triglyceride	below 150 mg/dL (1.7 mmol/L)
If any of the levels are elevated, it is important to discuss with your physician.	

annually. Desired levels are given in Table 2 of Chapter 11.

- Medications (the "statins") that block our body's cholesterol synthesis are available for people who have very high cholesterol or LDL levels. The statins have been shown to decrease the risk for heart attacks.
- Blood pressure should be checked at regular clinic visits. Increases in blood pressure should be treated early.
- People with diabetes should not use tobacco!
- Exercise is important to maintain a healthy weight and improve insulin sensitivity.

Sexual Function

✔ Some males with diabetes have problems with penile erections. The cause of this problem is believed to be related in part to microvascular disease. It is also related to autonomic neuropathy. The medicines Viagra®, Levitra® and Cialis® may be helpful to some men with diabetes who have this problem.

5. JOINT CONTRACTURES

Some facts:

✔ Some people cannot touch the knuckles of the second joint in their fifth fingers (little fingers) when their hands are in a "praying" position.

✔ The joints of the other fingers or other joints in the body can also be involved.

✔ When other joints or fingers other than just the fifth finger are involved, there has usually been a period of very high sugar levels, and sugar has attached to the proteins in the skin over the joints.

✔ No pain or other problems are usually related to these changes.

✔ Some doctors believe the curvatures of the fifth fingers may be partly inherited.

6. BIRTH DEFECTS (discussed in more detail in Chapter 31)

This complication is primarily important to a woman who might get pregnant.

Some facts:

✔ IT IS VERY IMPORTANT TO TALK TO YOUR DIABETES PHYSICIAN BEFORE GETTING PREGNANT.

✔ Insulin pumps and intensive diabetes management must be considered PRIOR TO THE PREGNANCY.

✔ If diabetes is not well managed (e.g., high HbA1c), a pregnant woman with diabetes is more likely to have a baby with one or more birth problems or defects.

✔ The first few months of pregnancy are the most important in avoiding defects.

✔ A woman should not stop using birth control or decide to get pregnant until her HbA1c is in the desired range.

✔ If the HbA1c, blood pressure and kidney microalbumin levels are normal or low prior to the pregnancy, the likelihood of kidney deterioration during pregnancy is minimized.

✔ Diabetic eye changes do sometimes worsen during pregnancy, and it is wise to be followed more closely by one's retinal specialist during this time.

7. FOOT PROBLEMS

Some facts:

✓ Foot problems due to decreased blood flow and neuropathy do not occur in children. Some families who are educated by diabetes care-providers who care mainly for adults with diabetes will be told that children must "wash their feet daily" or "never go barefoot." Although it is nice to have clean feet for clinic visits, these precautions are NOT necessary for children.

✓ Foot problems, when they occur, are usually occur in older adults and may be related to poor circulation or to neuropathy.

✓ There is research suggesting that regular exercise may help to maintain normal foot circulation later in life (see Chapter 13).

✓ It is important for diabetes care-providers to do careful examinations of feet in post-pubertal patients.

✓ It is also important for a person to know to call the doctor if a foot sore does not heal well or if there is any sign of an infection (redness, warmth or pus) or ulcer.

✓ Ingrown toenails (an infection) occur with similar frequency in children with or without diabetes.

✓ The ingrown toenails are usually caused by toenails that are cut too short at the corners.

✓ The toenails should be cut straight across with a straight nail clipper and the length should be even with the end of the toe.

✓ Ingrown toenails are more of a problem in people with diabetes, as infections cause high sugar levels. The high sugar levels, in turn, support the infection.

✓ Warts are not more common in people with diabetes. The best way to remove them is with the use of liquid nitrogen.

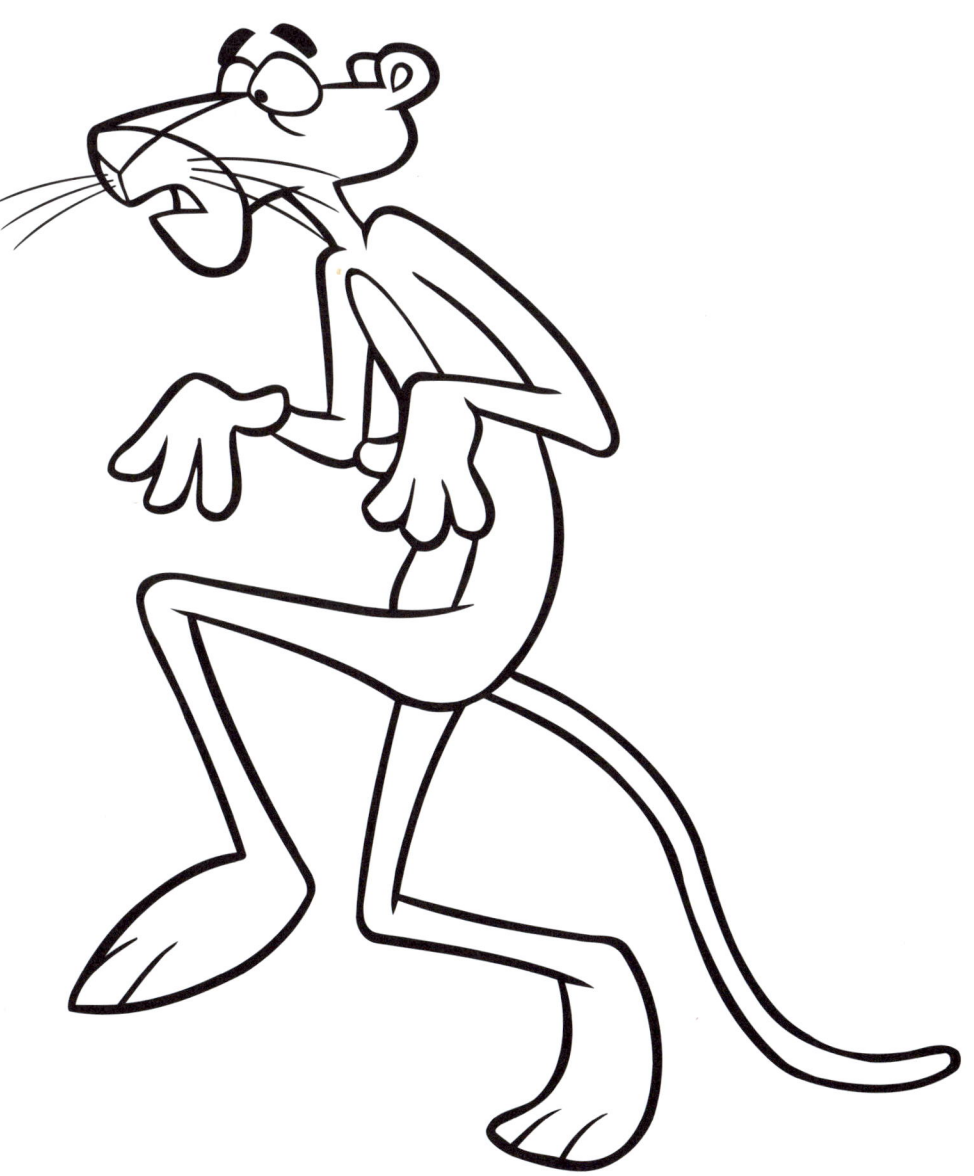

LONG-TERM COMPLICATIONS OF DIABETES

DEFINITIONS

Blood pressure: The blood pressure consists of a higher (systolic) pressure that reflects the pumping or working pressure of the heart and a lower (diastolic) pressure that reflects the resting pressure of the heart between beats. It is important to have the blood pressure checked regularly.

Blood Urea Nitrogen (BUN): A material in the blood normally cleared by the kidneys. It is elevated in advanced kidney disease as well as with dehydration.

Cataract: A density (clouding) in the lens that may cause spots, blurred or reduced vision.

Creatinine: A material in the blood normally cleared by the kidneys. The test to measure its clearance from the blood is called a creatinine clearance test.

DCCT: Diabetes Control and Complications Trial. A very large trial of people ages 13-39 years old, which showed that lower HbA1c values resulted in a lower risk for diabetic eye, kidney, nerve and heart problems. The trial ended in June 1993, but many of the people continued to be followed in the EDIC study.

Edema: Collection of fluid (swelling) under the skin.

Filter: To separate out or remove. The kidneys filter wastes from our blood.

Gastroparesis: Neuropathy involving the stomach and/or intestine.

Glomerulus: Small groups of blood vessels in the kidneys that filter the blood to remove wastes and water to make urine.

Hemorrhage: The breaking of a blood vessel. In the eye, this can occur in the retinal layer or, in more advanced cases, in the fluid (vitreous fluid) in front of the retina (vitreous hemorrhage).

Laser treatment: Using a very bright beam of light to destroy the new (proliferative) blood vessels in the retina, which are at high risk for hemorrhaging and causing a loss of vision.

Lens (see picture of eye in this chapter): The oval structure in the front of the eye that changes shape to allow the eye to focus on near or distant objects.

Microalbumin: A method to measure small amounts of a protein (albumin) in the urine to detect kidney damage from diabetes at a stage in which it might still be reversible.

Microaneurysm: A small dilatation (ballooning) of a blood vessel, which is a minor change that can be reversible. It is caused by diabetes.

Myoinositol: A compound that is reduced in nerves when sorbitol levels are elevated (in neuropathy).

Nephropathy: A generic name for kidney disease. It is usually used to indicate a more advanced stage of kidney involvement.

Neuropathy: A disease of the nerves. This is believed to happen in people with diabetes due to accumulation of sorbitol (formed from blood glucose), or possibly due to deficiency of another metabolite, myoinositol.

Ophthalmologist: The name for a doctor (MD) who specializes in eye diseases. The ophthalmologist may further specialize in the retinal layer in the back of the eye, which is affected by diabetes. The doctor is then called a "retinal specialist."

Optometrist: An eye doctor who is not an MD (although they are still important care-providers). They can screen for diabetic eye disease.

Podiatrist: A person who is specially trained in the care of the feet. They are not MDs (although they are still important care-providers).

Pre-proliferative or proliferative retinopathy: Terms for more advanced stages of eye involvement from diabetes (when a diabetes eye specialist needs to be seen more frequently).

Puberty: The time in a teen's life when adult sexual changes occur.

Retina (see picture of eye in this chapter): The layers of small blood vessels and nerves in the back of the eye that are very important for vision.

Retinal detachment: Separation of the retinal layer in the back of the eye from other layers in the eye.

Retinopathy: Changes in the retinal (small blood vessel) layer in the back of the eye from diabetes. These are more likely to occur after puberty in people who have had diabetes for a long time and who have had high HbA1c levels.

Vitreous fluid: The fluid between the lens and the retina. When retinal blood vessels break, they can bleed into the vitreous fluid (vitreous hemorrhage).

QUESTIONS AND ANSWERS FROM NEWSNOTES

Q: Is cigarette smoking unhealthy for someone with diabetes?

a: Yes. It is linked to lung cancer, high blood pressure and heart attacks in ALL people and is thus a poor choice for everyone. In addition, data from our Center has shown that smoking results in about a three-fold greater likelihood of diabetic kidney complications. Smoking also causes diabetic eye disease to progress more rapidly. The mechanism by which smoking does this is unknown, but as people who chew tobacco seem to have the same consequences, it may be from the absorption of nicotine into the body. HbA1c levels are often high in smokers with diabetes. Therefore, these effects had to be removed before a conclusion about smoking could be reached. Smoking results in higher HbA1c levels by increasing levels of other hormones, such as adrenaline, that raise the blood sugar. The heart rate and blood pressure also increase, and this may be related to the increased eye and kidney problems.

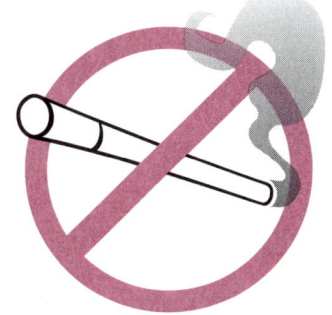

Q: How common is kidney disease in association with diabetes, and what can be done to reduce its likelihood?

a: Kidney problems occur in up to 30 percent of people with type 1 diabetes, although uncommon before the person reaches age 30 or 40 years. There are things that we can do now to help reduce the likelihood of kidney problems. These include optimal sugar management, keeping the blood pressure normal, prompt treatment of bladder and kidney infections and not smoking. It is very important to get the urine microalbumins checked yearly for people who have had type 1 diabetes for three or more years and who have reached puberty.

Q: Are contact lenses OK for a person with diabetes to use?

a: Yes, people with diabetes can wear contact lenses, but there are some extra precautions. The contact lens fits over the superficial layer of the eye called the cornea. The cornea needs a constant supply of oxygen and tears to keep it healthy. Thus, the contact lens must fit properly so that the cornea is not injured, and the tears are able to continue to flow. It is even more important for people with diabetes to follow the instructions for care and cleaning of the contact lenses than it is for other people. The corneas of people with diabetes are sometimes less sensitive to pain or irritation, so people may be less likely to feel discomfort when their contacts are causing problems. Infections may also not clear as quickly if they do occur. Thus, use the solutions and disinfectants exactly as your eye doctor recommends. Don't get lazy in cleaning or try to cut corners. Don't leave the contacts in any longer than recommended. Don't mix cleaning solutions.

MICROALBUMINS

Doctor: _____   Your Name: _____

A. INSTRUCTIONS FOR DOING THE OVERNIGHT URINE COLLECTIONS

COLLECTION #1
1. Empty your bladder at bedtime and discard this sample.
2. Save EVERY DROP of urine during the night.
3. Save EVERY DROP of the first morning sample.
   ALL urine from collection #1 should be placed in the same container.
4. Measure the volume of the total urine sample.

DATE: _____
TIME: _____
TIME: _____
TOTAL VOLUME: _____

COLLECTION #2
1. Empty your bladder at bedtime and discard this sample.
2. Save EVERY DROP of urine during the night.
3. Save EVERY DROP of the first morning sample.
   ALL urine from collection #1 should be placed in the same container.
4. Measure the volume of the total urine sample.

DATE: _____
TIME: _____
TIME: _____
TOTAL VOLUME: _____

B. IMPORTANT INFORMATION ABOUT YOUR COLLECTIONS

1. Label each container with your name and #1 or #2.
2. You may use any CLEAN container you have at home that will not leak to collect the sample. We do not provide containers.
3. Store part of each of the two collected and measured urine samples in a refrigerator until your visit (samples are good for one week if kept cold).
4. DO NOT mix collections #1 and #2 together in the same container.
5. DO NOT drink caffeinated or alcoholic beverages or use tobacco after 10 p.m. the evening of the collections.
6. DO NOT exercise strenuously for the four hours prior to bedtime.
7. DO NOT collect specimens during a menstrual period.
8. Failure to follow directions exactly may cause incorrect results.
9. If you have any questions, please call your healthcare-provider.

C. DIRECTIONS FOR MEASURING THE VOLUME

1. Have a measuring cup or (better) a cylinder – preferably marked in cc (mL). One cup is 240 cc. Urine is sterile and it is okay to use cooking measuring cups (just wash prior to next use for cooking).
2. Measure the total cc of each overnight sample and put the amounts in the blanks for step 4 for collections #1 and #2.
3. Put a sample of each urine collection in a clean tube. The rest may be discarded. Any clean red top tube from a doctor's office, clinic or hospital lab will work. Label which sample (#1 or #2) it is, put your name on the tube, and put the tube in a cup in the refrigerator until you get to your clinic. Bring this sheet with the times and total volumes with you.

CHAPTER 24

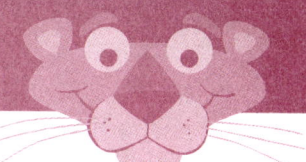

Associated Autoimmune Conditions of Type 1 Diabetes

INTRODUCTION

Other autoimmune (self-allergy) diseases are also associated with type 1 diabetes. This is due to the inheritance of genes increasing the risk for autoimmunity (type 1 diabetes also being partly due to autoimmunity). Some examples of autoimmune diseases seen more frequently in people with type 1 diabetes are discussed below:

THYROID DISORDERS (most common)

Some facts:

✔ Some thyroid enlargement occurs in about half of people with type 1 diabetes, although only about one in 10 ever needs treatment. The likelihood increases with increasing age. The reason for this is believed to be a similar "self-allergy" (autoimmune) type of reaction that causes both diabetes and the related thyroid enlargement.

✔ People who get diabetes often have an antibody (allergic reaction) in their blood against their pancreas (specifically, the islet cells in the pancreas, as discussed in Chapter 3). Likewise, people with diabetes who get thyroid problems usually have an antibody in their blood against the thyroid gland.

✔ Thyroid antibody tests can be done, although doctors frequently only measure thyroid function.

✔ It is important for the diabetes care-provider to always check the size of the thyroid gland at the time of clinic visits.

> **TOPICS:**
> **Monitoring Associated Autoimmune Diseases**
>
> **TEACHING OBJECTIVES:**
> The teacher will:
> 1. Present type 1 diabetes associated autoimmune diseases.
>
> **LEARNING OBJECTIVES:**
> Learner (parents, child, relative or self) will be able to:
> 1. List two autoimmune conditions associated with type 1 diabetes

✔ If the thyroid is not producing enough thyroid hormone, growth in height may be slowed and weight gain may be in excess.

✔ The person may feel tired or cold all of the time.

✔ If the gland is enlarged, specialized blood tests should be done (particularly a TSH level, as this is almost always the first test to become abnormal). If the TSH level is abnormal, it is wise to repeat the TSH level and to also evaluate other thyroid parameters.

✔ If the thyroid tests are abnormal, a thyroid tablet can then be taken once daily. Thyroid problems are not serious unless unrecognized or untreated. The treatment is excellent, easy, inexpensive, and involves taking pills (not shots).

✔ Sometimes the tablets can be discontinued (under a doctor's supervision) when the person is finished growing.

- ✔ Thyroid problems are common even in people who do not have diabetes (about one in 50 adults).
- ✔ Less frequently (≈ 1 percent), people with type 1 diabetes can also have an overactive thyroid gland that produces excess thyroid hormone (hyperthyroidism). This is important to diagnose and to treat.

CELIAC DISEASE (also common)

Celiac disease (also known as gluten sensitivity, gluten-enteropathy or celiac sprue) is an inherited disorder in which the small intestine is damaged by an autoimmune reaction to gluten, a protein found in grains like wheat, rye and barley. Celiac disease is more likely in youth diagnosed at a younger age, is more likely in girls than in boys, and may be associated with a lower height (close monitoring needed). The damage to the small intestine causes nutrients to be malabsorbed. When people are thought to have celiac disease, it is important to also work with the GI (gastro-intestinal) doctors.

Some facts:

- ✔ The risk for celiac disease is carried on one of the genes (DR types, DR3) that is also related to being at high risk for type 1 diabetes (see Chapter 3).
- ✔ Approximately one in 20 people with type 1 diabetes also has celiac disease (3.5 percent in a recent study of youth and 4.5 percent in average of many studies of all ages).

TABLE 1:
Grain, Seeds, Flours, and Cereals List for Celiac Disease

ALLOWED	USE WITH CAUTION	NOT ALLOWED
Amaranth	*Oats	Barley
Arrowroot		Bran
Buckwheat		Bulgur
Corn		Couscous
Flax		Durum
Hominy		Einkorn
Legume flours (bean, chickpea, garbanzo)		Emmer
Millet		Farina
Montina™ (Indian rice grass)		Farro
Nut flours (almond, hazelnut, pecan)		Graham
Potato flour		Kamut
Potato starch		Rye
Quinoa		Semolina
Rice		Spelt
Sorghum		Triticale
Soy and other beans		Wheat
Tapioca		Wheat germ
Teff		White flour
		Whole wheat

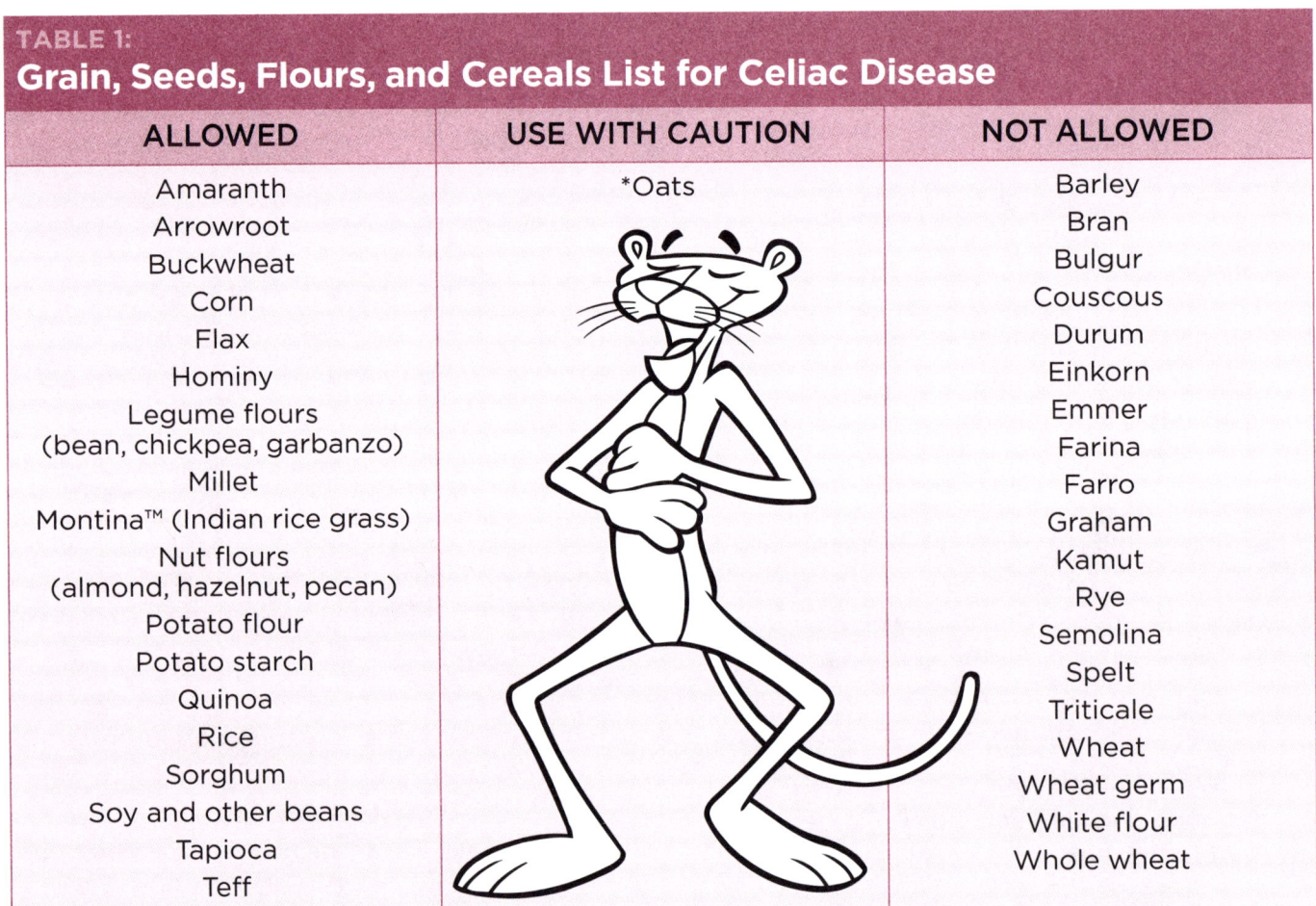

* Oats cannot be guaranteed to be gluten-free. Contamination can happen when oats are grown on the same field or processed in the same building as gluten-containing grains.

Table adapted from The Children's Hospital General Clinical Research Center's "Introduction to the Gluten-Free (GF) Diet" packet, Denver CO)

Reference List for Celiac Disease

CELIAC ASSOCIATIONS IN THE UNITED STATES

Celiac Disease Foundation
818-990-2354
13251 Ventura Blvd. #1
Studio City, CA 91604
www.celiac.org

Celiac Sprue Association/USA, Inc.
402-558-0600
877-CSA-4-CSA (Toll Free)
P.O. Box 31700
Omaha, NE 68131-0700
www.csaceliacs.org

Gluten Intolerance Group
253-833-6655
31214 124th Ave SE
Auburn, WA 98092
www.gluten.org

WEBSITES AND SUPPORT GROUPS:

www.celiac.com is an excellent site for safe/forbidden food additive lists, mainstream GF food products by brand name, GF recipes, discussion of controversial grains, etc. — just a good reference overall

www.celiachealth.org Children's Digestive Health and Nutrition Foundation. Can download: Gluten-Free Diet Guide for Families

www.glutenfreedrugs.com Lists gluten free drugs and vitamins and is maintained and run by clinical pharmacists. Lets you search a database of over 30,000 foods for gluten-free products, reads labels for you and gives you the gluten free status of each product

BOOKS:

Living Gluten-Free for Dummies by Danna Korn, For Dummies, 2010. www.amazon.com

Gluten-Free Diet: A Comprehensive Resource Guide by Shelly Case, Case Nutrition Consulting, 2010. www.glutenfreediet.ca

The Gluten-Free Gourmet Bakes Bread by Bette Hagman, Henry Holt, 2000. www.celiac.com

The Gluten-Free Gourmet Cooks Fast and Healthy by Bette Hagman, Henry Holt, 2000. www.amazon.com or www.celiac.com

Wheat-Free, Gluten-Free Cookbook for Kids and Busy Adults by Connie Sarros, McGraw Hill, 2010. www.amazon.com or www.celiac.com

Pocket Dictionary: Acceptability of Foods and Food Ingredients for the Gluten-Free Diet Canadian Celiac Association. www.celiac.ca

MAGAZINES:

Gluten-Free Living: The Resource for People with Gluten Intolerance. A newsletter available by contacting Gluten-Free Living, P.O. Box 105, Hasting-on-Hudson, NY 10706.

Living Without: A Lifestyle Guide for People with Allergies and Food Sensitivities. www.livingwithout.com

✔ As other family members who do not have diabetes may also have the DR3 genetic type, they are also more likely to have celiac disease (even though they do not have diabetes).

✔ It can be diagnosed using a blood antibody test (transglutaminase and/or anti-endomysial antibodies). At present, an intestinal biopsy is often also done to confirm the diagnosis.

Symptoms may include:

- Stomach pain
- Gas
- Diarrhea or constipation
- Decreased height or weight gain in children
- Iron deficiency anemia
- Irritability
- Dental enamel defects
- Osteoporosis (loss of calcium in bone)

The symptoms, the abnormal blood tests and the intestinal biopsy changes may return to normal within a few months after treatment is begun.

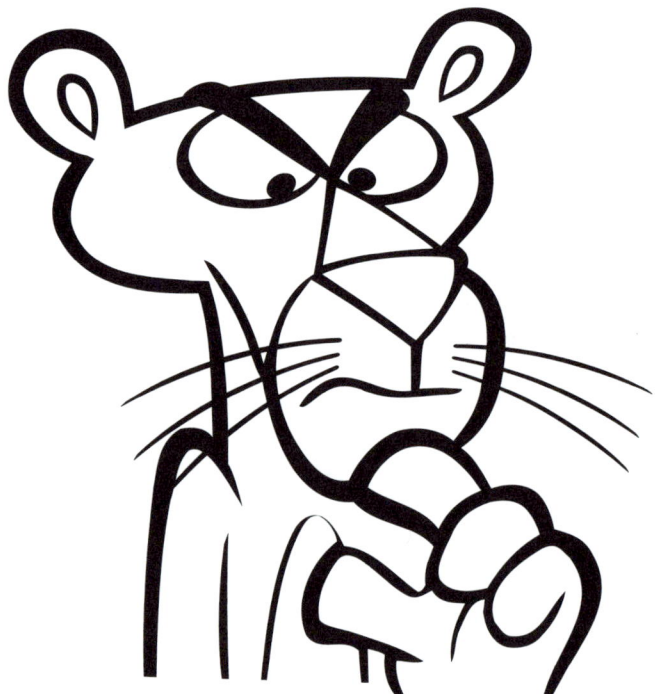

Treatment:

✔ The only current acceptable treatment for celiac disease is strict adherence to a 100 percent gluten-free diet for life.

✔ Remove all wheat, rye, and barley products from the diet and any ingredient that contains these grains. Oats and oat products may also be removed from the diet initially.

✔ Many foods are naturally gluten-free and are allowed in the diet, such as rice, corn, potatoes, fruits, vegetables, meats and dairy products. (See Table 1 for grains that are allowed.)

The National Institutes of Health Consensus Development Conference in 2004 came up with some elements needed in the management of celiac disease:

C Consultation with a skilled dietitian.

E Education about the disease.

L Lifelong adherence to a gluten-free diet.

I Identification and treatment of nutrition deficiencies.

A Access to an advocacy group.

C Continuous long-term follow-up by a multidisciplinary team.

(NIH Consensus Statement on Celiac Disease. NIH Consens State Sci Statements. 2004 Jun 28-30 [1] 1-22.)

ADRENAL DISORDERS (AUTOIMMUNE ADRENAL INSUFFICIENCY, ADDISON'S DISEASE)

Some facts:

✔ Autoimmunity against the adrenal gland can also occur.

✔ As with thyroid disease, initial screening for an antibody may indicate who is at risk. It is an antibody against an enzyme, 21-hydroxylase, and is called 21OH-autoantibody.

- It is quite rare (about one in 500 people with type 1 diabetes), but it is important to diagnose and treat, as it can result in death if untreated. Cortisol, the hormone the body is unable to produce in Addison's disease, is especially important during stress. If Addison's disease develops, additional teaching will be required. President Kennedy is an example of a famous person who had autoimmune adrenal insufficiency.

Some early signs for someone with diabetes may be:

- An increased frequency of severe low blood sugars.
- Episodes of feeling weak or faint (with normal blood sugars - but sometimes low blood pressure).
- Two electrolytes in the blood, sodium (Na+) and potassium (K+), may be low and high, respectively.
- Later, darker skin coloring over the back of the hands (or knuckles or elbows) may occur.
- Initial screening may be for an antibody against the adrenal gland.
- Eventually, morning ACTH and cortisol (cortisone) blood levels (and eventually an ACTH stimulation test) should be obtained. In follow-up, an annual random ACTH level should be done, with further testing if the level is above 50 pg/mL (11 pmol/L).
- The treatment (as with thyroid disease) is with tablets. Treatment includes training the person (or family) to increase the tablets during periods of stress (as with an infection or with surgery).

SKIN PROBLEMS

Some facts:

- A rare condition called **dermatitis herpetiformis** is also related to a sensitivity to the protein gluten (see celiac disease). It is characterized by blisters on the elbows, buttocks and knees. Like celiac disease, it responds to a gluten-free diet.
- Areas of loss of skin pigmentation (vitiligo) occur in about 2.4 percent of people with type 1 diabetes.
- Yellow fatty deposits (**necrobiosis**) can collect in the skin over the front of the lower legs. No one knows what causes these fat deposits, although they are most likely due to autoimmunity.

SUMMARY

In summary, much is now known about autoimmune problems associated with diabetes. Screening and treatment are now available for most conditions.

DEFINITIONS

Adrenal gland: A hormone-producing gland located above each kidney, which has the function of making cortisol, salt-retaining hormones and other hormones.

Autoimmunity (self-allergy): As defined in Chapter 3, this involves forming an allergic reaction against one's own tissues. This happens in type 1 diabetes and can happen in thyroid disorders and, more rarely, with the adrenal gland.

Celiac disease (sprue, gluten-enteropathy): An inherited disorder in which the small intestine is damaged by an autoimmune reaction to gluten, a protein found in grains like wheat, rye and barley.

Gluten: The protein found in wheat to which people are allergic if they have celiac disease.

Necrobiosis: The name for yellow fatty deposits that can occur over the lower legs in people with diabetes.

Thyroid: A hormone-producing gland in the lower front of the neck on each side of the windpipe (trachea). The hormone is called thyroid hormone.

QUESTIONS AND ANSWERS FROM NEWSNOTES

Q Are thyroid problems more common in children with diabetes, and if so, why?

a Yes, thyroid problems are more common in children with diabetes. They are caused by an "autoimmune" or allergic-type reaction that is very similar to the allergic-type reaction that is believed to be important in causing diabetes. Thus, most people with new-onset diabetes have islet cell antibodies (an allergic reaction against the islet cells that make the insulin) at the time of diagnosis of type 1 (but not type 2) diabetes. Likewise, many of the people with diabetes who develop thyroid problems have an antibody in their blood against the thyroid gland. The pancreas and the thyroid are endocrine glands that make insulin and thyroid hormone, respectively. Thus, the two glands have much in common. Some physicians recommend thyroid blood tests yearly or every other year in children with diabetes. The practice in our Clinic is to do the tests more frequently if the thyroid gland is large or if there is a special indication, such as a fall-off in growth. Fortunately, when low thyroid function is detected, it can be treated with a tablet. Also, the pills can sometimes be discontinued after growth is complete.

Q My doctor has found my child to have high transglutaminase antibodies that are associated with celiac disease. Does my child need to have an intestinal biopsy before considering a gluten-free diet?

a Children with type 1 diabetes are at higher risk for celiac disease, an illness in which gluten in the diet from a number of sources (e.g., wheat) causes the body's immune system to attack the inner wall of the intestine. When children have severe celiac disease associated with weight loss and diarrhea, avoiding gluten usually makes the symptoms go away and allows the child to grow normally. Nowadays, we screen for celiac disease with a simple blood test for an antibody that appears in the blood, termed transglutaminase. If high levels of the antibody are found, and the person has symptoms, we usually recommend a biopsy to confirm the diagnosis. Celiac disease is a life-long diagnosis, and no single test is diagnostic. The biopsy is usually done with anesthesia so the child is not conscious during the procedure. A tube with a camera is swallowed, and at the first part of the small intestine several pieces of the intestine are taken through the swallowed tube, each about the size of a pencil tip. The biopsy is then analyzed by the doctors under a microscope to confirm a diagnosis of celiac disease and determine the amount of intestinal damage, if any.

Many children do not have symptoms of celiac disease, even though they have antibodies in the blood. High levels of antibodies usually indicate that there is damage to the intestine, and in general we recommend biopsy only when the antibody levels are high, unless there are also celiac disease symptoms. In some children without symptoms, with high levels of the antibody, there is severe damage to the intestine. It is remarkable, but even with severe damage, with a gluten-free diet, the intestine can grow back and be normal as long as gluten is avoided. In general, with a diagnosis of celiac disease we recommend life-long avoidance of gluten. It is very important to have a firm diagnosis for people with symptoms or high levels of antibodies, and thus the recommendation for confirmation through a biopsy.

CHAPTER 25

The School and Diabetes: A Standard of Care

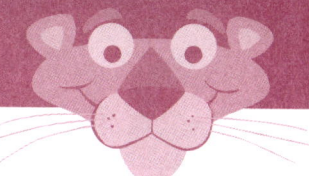

H. Peter Chase, MD
Leah Wyckoff, MS, BSN, RN, NCSN
Brigitte I. Frohnert, MD, PhD

INTRODUCTION

The first and main job of parents in relation to school is to ensure that those who will be working with the child at school are educated about diabetes. Ideally, this education would be done in partnership with the school nurse when there is a school nurse available. It is important NOT to leave it up to the child to inform and educate the school. Parents want to feel that their child is in safe hands while at school (often the place where the majority of the child's waking hours are spent). Parents also want to make sure their child is not treated differently because of having diabetes. Permission is granted to copy this chapter and/or the tables as often as wished. It is wise for the parent to phone the school nurse, teacher or principal to discuss the best way to inform all of the necessary people. The week before classes start is usually the best time. A checklist is provided in Table 1 to remind parents of their responsibilities. A tiered diabetes training model (three levels of education) for school personnel is available in reference 4 of the Additional Resources at the end of this chapter.

This chapter may also be helpful in educating co-workers of a person with diabetes in the workplace.

TOPICS:
Monitoring (checking blood/CGM sugar and ketones, giving insulin)
Prevent, Detect and Treat Acute Complications
Psychosocial Adjustment

TEACHING OBJECTIVES:
The teacher will:
1. Assess who will educate school/work personnel about diabetes.
2. Identify supplies needed to reduce the likelihood of acute complications at school/work.
3. Develop a "health action plan" for school/work.
4. Provide basic information on insulin pump and continuous glucose monitor (CGM) use, if relevant.

LEARNING OBJECTIVES:
Learner (parents, child, relative or self) will be able to:
1. Define who will educate school/work personnel about diabetes.
2. List all supplies needed at school/work to reduce the likelihood of acute complications.
3. Design a health action plan for school/work with healthcare provider(s).
4. Explain the basics of insulin pump and CGM use in the school, if relevant.

- The terms "glucose" and "sugar" are used interchangeably.
- The term "blood/CGM" means a glucose level from either a fingerstick blood sugar or a continuous glucose monitor (CGM).

It is essential for the family and school nurse to educate the following people:

- ✓ teacher(s), including gym, art and music
- ✓ health aide
- ✓ bus driver
- ✓ lunchroom workers
- ✓ playground aides
- ✓ others involved with their child at school

Sometimes the school nurse or the parent will help educate other staff such as substitute teachers, coaches or activity directors. It is very important that when a substitute teacher is at school, the substitute knows that a child in the classroom has diabetes and how to respond when the child is experiencing hypo- or hyperglycemia (see Substitute Teachers section below).

A second job of parents is to keep an adequate supply of items at school for the treatment of low blood sugars. Suggested items are included in Table 1.

The supplies should be kept in a container in the classroom, or in the teacher's, principal's or nurse's office. The container should be clearly labeled with the child's name and a set of instructions with contact phone numbers. They should be readily available to the child at all times. They shouldn't be locked in the young person's locker. The child may not remember their own locker combination if hypoglycemic.

There is often a special anxiety about a young child starting preschool.

This anxiety is due to a young child who will need extra help, and who:

- ✓ may not yet be able to recognize low blood sugars
- ✓ will not be mature enough to help remember snacks, blood/CGM sugar checks, or insulin doses.
- ✓ might not have been away from the care of the parents for any significant period of time prior to starting preschool

Separation may be difficult for the parents and the child, and yet, preschool may be important for the child in learning social and other skills. It is important to allow participation just as one would if the child did not have diabetes.

SCHOOL HEALTH PLANS

Most schools now require a Diabetes Medical Management Plan (**DMMP**; see provider orders, Table 5 or 6) to provide guidance for the individual student's diabetes care. Some schools use a basic "Standard of Care" to guide management of diabetes at school or in a child-care setting. An example of a "Standard of Care" can be found at www.coloradokidswithdiabetes.org. There is also a place for the parent to sign at the end of the chapter if they wish to use this chapter, and/or the directions in this chapter for hypo- and hyperglycemia and exercise, as a Standard of Care. The family and the school nurse collaborate to complete the "**Individualized Health Plan (IHP): Student with Diabetes**," using either Table 2 for insulin injections or Table 3 for an insulin pump. A checklist for the school nurse to follow in relation to the IHP is shown in Table 4.

Directions for accessing a Section 504 plan online are included in the Legal Rights section below. This plan addresses accommodations for the child with diabetes to have equal access to education. This plan is often used when other means have failed.

TABLE 1:
School Diabetes Management and Supply Checklist for Parents

_____ Discuss specific care of your child with the teachers, school nurse, bus driver, coaches and other staff who will be involved.

_____ Complete the Individualized Health Plan (IHP) in collaboration with the school nurse, school staff, and the diabetes care staff (see Table 2 or 3); also complete your child's Diabetes Medical Management Plan (DMMP) with your diabetes care-provider (Table 5 or 6).

_____ Make sure your child understands the details of who will help him/her with blood/CGM sugar checking, shots and treatment of high or low blood sugars at school, and where supplies will be kept. Supplies should be kept in a place where they are always available if needed (not in a locker).

_____ Make arrangements for the school to send home blood sugar records weekly.

_____ Keep current phone numbers where you can be reached. Collect equipment for school: meter, strips and finger-poker, lancets, insulin, insulin syringes or pen, biohazard container, logbook or a copy of blood sugar record form, extra insulin pump supplies, ketone strips, photo for substitute teacher's folder.

_____ Food and drinks; parents need to check intermittently to make sure the following supplies are available:

▼ juice cans or boxes (approximately 15g of carb each)

▼ glucose tablets (and instructions to give four tablets for low blood sugar)

▼ instant glucose or cake-decorating gel

▼ snacks, such as Fruit Roll-Ups, dried fruit, raisins, crackers, granola bars or other snacks

▼ quarters to buy sugar pop (soda) if needed

▼ provide a box with the child's name to store these food and drink items

▼ intranasal glucagon (3 mg) if available or injectable glucagon

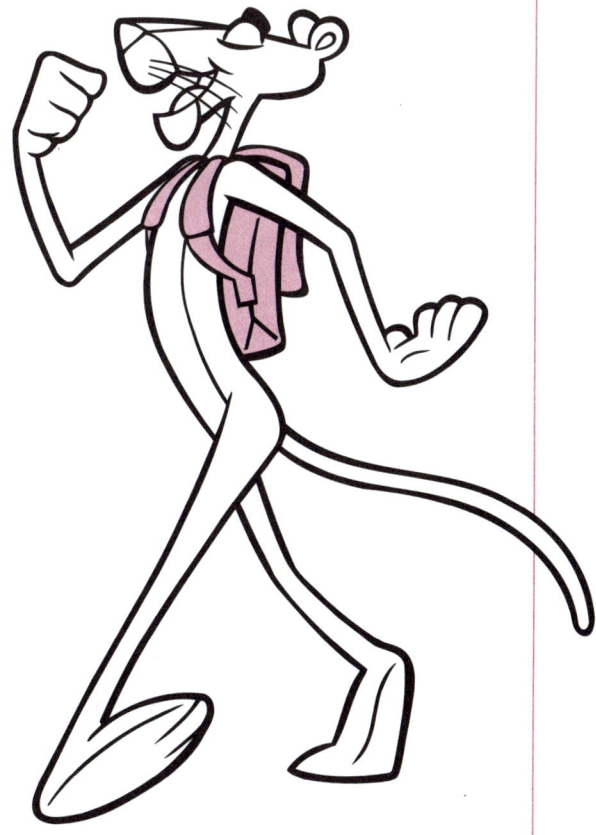

THE SCHOOL AND DIABETES: A STANDARD OF CARE

TABLE 2:
Individualized Health Plan (IHP) for Student with Diabetes Using Injections

Student: _____ DOB: _____ School: _____ Grade: _____
Physician: _____ Phone: _____
Diabetes Educator: _____
Parent name(s) and phone number(s) _____
_____

WHEN TO CHECK BLOOD/CGM GLUCOSE: *For provision of student safety while limiting disruption to learning*
✔ **ALWAYS** when signs & symptoms of low/high blood glucose, when does not feel well, and/or if behavior concerns. Also check:
☐ Before-School Program ☐ Before Snack ☐ Mid-morning ☐ After-School Program/Extracurricular Activity
☐ Before Lunch ☐ After Lunch ☐ Recess ☐ Before PE ☐ After PE
☐ School Dismissal ☐ Before riding bus/walking home ☐ 2 hrs after correction
☐ Other: _____

GLUCOSE TARGET RANGE – Blood Glucose: _____ to _____
☐ (suggested for <6 y.o.) ☐ (suggested for 6 – 17 y.o.) ☐ (suggested for >17 y.o.)
70-150 mg/dL (3.9-8.3 mmol/L) 70-130 mg/dL (3.9-7.2 mmol/L) 70-130 mg/dL (3.9-7.2 mmol/L)
Notification to Parents if blood/CGM glucose is less than _____ or greater than _____
The following devices may be used for blood glucose in place of finger stick:
☐ Dexcom G5/G6 ☐ Freestyle Libre ☐ Other: _____

HYPOGLYCEMIA (also see section in text and Table 7):
Student should be accompanied to health office if symptomatic or glucose level below _____.
- If symptomatic but glucose/CGM meter not available, treat as indicated for mild symptoms below.
- If blood glucose in range _____ – _____ but symptomatic, treat with 10 to 15g carbohydrate snack.
- **If mild symptoms** (e.g., shaky, hungry, pale) check blood/CGM glucose and if below _____, treat with juice, glucose tabs, etc. every 10-15 min until blood sugar above _____. Then give 10-15g carb snack or give lunch.
- Do not give insulin for glucose used to treat hypoglycemia. If at lunchtime, wait to give meal insulin until after the meal.
- **If moderate symptoms** (e.g., not thinking clearly), they may be unable to drink independently. Check blood/CGM glucose and administer sugar drink or glucose gel. If unable to administer, may use intranasal glucagon (3 mg) if available. Re-check every 15 minutes until blood sugar above _____. Then give a snack that includes 10-15g carbs, or lunch.
- **If severe reaction** (seizure, unconscious), check glucose level and inject glucagon _____ units (_____cc/mL); or, if available, intranasal spray glucagon (Baqsimi, 3 mg) may be used instead. ***Give nothing by mouth! CALL 911 AND PARENT.***
- Other: _____

HYPERGLYCEMIA AND KETONE TESTING (also see section in text and Table 8):
- If blood/CGM glucose is above the target range, and it has been over 3 hours since the last dose of insulin, provide insulin for glucose correction as indicated in the orders below. If at lunchtime, include the insulin to cover the meal carbohydrates, as in the orders below.
- The school nurse should take into consideration upcoming activities, including PE, lunch dosing, walking home, after-school activities, etc., when giving insulin corrections for high glucose (for both injections and pumps). *If the correction factor is not available, or there is not a sliding scale for insulin dosage, contact the diabetes care-provider for a one-time order.*
  - If glucose greater than 300 mg/dL (16.7 mmol/L) after two consecutive checks (1-2 hours apart), or illness, such as nausea/vomiting, CHECK KETONES. Check one: ☐ blood ☐ urine
  - If no method to check ketones is available, call parents to come to do the ketone check or to take student home to monitor and treat.
  - If ketones are below moderate in urine or 1.0 mmol/L in blood, student may require insulin injection. First, contact parent. If parents are not available, call diabetes care-provider for further instructions.

CONTINUED

TABLE 2: IHP FOR STUDENT USING INJECTIONS (CONTINUED)

- Recommend student be released to parents when ketones are moderate or large in urine or above 1.0 mmol/L in blood, **OR** if student has symptoms of illness (e.g., nausea, vomiting), in order to be treated and monitored more closely by parent/guardian.
- If ketones present, provide water and keep student from exercise.
- Other: _____

CONTINUOUS GLUCOSE MONITOR (CGM)
- Parents will set alarms for CGMs sparingly to avoid unnecessary disruption of school activities (i.e., set alarms for glucose levels that require immediate action). Parents will notify school nurse of the parameters (e.g., alarm set for glucose lower than 70 mg/dL [3.9 mmol/L] or above 300 mg/dL [16.7 mmol/L]).

Alarms set for this student: Lower limit: _____   High glucose alarm: _____

INSULIN DOSING ORDERS (Insulin-to-Carb Ratios Plus the High Sugar Correction):

Insulin Dosage Injection at: ☐ Breakfast   ☐ Snack   ☐ Lunch   ☐ Other:
Bolus for carbohydrates should occur: ☐ Approximately 20 minutes prior to lunch/snack
☐ Immediately before lunch/snack   ☐ Immediately after lunch/snack   ☐ Split ½ before lunch & ½ after lunch
Other: _____

Insulin to Carbohydrate (I/C) ratio dose (to use if food to be consumed):

Time	Carbohydrate Ratio
_____ to _____	Give 1 unit of insulin per _____ grams of carbohydrate
_____ to _____	Give 1 unit of insulin per _____ grams of carbohydrate
_____ to _____	Give 1 unit of insulin per _____ grams of carbohydrate
_____ to _____	Give 1 unit of insulin per _____ grams of carbohydrate

☐ Parent/guardian authorized to increase or decrease insulin to carb ratio 1 unit/5 grams of carbohydrates

Sensitivity/Correction Factor Bolus for High Blood Sugar:

Time	Correction Dose
_____ to _____	Give _____ units of insulin for every _____ above _____
_____ to _____	Give _____ units of insulin for every _____ above _____
_____ to _____	Give _____ units of insulin for every _____ above _____
_____ to _____	Give _____ units of insulin for every _____ above _____

OTHER INSULIN/MEDICATIONS:
Basal Insulins: _____ units of _____ given at _____ Administered @ ☐ Home ☐ School
Intermediate Insulins (e.g., NPH): _____ units of _____ given at _____ Administered @ ☐ Home ☐ School
Oral Medications: _____ mg of _____ given at _____ Administered @ ☐ Home ☐ School

Student's Self Care: (Ability level determined by school nurse and parent with input by healthcare-provider)

Independently monitors blood/CGM glucose	☐ Yes	☐ No
Independently treats mild hypoglycemia	☐ Yes	☐ No
Independently counts carbohydrates	☐ Yes	☐ No
Independently checks urine/blood ketones	☐ Yes	☐ No
Self-injects with verification of dosage	☐ Yes	☐ No Injections to be done by trained staff.

Additional Information/Comments:

Signatures:
My signature below provides authorization for the written orders above and exchange of health information to assist the school nurse. I understand that all procedures will be implemented in accordance with state laws and regulations and may be performed by unlicensed designated school personnel under the training and supervision provided by the school nurse. This order is for a maximum of one year.

Parent: _____   Date: _____

School Nurse: _____   Date: _____

TABLE 3:
Individualized Health Plan (IHP) for Student with Diabetes Using Insulin Pump

Student: _____ DOB: _____ School: _____ Grade: _____
Physician: _____ Phone: _____
Diabetes Educator: _____
Parent name(s) and phone number(s) _____
_____

WHEN TO CHECK BLOOD/CGM GLUCOSE: *For provision of student safety while limiting disruption to learning*
✔ **ALWAYS** when signs & symptoms of low/high blood glucose, when does not feel well, and/or if behavior concerns. Also check:
☐ Before-School Program ☐ Before Snack ☐ Mid-morning ☐ After-School Program/Extracurricular Activity
☐ Before Lunch ☐ After Lunch ☐ Recess ☐ Before PE ☐ After PE
☐ School Dismissal ☐ Before riding bus/walking home ☐ 2 hrs after correction
☐ Other: _____

GLUCOSE TARGET RANGE – Blood/CGM Glucose: _____ to _____
☐ (suggested for <6 y.o.)   ☐ (suggested for 6 – 17 y.o.)   ☐ (suggested for >17 y.o.)
70-150 mg/dL (3.9-8.3 mmol/L)   70-130 mg/dL (3.9-7.2 mmol/L)   70-130 mg/dL (3.9-7.2 mmol/L)
Notification to Parents if blood/CGM glucose is less than _____ or greater than _____
The following devices may be used for blood glucose in place of finger stick:
☐ Dexcom G5/G6   ☐ Freestyle Libre   ☐ Other: _____

HYPOGLYCEMIA (also see section in text and Table 7):
Student should be accompanied to health office if symptomatic or blood/CGM glucose level below _____.
- If symptomatic but CGM/glucose meter not available, treat as indicated for mild symptoms below.
- If blood glucose in range _____ – _____ but symptomatic, treat with 10 to 15g carbohydrate snack.
- **If mild symptoms** (e.g., shaky, hungry, pale) check blood/CGM glucose and if below _____, treat with juice, glucose tabs, etc. every 10-15 min until blood sugar above _____. Then give 10-15g carb snack or give lunch.
- Do not give insulin for glucose used to treat hypoglycemia. If at lunchtime, wait to give meal insulin until after the meal.
- **If moderate symptoms** (e.g., not thinking clearly), they may be unable to drink independently. Check blood/CGM glucose and administer sugar drink or glucose gel. If unable to administer, may use intranasal glucagon (3 mg) if available. Re-check every 15 minutes until blood sugar above _____. Then give a snack that includes 10-15g carbs, or lunch.
- **If severe reaction** (seizure, unconscious), check glucose level and inject glucagon _____ units (____cc/mL); or, if available, intranasal spray glucagon (Baqsimi, 3 mg) may be used instead. **Give nothing by mouth! SUSPEND OR DISCONNECT PUMP. CALL 911 AND PARENT.**
- Other: _____

HYPERGLYCEMIA (also see Pump Insulin Dosing orders below and section in text and Table 8):
- If blood/CGM glucose is above the target range, and it has been over 3 hours since the last dose of insulin, provide insulin for the correction as indicated in the orders below. If at lunchtime, include the insulin to cover the meal carbohydrates, as in the orders below.
- The school nurse should take into consideration upcoming activities, including PE, lunch dosing, walking home, after-school activities, etc., when giving insulin corrections for high blood/CGM glucose (for both injections and pumps). *If the correction factor is not available, or there is not a sliding scale for insulin dosage, contact the diabetes care-provider for a one-time order.*
  - If blood/CGM glucose greater than 300 mg/dL (16.7 mmol/L) even once, or with illness, such as nausea/vomiting, CHECK KETONES. Check one: ☐ blood   ☐ urine

CONTINUED

TABLE 3: IHP FOR STUDENT USING INSULIN PUMP (CONTINUED)

- If no method to check ketones is available, call parents to come to do the ketone check or to take student home to monitor and treat.
- If ketones are below moderate in urine or 1.0 mmol/L in blood, student may require insulin injection. First, contact parent. If parents are not available, call diabetes care-provider for further instructions.
- Recommend student be released to parents when ketones are moderate or large in urine or above 1.0 mmol/L in blood, **OR** if student has symptoms of illness (e.g., nausea, vomiting), in order to be treated and monitored more closely by parent/guardian.
- If ketones present, provide water and keep student from exercise.

- *Potential pump malfunction*: The concern for a student on a pump is the possibility of prolonged hyperglycemia due to blocked insulin tubing, and the consequent risk of going into diabetic ketoacidosis (DKA). This can happen after 2 or 3 hours without insulin. Unlicensed assistive personnel should contact school nurse or diabetes care-provider for further instructions regarding insulin by injection or new infusion set by parent or independent student.
- Other: _____

PUMP INSULIN DOSING ORDERS (High Blood Sugar Correction Factor and Insulin-to-Carb Ratio):

- Enter glucose level and approximate grams of carbs to be eaten. A suggested insulin dose will appear. Then just press "accept" or "enter" to give bolus.

Insulin Pump: (Type of pump: _____; type of insulin in pump: _____)

- Pump settings are established by the student's healthcare-provider and should not be changed by the school staff. All setting changes to be made at home or by student authorized to provide self-care.
- Parents will set alarms for pumps and CGMs conservatively to avoid unnecessary disruption of school activities (i.e., set alarms for blood glucose levels that require immediate action). Parents will notify school nurse of the parameters (e.g., alarm set for glucose levels below 70 mg/dL [3.9 mmol/L]). Alarms set for this student: Lower limit _____ High glucose _____

Sensitivity/Correction Factor Bolus for High Blood Sugar:

Provide correction bolus per pump calculator. Corrections should not be given more frequently than every 2 hours. The sugar level should be entered into the pump for calculation of pump-calculated correction bolus. Press "enter" or "accept" to give the bolus.

The correction factor below is to be used only if pump is not working.

Time	Correction Dose
_____ to _____	Give _____ units of insulin for every _____ above _____
_____ to _____	Give _____ units of insulin for every _____ above _____
_____ to _____	Give _____ units of insulin for every _____ above _____
_____ to _____	Give _____ units of insulin for every _____ above _____

Carbohydrates and Insulin Dosage per pump at: ☐ Breakfast ☐ Snack ☐ Lunch ☐ Other:
Bolus for carbohydrates should occur: ☐ Approximately 20 minutes prior to lunch/snack
☐ Immediately before lunch/snack ☐ Immediately after lunch/snack ☐ Split ½ before lunch & ½ after lunch
Other: _____

Insulin to Carbohydrate (I/C) ratio dose (to use if food to be consumed; typically programmed into pump):

Time	Carbohydrate Ratio
_____ to _____	Give 1 unit of insulin per _____ grams of carbohydrate
_____ to _____	Give 1 unit of insulin per _____ grams of carbohydrate
_____ to _____	Give 1 unit of insulin per _____ grams of carbohydrate
_____ to _____	Give 1 unit of insulin per _____ grams of carbohydrate

☐ Parent/guardian authorized to increase or decrease insulin to carb ratio 1 unit/5 grams of carbohydrates

CONTINUED

TABLE 3: IHP FOR STUDENT USING INSULIN PUMP (CONTINUED)

Insulin Pump Basal Rates:
(The pump gives these doses automatically and they are included only for information.)

Start Time:	Units Per Hour:

PUMP MALFUNCTIONS:
Disconnect pump when malfunctioning (usually due to plugged pump tubing).
- Check ketones if needed (see Hyperglycemia and Ketone Testing section above)
- If ketones are moderate/large (urine) or greater than 1.0 mmol/L (blood), follow instructions in Hyperglycemia and Ketone Testing section above.
- If pump calculator is operational, the insulin dosing should be calculated by using the pump bolus calculator and then insulin given by injection.
- If pump calculator is not operational, give insulin by injection using Insulin to Carbohydrate Ratio and Correction Factor above.

Student's Self Care: (Ability level determined by school nurse and parent with input by healthcare-provider)

Independently monitors blood/CGM glucose	☐ Yes	☐ No	
Independently treats mild hypoglycemia	☐ Yes	☐ No	
Independently counts carbohydrates	☐ Yes	☐ No	
Independently checks urine/blood ketones	☐ Yes	☐ No	
Independentlly manages pump boluses	☐ Yes	☐ No	Needs assistance with pump management.
Self-injects with verification of dosage	☐ Yes	☐ No	Injections to be done by trained staff.
Independently inserts infusion sets	☐ Yes	☐ No	Needs assistance
Troubleshoots all alarms	☐ Yes	☐ No	Needs assistance with pump management.

Additional Information/Comments:

Signatures:
My signature below provides authorization for the written orders above and exchange of health information to assist the school nurse. I understand that all procedures will be implemented in accordance with state laws and regulations and may be performed by unlicensed designated school personnel under the training and supervision provided by the school nurse. This order is for a maximum of one year.

Parent: _____ Date: _____

School Nurse: _____ Date: _____

TABLE 4:
Individualized Healthcare Plan Checklist for the School Nurse

Student: _____ DOB: _____

Student #: _____ School: _____ Date: _____

1. Enter completion date and initial each step listed below.
2. File completed checklist in the student's health file.

Date and Initial

1. Healthcare Plan developed with _____ ± _____
                                          parent or guardian   area nurse consultant

2. Parents signature needed? ☐ Yes ☐ No

3. School staff information and copy of Healthcare Plan to the following:
   - ☐ Clinic aide
   - ☐ Secretaries
   - ☐ Classroom teacher(s)
   - ☐ Admin.
   - ☐ P.E.
   - ☐ Art
   - ☐ Music
   - ☐ Cafeteria
   - ☐ Transportation

   Others: _____
                               List Names

4. Copies of signed plan in ☐ Clinic Healthcare Plan Book
                              ☐ Substitute Folder
                              ☐ With student information/emergency page

5. Original plan with signatures in health file

6. Classroom presentation requested: ☐ No ☐ Yes Who requested: _____

7. Inservice: ☐ No ☐ Yes Who requested: _____

8. Training/delegation needed: ☐ No ☐ Yes

   Procedure: #1 _____

   Staff: Name:_____ Position: _____ Date: _____

   Staff: Name:_____ Position: _____ Date: _____

   Staff: Name:_____ Position: _____ Date: _____

   Procedure: #2 _____

   Staff: Name:_____ Position: _____ Date: _____

   Staff: Name:_____ Position: _____ Date: _____

   Staff: Name:_____ Position: _____ Date: _____

ALL HEALTHCARE PLANS ARE CONFIDENTIAL
(Information to be shared on a need-to-know basis only!)

TABLE 5:
Diabetes Medical Management Plan (DMMP) for Student with Diabetes on Injections/Oral Medication To be completed by the healthcare-provider

Student: _____ DOB: _____ School: _____ Grade: _____

Physician/Provider: _____ Phone: _____

Diabetes Educator: _____ Phone: _____

TARGET RANGE – Blood Glucose: _____ mg/dL to _____ mg/dL
☐ <5 years old   ☐ 5-8 years old   ☐ 9-11 years old   ☐ 12-18 years old   ☐ >18 years old
    80-200 mg/dL   80-200 mg/dL   70-180 mg/dL   70-150 mg/dL   70-130 mg/dL

Notification to Parents:
Low < <u>target range</u> and High ><u>300 mg/dl</u> or less than _____ mg/dL and greater than _____ mg/dL

☐ Other: _____

Continuous glucose monitoring: Always confirm glucose level with a fingerstick/meter prior to treatment unless student has a Dexcom G5 or G6 or the FreeStyle Libre, which may be used for dosing and treatment.

Hypoglycemia:
Per ☐ IHP and/or ☐ Standards of Care from School chapter or ☐ www.coloradokidswithdiabetes.org
For Severe Symptoms: **Call 911 & Administer Glucagon:**
Injection Dose: _____ mg (Intramuscular or Sub-Q), OR BAQSIMI nasal spray: one device (3 mg) in one nostril

Hyperglycemia:
Per ☐ IHP and/or ☐ Standards of Care from School chapter or ☐ www.coloradokidswithdiabetes.org

Ketone Testing:
Per ☐ IHP and/or ☐ Standards of Care from School chapter or ☐ www.coloradokidswithdiabetes.org
    ☐ Other: _____

When to Check Blood Glucose: *For provision of student safety while limiting disruption to learning*
☐ Always for signs & symptoms of low/high blood glucose, when does not feel well and/or behavior concerns
☐ Check before meals and as mutually agreed upon by parent and school nurse
☐ Other: _____

CONTINUED

TABLE 5: DMMP FOR STUDENT USING INJECTIONS/ORAL MEDS (CONTINUED)

Sensitivity/Correction Factor Bolus for High Blood Sugar:
Sensitivity/Correction Factor: _____ unit insulin for every _____ mg/dL above _____ starting at _____ mg/dL
- **Use Rapid-Acting/Short-Acting Insulin Type:** *Injections should be given subcutaneously & rotated*
- **Lunchtime Correction:** Give ☐ Prior to lunch ☐ Immediately after lunch ☐ Split ½ before lunch & ½ after lunch

  ☐ Other: _____

- Insulin Dosing may also be in the Individualized Health Plan (IHP)
- Alternatively, the scale below may be used ☐:

Blood Glucose Range: _____ mg/dL to _____ mg/dL → Administer: _____ units → Check ketones ☐

Blood Glucose Range: _____ mg/dL to _____ mg/dL → Administer: _____ units → Check ketones ☐

Blood Glucose Range: _____ mg/dL to _____ mg/dL → Administer: _____ units → Check ketones ☐

Blood Glucose Range: _____ mg/dL to _____ mg/dL → Administer: _____ units → Check ketones ☐

Parent/guardian authorized to increase or decrease sliding scale +/- 2 units of insulin.

When hyperglycemia occurs other than at lunchtime:
If it has been greater than **3 hours** since the last dose of insulin, the student may be given insulin via injection using the above correction factor ☐, or the scale above ☐ **if approved by the school nurse and parent is notified.**

Alternatively, contact Healthcare-Provider for One-time order

Insulin Dosage for Carbohydrates when eating: ☐ Breakfast ☐ Snack ☐ Lunch
Insulin to Carbohydrate Ratio: _____ unit(s) for every _____ grams of carbohydrate to be eaten
(or dosing as in IHP)

☐ Other: (To be given in conjunction with the correction dose as indicated) _____

☐ Parent/guardian authorized to increase or decrease insulin to carb ratio 1 unit +/- 5 grams of carbohydrates

☐ **Oral Medication** _____ _____ mg Time: _____

☐ **NPH or Other Medicine** _____ Dose: _____ units SQ Time: _____

Student's Self Care:
☐ No supervision ☐ Full supervision ☐ Requires some supervision: ability level to be determined
by school nurse and parent unless otherwise indicated here:

Additional Information:

Signatures:
My signature below provides authorization for the written orders above and exchange of health information to assist the school nurse an Individualized Health Plan. I understand that all procedures will be implemented in accordance with state laws and regulations and may be performed by unlicensed designated school personnel under the training and supervision provided by the school nurse. This order is for a maximum of one year.

Physician: _____ Date: _____

Parent: _____ Date: _____

School Nurse: _____ Date: _____

TABLE 6:
Diabetes Medical Management Plan (DMMP) for Student with Diabetes on Insulin Pump To be completed by the healthcare-provider

Student: _____ DOB: _____ School: _____ Grade: _____
Physician/Provider: _____ Phone: _____
Diabetes Educator: _____ Phone: _____

TARGET RANGE – Blood Glucose: _____ mg/dL to _____ mg/dL

☐ <5 years old	☐ 5-8 years old	☐ 9-11 years old	☐ 12-18 years old	☐ >18 years old
80-200 mg/dL	80-200 mg/dL	70-180 mg/dL	70-150 mg/dL	70-130 mg/dL

Notification to Parents:
Low < target range and High >300 mg/dl or less than _____ mg/dL and greater than _____ mg/dL
☐ Other: _____

Continuous glucose monitoring: Always confirm glucose level with a fingerstick/meter prior to treatment unless student has a Dexcom G5 or G6 or the FreeStyle Libre, which may be used for dosing and treatment.

Hypoglycemia:
Per ☐ IHP and/or ☐ Standards of Care from School chapter or ☐ www.coloradokidswithdiabetes.org
For Severe Symptoms: Call 911, Disconnect Pump, and Administer Glucagon:
Injection Dose: _____ mg (Intramuscular or Sub-Q), OR BAQSIMI nasal spray: one device (3 mg) in one nostril

Hyperglycemia:
Per ☐ IHP and/or ☐ Standards of Care from School chapter or ☐ www.coloradokidswithdiabetes.org

Ketone Testing:
Per ☐ IHP and/or ☐ Standards of Care from School chapter or ☐ www.coloradokidswithdiabetes.org
  ☐ Other: _____

When to Check Blood Glucose: *For provision of student safety while limiting disruption to learning*
☐ Always for signs & symptoms of low/high blood glucose, when does not feel well and/or behavior concerns
☐ Check before meals and as mutually agreed upon by parent and school nurse
☐ Other: _____

CONTINUED

TABLE 6: DMMP FOR STUDENT ON INSULIN PUMP (CONTINUED)

Insulin Pump:
Follow Guidelines for Insulin Administration by School Staff, Diabetes Resource Nurses February 2013
- Pump settings are established by the student's healthcare-provider and should not be changed by the school staff. All setting changes to be made at home or by student providing self care as indicated on IHP.
- Internal safety features for the insulin pump should be active at all times while the student is at school - (Alarms set conservatively).

Insulin Pump Brand: _____   Type of Insulin in Pump _____

Blood Glucose Correction Factor Insulin Bolus (for high blood sugar):
Provide Correction bolus per pump calculator. All BG levels should be entered into the pump for administration of pump-calculated corrections unless otherwise indicated on the provider orders.

Sensitivity/Correction Factor: _____ unit insulin for every _____ mg/dL above _____ starting at _____ mg/dL
- Or Insulin Dosing may also be in the Individualized Health Plan (IHP)

When hyperglycemia occurs other than at lunchtime:
If it has been greater than **3 hours** since the last dose of insulin, the student may be given insulin via injection using the indicated correction factor on the provider orders **if approved by the school nurse and parent is notified, or contact Healthcare-Provider for One-time order**

Insulin Dosage for Carbohydrates when eating: ☐ Breakfast ☐ Snack ☐ Lunch
- **Enter blood sugar and approximate grams of carbs into pump and accept dose.**
- Or, insulin dosing may also be in the Individualized Health Plan (IHP)
- **Insulin to Carbohydrate Ratio:** _____ unit(s) for every _____ grams of carbohydrate to be eaten

Bolus for carbohydrates should occur:
☐ Prior to lunch/snack   ☐ After lunch/snack   ☐ Split ½ before lunch & ½ after lunch
☐ Parent/guardian authorized to increase or decrease insulin to carb ratio 1 unit +/- 5 grams of carbohydrates
☐ If blood glucose is less than _____ mg/dL, wait to give meal bolus until after meal

Pump Malfunctions: Disconnect pump when malfunctioning
If pump calculator is operational: then the insulin dosing should be calculated by using the pump bolus calculator and then insulin given by injection

If pump calculator is not operational: School Nurse or Parent to give insulin according to Insulin to Carbohydrate Ratio and/or Correction Factor
Call Parent and Healthcare-Provider (for orders)

Student's Self Care:
☐ No supervision   ☐ Full supervision   ☐ Requires some supervision: ability level to be determined by school nurse and parent unless otherwise indicated here:

Additional Information:

Signatures:
My signature below provides authorization for the written orders above and exchange of health information to assist the school nurse an Individualized Health Plan. I understand that all procedures will be implemented in accordance with state laws and regulations and may be performed by unlicensed designated school personnel under the training and supervision provided by the school nurse. This order is for a maximum of one year.

Physician: _____ Date: _____

Parent: _____ Date: _____

School Nurse: _____ Date: _____

BLOOD SUGARS IN THE SCHOOL

All children must have at school:

✔ a blood sugar meter; it should NOT be kept in the child's locker (for youth with a CGM, this will be a "back-up" in case the CGM is not working or is having questionable values)

✔ strips for the meter

✔ a lancing device (finger poker) and lancets

✔ urine or blood ketone strips

At a minimum, a blood/CGM sugar must be checked whenever the child is feeling low. Most physicians and parents also ask that a blood/CGM sugar be checked routinely prior to lunch or snacks.

Often children carry their own meter in their backpack. Other children are now wearing a continuous glucose monitor (**CGM**), which gives the current glucose level (Chapter 29). As a result, blood sugar measurements may not be needed as frequently. This should then be noted in the IHP (Table 2 or 3).

We prefer that the child be allowed to check the blood/CGM sugar in the classroom. Less school time is missed when this is allowed. If done in the classroom, an adult may need to look at the result. The adult can determine whether a low blood sugar has occurred. A disadvantage of checking the sugar in the classroom is that the teacher may have many other responsibilities and may not have time to supervise a young child. Another disadvantage is that the teacher may be very busy and unable to deal with possible problems. Also, the hands cannot be washed first if there isn't a sink. A trace of sugar on the finger can cause a high reading. If alcohol is used to clean the finger, be sure to let it dry completely before lancing. An option for routine glucose checks, is to have a health assistant come to the classroom to assist the child.

The FDA has approved the use of the Dexcom G5 and G6 and the FreeStyle Libre Flash CGMs for deciding on insulin dosages (see Table 2 or 3) without the need for a finger-stick blood sugar. However, fingerstick blood sugars may still need to be done, even if using a CGM. Many physicians recommend checking a fingerstick blood sugar with hypoglycemic episodes or anytime the CGM value is out of range (e.g., above 250 mg/dL [13.9 mmol/L] or below 70 [3.9]). This is done for verification. It is important to remember that with certain CGMs, the readings may not be accurate if the person has recently received a medicine containing acetaminophen (e.g., Tylenol). This is not a problem with the Dexcom G6 or the Libre Flash.

It should be noted, **IF THE CHILD FEELS LOW AND NO BLOOD SUGAR EQUIPMENT IS AVAILABLE, TREAT THE LOW WITH A SOURCE OF CARBOHYDRATE.** Also, a reminder that **a person who has a possible low sugar must never be allowed to leave the classroom alone.**

INSULIN IN THE SCHOOL

If insulin is to be given at school, the parent and the child's physician must sign a DMMP (see Table 5 or 6). It must specify when the insulin is to be given and the dose. This "physician order" is usually mandatory in order for the school nurse to deliver a dose of insulin at school. Individual state laws often dictate how this dose can be delivered. In some states, only a school nurse, the child, or the child's parent/guardian may administer the insulin. In other states, the nurse or principal may delegate this task to a layperson(s) in the school setting. If a child is drawing up the insulin and giving their own dose, it is recommended to have an adult check the amount. On other occasions, the parent may need to come in and give the injection (e.g., a private or a religious school). If a layperson will be responsible for the injection, it's important that there be at least two people trained (in the event one is absent). These delegates should be supervised and recertified routinely and their names recorded in the child's care plan. Insulin pens are often a great tool for injections at school. They are very convenient, more accurate and leave less room for error when drawing up the dose at school. Unfortunately, insurance may not cover their cost.

LOW BLOOD SUGAR ("Insulin Reaction" or "Hypoglycemia"; Table 7)

This is the only emergency likely to occur at school. The severity of the low blood sugar is not determined by the glucose value but rather by signs and symptoms. Hypoglycemia is most likely to occur before lunch or during or after gym class. Possible causes include too much insulin, extra exercise, a missed snack, or less food at a meal than is usually eaten. Field days or field trips with extra exercise and excitement may result in reactions (see below). If a child is sent to the office, he/she must always have a responsible person accompany him/her. The child may become confused and not make it to the office if he/she is alone. Treatment for different levels of hypoglycemia is outlined in Table 7.

TABLE 7: Treatment for Different Levels of Hypoglycemia

Levels of Hypoglycemia	Action
Student reports feeling "low," and/or symptoms are noted by staff, or CGM is alarming. ➡⬇	• Check blood glucose (BG) with glucometer or use Dexcom G5, G6 or FreeStyle Libre CGM (if BG <70, check fingerstick). If Dexcom G5/G6 or FreeStyle Libre reads "LO," then check fingerstick. • If no meter/sensor is available, assume BG is low and treat per symptoms.
BG below target range and/or Mild Symptoms: Dizziness, irritability, moodiness, anxiety, hunger, shakiness, sweating (usually cold sweat), and/or rapid heartbeat	• If <5 y.o. treat with ~7.5g fast-acting carbohydrates*. • If >5 y.o. treat with ~15g fast-acting carbohydrate*. • Do not give insulin for these carbohydrates. • Recheck BG in 10-15 min. • If still below Target Range, repeat steps until within target range. • Once in Target Range, consider following with ~15g solid food snack, or have someone take to lunch/meal. • Follow **Snack/Meal Protocol**** (See below).
BG below target range and/or Moderate Symptoms: Confusion, headache, poor coordination	• Check BG with glucometer if available. • If unable to drink juice, administer glucose gel/cake icing. • Recheck BG in 10-15 min. • Re-treat until within Target Range. • Follow **Snack/Meal Protocol**** (See below).
BG below target range and/or Severe Symptoms: Severe drowsiness, fainting, loss of consciousness, seizures, unable or unwilling to eat or drink or take glucose gel	• **Call 911!** • Check BG with glucometer if available. • Administer glucagon, intranasal if available, per orders/DMMP. • Trained personnel should be available for administration of glucagon. • Contact/Notify parent. Note: In all cases, notify parents after student has been treated.

*Fast-acting carbohydrates can include juice, glucose tablets, Skittles, sugar pop, etc. (see Chapter 6).
Snack/Meal Protocol: Do not give insulin (do not enter carbs in pump) for carbohydrates given to treat low blood glucose per IHP.
At mealtime, after BG is within target range, send the student to lunch/meal and give insulin after eating, based on the grams of meal carbs only, unless otherwise indicated on DMMP orders. For Pumps: After eating, enter into pump the grams of meal carbs only, and use the pump calculator to determine the amount of insulin to be given.

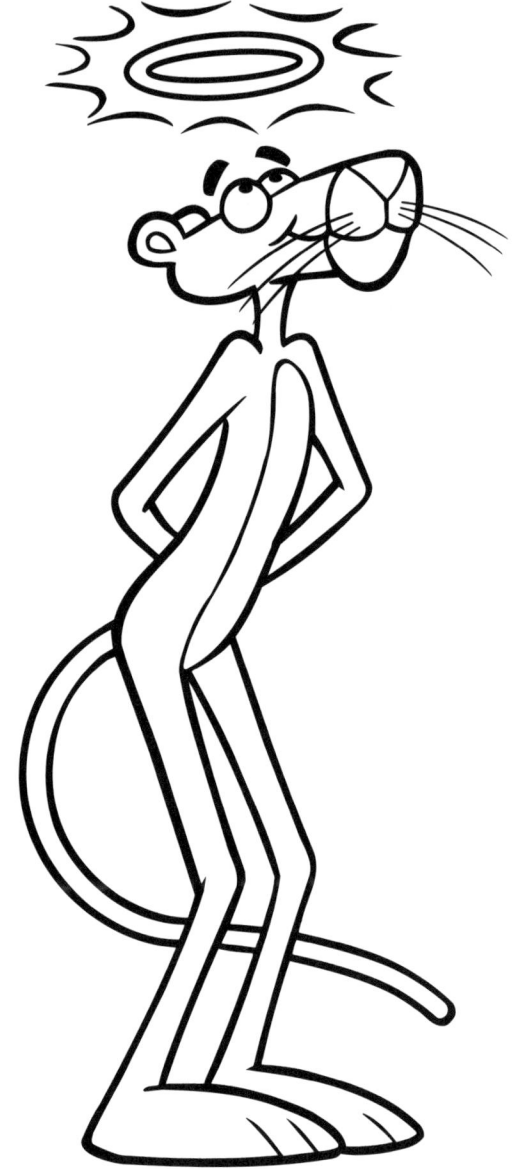

GLUCAGON

As discussed in Chapter 6, glucagon is a hormone with the opposite effect of insulin. It raises the blood sugar, but it is not sugar. Glucagon is used for emergencies when a person becomes unconscious, has a seizure or is unable to safely drink a liquid carbohydrate due to low blood sugar. **Glucagon is very safe to give and results in a rapid rise in blood sugar.** The appropriate dose of glucagon in the school can be found in Table 2 or 3 under Hypoglycemia. Glucagon can now be given by injection or nasal administration. Injectable glucagon may be pre-mixed or may need to be mixed with a liquid before it can be injected. It can be injected under the skin into the subcutaneous fat, just like insulin, or deeper into muscle. It works just as well either way. Since glucagon is considered an emergency medication, many states allow it to be administered by a trained layperson. In states that do not allow glucagon to be given by unlicensed personnel, physicians, schools and families may work out a way that the glucagon can be given at the school in case of an emergency. (The physician must give orders [Tables 5 or 6] for the dose and when to give it.) If the family lives in a rural area, where emergency personnel are not immediately available (we have heard of responses taking as long as 40 minutes), glucagon must be kept in the school. It may have to be administered by a layperson, but most parents are lay people, and they administer glucagon. At least two people should be trained. The school nurse must arrange for routine recertification of these skills for the school staff members assigned to do this task. The instructions from Chapter 6 should be taped to the box.

If available, intranasal spray glucagon (Baqsimi, 3 mg) may be used instead of injected glucagon.

HIGH BLOOD SUGAR (± KETONES) (Table 8)

People with diabetes may have high blood/CGM sugars and spill extra sugar into the urine on some occasions. These occasions include periods of stress, illness, missed insulin, overeating and/or lack of exercise. High sugars are generally NOT an emergency (unless accompanied by elevated ketones and vomiting).

When the sugar is high, the child will have to drink more and urinate more frequently. **It is essential to make bathroom privileges readily available.** If the teacher notes that the child is going to the bathroom frequently over a period of several days, a parent should be notified. The family or diabetes care-provider can then adjust the insulin dose. Treatment for high blood/CGM sugar (with or without ketones) is outlined in Table 8.

TABLE 8:
Treatment for Hyperglycemia (High Blood Sugar with or without Ketones)

Hyperglycemia: Blood glucose (BG) higher than target, as indicated in DMMP orders.
Definition of *Symptomatic* as used below: experiencing flu-like symptoms; nausea and/or vomiting; abdominal pain; severe drowsiness; rapid, shallow or deep breathing; confusion.

Blood Glucose (BG) Levels ➔	Action With Injections (No Pump)	Action With Pump
BG above target, but <300 mg/dL once prior to lunch (Note: to convert mg/dL to mmol/L, divide by 18.)	• Provide correction as indicated in DMMP orders. • Recheck in 3 hrs; if >300 mg/dL – contact school nurse and follow instructions below under "BG >300 mg/dL twice in a row."	• Provide correction per pump calculator. • Recheck in 2 hrs; if greater than 300 mg/dL, contact school nurse and follow instructions below "BG>300 mg/dL twice in a row."
Hyperglycemia (>180 mg/dL but less than 300 mg/dL) other than lunchtime and >3 hours since last insulin dose *Note: Do not give extra correction if student on a sliding scale – contact provider for assistance and notify parent.* *Note: In general, children without mod-large ketones should get corrections no more often than every 3 hours, unless specifically indicated by provider on DMMP.*	• Contact school nurse/child-care health consultant for approval; provide insulin via injection, using indicated correction factor on DMMP orders. • If not available, contact diabetes healthcare-provider for one-time orders. • Contact/Notify parent of correction dosing. • To avoid excess insulin accumulation: o If lunch is within 30 minutes at the time of hyperglycemia, wait for lunch and recheck BG prior to dosing. • If > than 30 minutes until lunch, give correction now. Then at lunchtime give ONLY insulin for carbs eaten and NO insulin for correction.	• ← Follow "Action With Injection" protocol but provide correction per pump calculator. • If unable to use pump calculator use correction formula provided on DMMP orders • If no orders available, RN should contact diabetes healthcare-provider for one-time orders. • Contact/Notify parent if available.
BG >300 mg/dL once and non-symptomatic	• Provide correction as indicated in DMMP orders if greater than 3 hrs since last insulin dose. • If <3 hrs since last dose, recheck at 3 hrs unless symptomatic (see below if symptomatic).	• Check for ketones. • If mod-large ketones, follow instructions below for "BG>300 mg/dL twice in a row." • Possible pump malfunction: see below and Chapter 28.
BG >300 mg/dL twice in a row (> than 2 hours apart) **OR symptomatic as described above** Note: Do not give extra correction if student on a sliding scale; contact provider for assistance and notify parent.	• Check for ketones. • Provide water. • If mod-large ketones, contact parent/guardian, as child should be treated at home. If unable to contact parent, monitor and call healthcare-provider for assistance. • If <3 hrs since last insulin dose, recheck BG when >3 hours, then give correction dose per DMMP orders. • If >3 hrs since last insulin dose and no ketones, contact school nurse –may give correction per DMMP orders.	• This may indicate pump/site malfunction (see Chapter 28). • Pump site will need to be changed by parent/guardian or independent student. • ← Follow "Action With Injection" protocol. • Insulin should be given by injection.

If at any time a child (with or without a pump) has moderate – large ketones or blood ketones ≥1.0 and/or the student has labored breathing, change in mental status or is dehydrated, call parent to take child home; if unavailable, call 911.

INSULIN PUMPS IN THE SCHOOL
(also see Table 3 and Chapter 28)

Many children are now using insulin pumps, some of which, when connected to a CGM, have artificial pancreas features (see Chapter 30). The pumps allow sugar control to be more like that of a person who does not have diabetes. Below are listed some of the special issues of insulin pump use in the school:

- Hypo- and hyperglycemia instructions are in the boxes above and in Tables 3 and 5.

- The computerized features/calculator in the pump should be used for insulin boluses.

- **All** blood glucose values and carbohydrate grams to be eaten (with the exception of treatment for hypoglycemia) must be entered into the pump for delivery of pump-recommended boluses.

- Parents/guardians are responsible for ensuring all pump settings align with orders.

- The pump bolus calculator should only rarely be overridden (e.g., in dosing changes). Encourage parents to follow up with their healthcare-provider for insulin pump dose adjustments if frequent overrides are being requested.

- Delegated staff should always get approval from their school nurse to override pump insulin calculations.

- Potential pump malfunction: The concern for a student on a pump is the possibility of prolonged hyperglycemia due to blocked insulin tubing and the risk of going into diabetic ketoacidosis (DKA). This can happen after 2 or 3 hours without insulin. Unlicensed assistive personnel should contact the school nurse for further instructions regarding insulin by injection or new infusion set by parent or independent student.

- For more information on new pump technologies, see www.coloradokidswithdiabetes.org.

CONTINUOUS GLUCOSE MONITORS
(**CGM;** also see Chapter 29)

- CGM systems use a tiny sensor inserted under the skin to monitor glucose levels (ongoing or short term) in interstitial fluid. Some CGMs need to be calibrated using a finger-stick glucose reading when readings are stable, approximately two-three times/day, typically outside of school. Parents/independent children are responsible for changing sensor/site. Calibration may need to occur in school if prompted by the CGM and should ideally occur when the blood glucose levels are stable (not rising or falling rapidly), typically before meals and not after meals.

- In the school setting, delegated school staff should respond to low and high BG alarms rather than the constantly fluctuating trends and numbers.

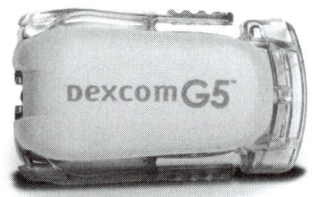 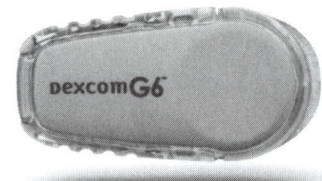

- The FDA has approved use of the **Dexcom G5** (requires calibration 2x/day), and the **Dexcom G6 CGM** and **Freestyle Libre CGM** (neither needs calibration) to make treatment decisions without needing to validate with finger-stick values. Please refer to the *Collaborative Guidelines for Dexcom G5 Non-Adjunctive Dosing in the School Setting 2019,* www.coloradokidswithdiabetes.org. if more information is needed.

- The **benefits of a CGM** in the school/child-care setting include real-time glucose information, which enhances the safety of the child and their diabetes control. The school nurse/child-care health consultant should support the use of CGMs and establish parameters so that there is little disruption to the student's school activities, thereby enhancing their education. The use of the CGM in the school setting includes using alarms sparingly and setting alarms for blood glucose levels that require an immediate action/response. This will help the child avoid alarm fatigue and enhance learning by avoiding unnecessary disruption to their learning in the classroom. Alarms should be set for low and high sugar levels when treatment/action is needed (for example: sensor glucose is <70 mg/dL [3.9 mmol/L] or >300 mg/dL [16.7 mmol/L]).

- School and childcare staff are responsible for keeping all children safe in the school setting. School staff do not have the staffing capacity to support unique requests for frequent glucose pattern management techniques at school. Diabetes care at school will be provided in accordance with the regimen prescribed in the child's medical orders.

- Remote monitoring of the CGM in the school/child-care setting by school/child-care staff is generally not required, as the child is usually supervised by trained staff, and alarms are used to identify urgent glucose levels requiring action. However, in certain unique cases (e.g., preschool age, non-verbal, impaired cognition, severe hypoglycemia unawareness) monitoring/remote monitoring may be appropriate, and the school nurse/child-care health consultant, along with the Section 504 Team, will do an assessment and determine the accommodations based on the child's individual need(s) and the IHP. When determined appropriate, the school nurse/child-care health consultant will indicate these accommodations on a Section 504 plan and the Individualized Health Plan.

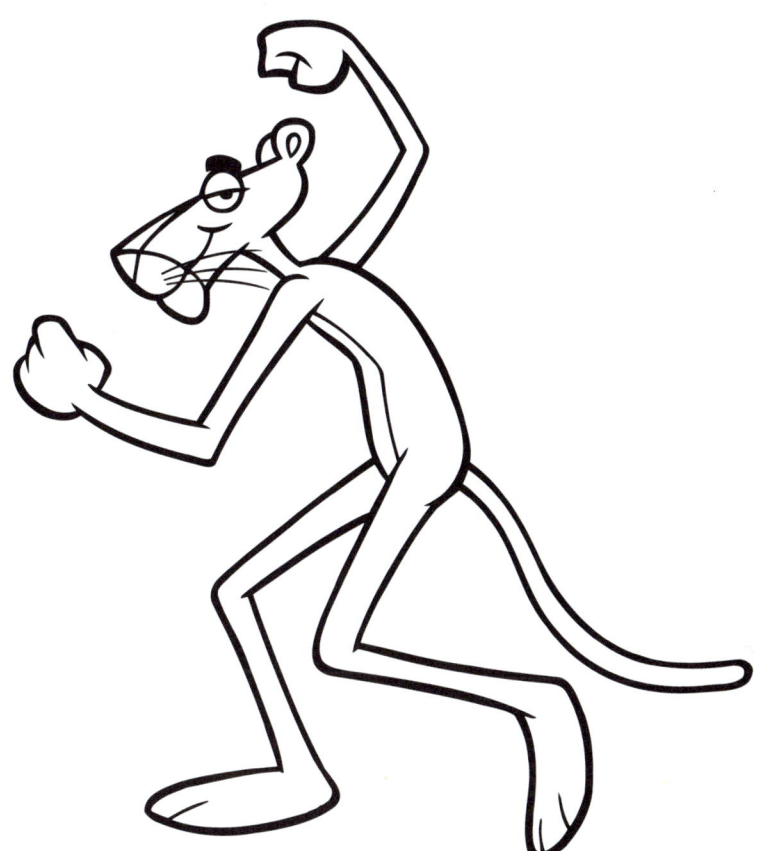

- Trend Arrows: The healthcare-provider may indicate on the DMMP how to use trend arrows in determining insulin dosing/treatment. If not indicated, for the Dexcom G5 & G6 CGMs, these trend arrows may be used in treatment decisions (as agreed upon by the school nurse and parent or per DMMP):

  - CGM 70-80 mg/dL (3.9-4.5 mmol/L) with 1 arrow facing down: give 7.5g of carbohydrates *
  - CGM 70-80 with 2 arrows facing down: give 15g of quick sugar *
  - CGM 70-80 with level arrow: consider giving complex carb snack (10-15g of carbs)*

*Without insulin injection/bolus for these carbs

EXERCISE AND SCHOOL ATTENDANCE (Table 9)

Exercise is important for all students, with or without diabetes. It is particularly important for the gym teacher or coach also to have a copy of the school health plan. Low sugars may occur during exercise, and a source of instant sugar should be readily available. Often a snack is recommended before gym. The child should get the snack early enough to help them be on time. Exercise is even more important for children with diabetes than for other children. They should not be excluded from gym or sports activities. If the child is wearing an insulin pump and disconnects during PE, provision must be made for the pump to be stored in a safe place. However, if the student has elevated blood/CGM glucose levels or symptoms*, exercise may need to be regulated as in Table 9.

CLASS PARTIES

If the class is having a special snack, the child with diabetes should also be given a snack. Parents should be notified ahead of time so that they can decide whether the child may eat the same snack as the other students, or they may want to provide an alternate food.

If an alternate snack is not available, the student should be given the same snack as the other children. A plan on whether to give an extra dose of insulin for the snack can be worked out with the family.

BUS TRAVEL

It is important for the child with diabetes to take some food with him/her on the bus. If the child feels low, he/she must be allowed to eat the food. At times, bus rides take longer than usual due to bad weather or delays, and the child needs to have a snack available and permission from the bus driver to eat it if necessary. Bus drivers should be trained in the basics of diabetes care and the response to hypoglycemia on the bus.

SUBSTITUTE TEACHERS

Ask to have a copy of the school health plan (Table 2 or 3) placed in the substitute teacher's folder and the attendance register so that a substitute would know:

- which child in the class has diabetes (attach a photo)
- when he/she usually eats a snack

TABLE 9:
Exercise and School Attendance (for children on insulin injections or pump)

IF Child's Symptoms & BG Level are...	and Ketone Level is ... then	Exercise	Stay in School
≥300 mg/dL first time, no symptoms	Not required unless on pump	Yes	Yes
≥300 mg/dL - 2 consecutive times (over 2 hours apart), no symptoms	Negative to small	Yes**	Yes
≥300 mg/dL **with symptoms***	Negative or greater	No	No
≥300 mg/dL, with or without symptoms	Urine: Moderate-Large or Blood ketones ≥1.0	No	No
≥300, 2 consecutive times, *no symptoms*	Unable to check ketones	No	Call parent
≥300 mg/dL, with symptoms*	Unable to check ketones	No	No

* Moderate to Severe symptoms include stomachache, nausea, vomiting, labored breathing, slurred speech, change in mental status, and possible dehydration.

**School Nurse/Child-care health consultant should determine if type of exercise is appropriate.

Note: always check blood glucose and ketones before exercise if the child is not feeling well.

- symptoms and treatment of an insulin reaction
- who to contact for assistance if the student is having symptoms of hypo/hyperglycemia
- where the treatment supplies are kept

AFTER-SCHOOL DETENTION

Children with diabetes should not be singled out or treated differently from the rest of the class. However, if required to remain after school (at noon or in the afternoon) for a longer time than usual, the child should have access to blood/CGM sugar supplies and snacks as needed. Most parents will have packets of cheese and crackers, peanut butter and crackers or some such snack available in the classroom. This is a common time of the day for the morning or noon insulins to be peaking.

SPECIAL DAYS (FIELD TRIPS, FIELD DAYS)

Field trips or field days usually involve extra excitement and exercise. Either of these can result in an increased chance of low blood sugars. The parents should ask to be notified beforehand so that they can reduce the dose of insulin. They may also wish to send extra snacks (granola bars, Fruit Roll-ups, etc.). It is important for parents to be aware that in the public school system, the child's diabetes should never be a cause for the school to exclude him or her from any school-sanctioned activity, whether during or after regular school hours. This includes overnight field trips and band or sporting activities away from the school. If the child would be allowed to participate without diabetes, the school must accommodate the needs of the child with diabetes.

MEDICAL RELEASE

It is important for the parent or legal guardian to give the school written permission to contact the child's healthcare-provider. This may be necessary in the event of an emergency. Without this "medical release" in place, the doctor or care-provider may not discuss or give advice pertaining to the child's care. This permission is included in the last paragraph of the IHP (Table 2 or 3).

LEGAL RIGHTS

It is our experience that schools, principals, teachers, and staff want to do their best to help families care for their child with diabetes. Most misunderstandings can be solved with education. Sometimes, implementation of federal law is needed:

Section 504 of the Rehabilitation Act of 1973 prohibits recipients of federal funds from discriminating against people on the basis of a disability (including diabetes). A formal contractual healthcare plan outlining all accommodations necessary to care for the child with diabetes during school is known as a "504" plan. Putting this plan together usually involves meetings between the parents, child, school staff (nurse, teachers, principal, special education facilitator) and/or diabetes healthcare-providers. The child is protected from discrimination by this law not only during the school day but on any school-sanctioned activity as well. In our experience, the parents and school staff are usually able to agree on a School Healthcare Plan (Table 2 or 3).

The 504 plan addresses accommodations for the child with diabetes to have equal access to their education. The accommodations on the 504 plan may include access to cell phones for continuous glucose monitoring, blood glucose testing at school, and accommodations for standardized testing such as college entrance exams (SAT, ACT). These 504 accommodations may go with the child to college as needed.

A child with diabetes has the right to a free and appropriate public education, including accommodations to manage their diabetes at school. The child may also need special accommodations under the "Individuals with Disabilities Education Act" (IDEA). This law protects children who may be experiencing learning difficulties due to their disability. In the case of diabetes, this may arise as a result of reoccurring high or low sugars, impacting the ability to learn or think clearly on exams. If the child must leave the classroom frequently to do blood sugars, eat snacks or inject insulin, and misses lesson time, this may also impact their ability to learn. Accommodations for any of these must be made to assist the child to learn. This may mean, for example, making provision for the child to do blood sugars in the classroom so as not to miss teaching time. It may also provide for the child to check a blood sugar level before exams in order to bring sugar levels to the appropriate target prior to sitting for an exam. The plan outlining what provisions must be made to assist the child to learn is called an IEP (individualized education program). It will be put together through the school's special education program in conjunction with the parents, child and healthcare providers. You can review these rights on the ADA website, www.diabetes.org. The ADA also has a brochure and section on their website called "Safe at School."

Additional resources are:

1. The Law, Schools and Your Child with Diabetes at
   http://www.childrenwithdiabetes.com/d_0q_600.htm (please note the underscores)
   This website allows access to www.diabetes.org/safeatschool, from the American Diabetes Association, which discusses the legal obligations of school systems under Section 504 of the Rehabilitation Act of 1973 and the Education for All Handicapped Children Act of 1975, amended in 1991.
   It also has a section, How to Write an IEP, a book designed to help parents who have children with disabilities succeed in school; www.childrenwithdiabetes.com/504

2. The National Information Center for Children and Youth with Disabilities (NICHCY) is a U.S. Government-sponsored clearinghouse that provides information about disabilities, including information about obtaining assistance at school.

3. The U.S. Department of Education website (www.ed.gov) includes:
   The Individuals with Disabilities Education Act, with detailed information about IDEA.
   IDEA: The Law contains links to downloadable versions of the law.

4. Helping the Student with Diabetes Succeed (A Guide for School Personnel). This is a 76-page primer that can be downloaded from: https://www.niddk.nih.gov/health-information/professionals/clinical-tools-patient-management/diabetes/helping-student-diabetes-succeed-guide-school-personnel.

5. www.diabetes.org/safeatschool

6. Diabetes Care Tasks @ School: What Key Personnel Need to Know. Eighteen PowerPoint presentations online at https://www.diabetes.org/resources/know-your-rights/safe-at-school-state-laws/training-resources-school-staff/diabetes-care-tasks-school

7. Living with Diabetes: Tips for Teachers is a 19-minute DVD available from Maxishare. Call for prices. Their address is: Maxishare, P.O. Box 2041, Milwaukee, WI 53201. Phone: 1-800-444-7747, Fax: 414-266-1540. A customer service representative for Maxishare can be contacted at 414-266-3428. Hospitals can pay for this video with purchase orders, and individuals can pre-pay with a check or credit card. Some clinics have copies of these videos that can be loaned to parents to take to their school. www.maxishare.com

8. Diabetes Management in School and Child Care RN Instructor Guide.
   www.coloradokidswithdiabetes.org/training

I agree with use of this chapter as a Standard of Care for my child:

Parent signature(s): _____ Date: _____

_____ Date: _____

CHAPTER 26

Child-Sitters, Grandparents and Diabetes

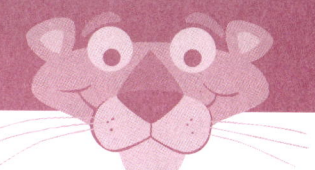

INTRODUCTION

The time required to instruct a sitter or grandparent will depend on how long he/she will be with your child. A person helping for a few hours will generally do fine after you teach him/her "the basics" in this handout. A person staying with a child for a longer time or day-sitting for many weeks will require more time to learn to give insulin and to gain other knowledge. More than half of young children with diabetes in the U.S. are now using a continuous glucose monitor (CGM) and/or an insulin pump. Thus, some knowledge in these areas may be needed. You are welcome to bring the sitter or grandparent along to diabetes clinic visits. In some cities, child-care courses are offered to teach people diabetes-related skills.

Our Center offers a one-day course several times each year for grandparents and other caregivers of children with diabetes. It is important for grandparents to have a normal relationship with their grandchildren. This includes having the children for a day or, when parents are away, caring for them for a longer period. This requires having some knowledge and skills in many areas of diabetes management. Certainly, recognizing low blood sugars and knowing how to treat them is essential. Checking blood/CGM glucose levels (Chapter 7) and, if the child is going to spend more than the day, knowing how to draw and give insulin (Chapter 9) is also essential. Grandparents do not usually need to know how to manage illness or how to adjust insulin doses. They should be in contact with the parents or healthcare team if the child is ill or has high

TOPICS:
Prevent, Detect and Treat Acute Complications
Monitoring (blood sugars, ketones)
Psychosocial Adjustment

TEACHING OBJECTIVES:
The teacher will:
1. Present to caregivers the signs, symptoms and treatment of hypoglycemia.
2. Instruct caregivers about essential information for the care of the child (e.g., meals and activity).
3. Teach the skills needed for the care of the child (injections, blood sugar and ketone checking, etc.).
4. Encourage the utilization of child-sitters and grandparents for the occasional relief of parental and child stress.

LEARNING OBJECTIVES:
Learner (parents, child, relative or self) will be able to:
1. Describe three signs and symptoms of hypoglycemia with the appropriate treatment.
2. Define two factors important in the management of diabetes.
3. Demonstrate the necessary skills for the care of the child.
4. Formulate a "stress relief" plan for the family.

blood/CGM glucose levels for other reasons. Grandparents who take the time to learn about diabetes are showing love and support for their children and their grandchildren. Aunts, uncles, godparents and others close to the child are encouraged and welcome to attend if they will have the opportunity to care for the child.

WHAT DO ALL CAREGIVERS NEED TO KNOW?

How much training is needed will depend upon the amount of time the child will be with the caregiver and upon the age of the child.

All caregivers need:

- some information about signs of low blood sugar and how to treat a low. Being prepared for a low blood sugar is essential.
- some basic instruction on foods and diabetes. A handout is in this chapter which can be cut out or copied for the caregiver.
- emergency phone numbers in case the parents cannot be reached. This helps everyone feel better.
- knowledge on how to give shots or pump boluses, when to check for urine or blood ketones, and other more detailed information if the parents are to be away for a longer time period. It may be easier to learn to give the insulin(s) using an insulin pen.
- an extra supply of insulin, etc. (in case a bottle is dropped and broken). A glucagon kit (preferably intranasal) is also helpful.
- "smart phones" can be used to send texts or other information or to observe CGM sugar levels.

Please feel free to cut out/copy the following pages for the caregiver.

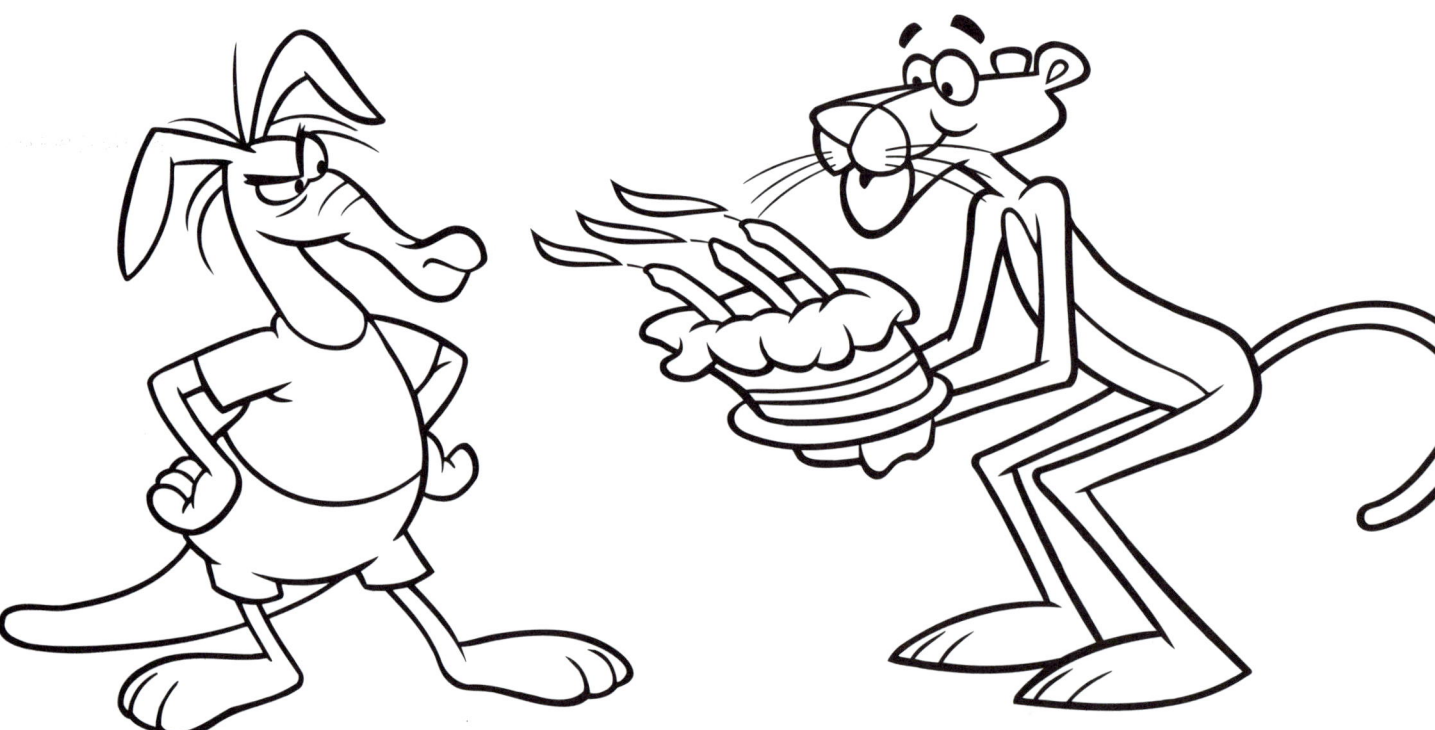

Information for the Sitter or Grandparent

Our child, _____, has diabetes.

Children with diabetes are generally normal and healthy. In a child who has diabetes, sugar cannot be used by the body because the pancreas no longer makes the hormone insulin. Because of this, daily insulin injections are needed. Diabetes is not contagious. Caring for a child with diabetes does require a small amount of extra knowledge.

LOW BLOOD SUGAR

The only emergency that could come on quickly is **LOW BLOOD SUGAR** (otherwise known as "hypoglycemia" or an "insulin reaction"). This can occur if the child gets more exercise than usual or does not eat as much as usual. Care-providers must be able to recognize the symptoms and be prepared to treat the low blood sugar as needed.

The warning signs of low blood sugar vary but include any of the following:
(They are discussed in greater detail in Chapter 6.)

1. Hunger
2. Paleness, sweating, shaking
3. Eyes appear glassy, dilated or the pupils are "big"
4. Pale or flushed face
5. Personality changes such as crying or stubbornness
6. Headaches
7. Inattention, drowsiness, sleepiness at an unusual time
8. Weakness, irritability, confusion
9. Speech and coordination changes
10. If not treated, loss of consciousness and/or seizure

The signs our child usually has are: _____
_____
_____

Blood Sugar: It is ideal to check the blood sugar (Chapter 7) if this is possible. It takes approximately 10-20 minutes for the blood sugar to increase after taking liquids with sugar. Thus, the blood sugar can even be done after taking sugar. If it is not convenient to check the blood sugar, go ahead with treatment anyway.

Treatment: Give SUGAR (preferably in a liquid form) to help the blood sugar rise.
You may give any of the following:

1. One-half cup of soft drink that contains sugar – **NOT a diet pop**
2. Three or four glucose tablets, sugar packets or cubes or a teaspoon of honey (if over age one year)
3. One-half cup of fruit juice
4. LIFE-SAVERS candy (FIVE or SIX pieces) if over three years of age
5. One-half tube of Insta-Glucose, or cake decorating gel (see below)

We usually treat reactions with: _____

If the child is having an insulin reaction and he/she refuses to eat or has difficulty eating, give Insta-Glucose, cake decorating gel (1/2 tube) or other sugar source. Put the Insta-Glucose, a little bit at a time, between the cheeks (lips) and the gums and tell the child to swallow. If he/she can't swallow, lay the child down and turn the head to the side so the sugar or glucose doesn't cause choking. You can help the sugar solution absorb by massaging the child's cheek.

CONTINUED

CHILD-SITTERS, GRANDPARENTS AND DIABETES

If a low blood sugar (insulin reaction) or other problems occur, please call (in order):

1. Parent: _____ at: _____
2. Physician: _____ at: _____
3. Other person: _____ at: _____

The child must have meals and snacks on time. The schedule is as follows:

	Time	Food to Give	Insulin to Give*
Breakfast	_____	_____	_____
Snack	_____	_____	_____
Lunch	_____	_____	_____
Snack	_____	_____	_____
Supper	_____	_____	_____
Snack	_____	_____	_____

* Can be drawn ahead of time by the parent.

Sometimes young children will not eat meals and snacks at exactly the time suggested. If this happens, DON'T PANIC! Set the food within the child's reach (in front of the TV set often works) and leave him/her alone. If the food hasn't been eaten in 10 minutes, give a friendly reminder. Allow about 30 minutes for meals.

BLOOD SUGARS

It may be necessary to check the blood sugar (particularly if a CGM is not used) or blood or urine ketones (Chapter 5).

The test supplies we use are: _____

The supplies are kept: _____

Please record any blood or urine results.

Time: _____ Result: _____ Time: _____ Result: _____

INSULIN PUMPS

Many young children now receive their insulin via an insulin pump. The needed depth of knowledge about pumps will depend on the time of stay. At a minimum, you must be able to turn the pump off (or disconnect the tubing) with a low blood/CGM sugar and to turn it back on when the blood/CGM sugar rises. Also, if a very high blood/CGM sugar occurs (± ketones), a new infusion set may be needed (or a temporary shot of insulin). Parents often stay in close contact (when possible) to help advise.

If the stay is to be more than a few hours, it may be necessary to know how to approximate the amount of carbohydrates (carbs) to be eaten and to enter the value in the pump. If the blood sugar meter or CGM does not communicate automatically with the pump, the sugar value will also need to be entered. An insulin dose is then suggested by the pump and only needs to be accepted.

SIDE TRIPS

Please be sure that if the child is away from home, with you or with friends, extra snacks and a source of sugar are taken along.

OTHER CONCERNS: _____
_____
_____

If there are any questions, or if our child does not feel good or vomits, please call us or the other people listed above.

Thank you.

QUESTIONS AND ANSWERS FROM NEWSNOTES

Q: What is the Grandparents' Workshop, and why does the Center have this?

A: The Center has the Grandparents' Workshop (usually two to four times per year based on need) so that grandparents can care for grandchildren and grandchildren can stay with grandparents. Both are very important to each other! I recently had a family tell me that when their five-year-old was diagnosed with diabetes, one set of grandparents jumped in and learned about diabetes, including how to check blood/CGM sugars, give insulin and the whole "ball of wax." The other set of grandparents was scared of the diabetes and never learned any of the needed diabetes skills. Needless to say, the first set of grandparents gained a grandchild, while the second set lost one; the grandchild lost the opportunity for a close relationship with the second set of grandparents.

For most grandparents, attending the one-day workshop and possibly reading the Center's short *First Book for Understanding Diabetes*, or the more-detailed educational book, *Understanding Diabetes* (see order form in back) results in enough skills to be able to have the child spend a night or a week with them like any other grandchild. Perhaps even more important, attending the workshop helps lessen the fears of diabetes, particularly involving hypoglycemia and giving insulin.

The child must not feel different or punished because of having diabetes. If siblings get to stay with the grandparents, the child with diabetes must have the same opportunity. It is also a chance for the child (and parents) to break inter-dependencies.

Finally, all parents need a break and an occasional vacation without the children. Grandparents are often the best possible solution and can sometimes be the only option. The chance to get to know one's grandparents better and to have memories of staying with them is something that is valued for many years to come.

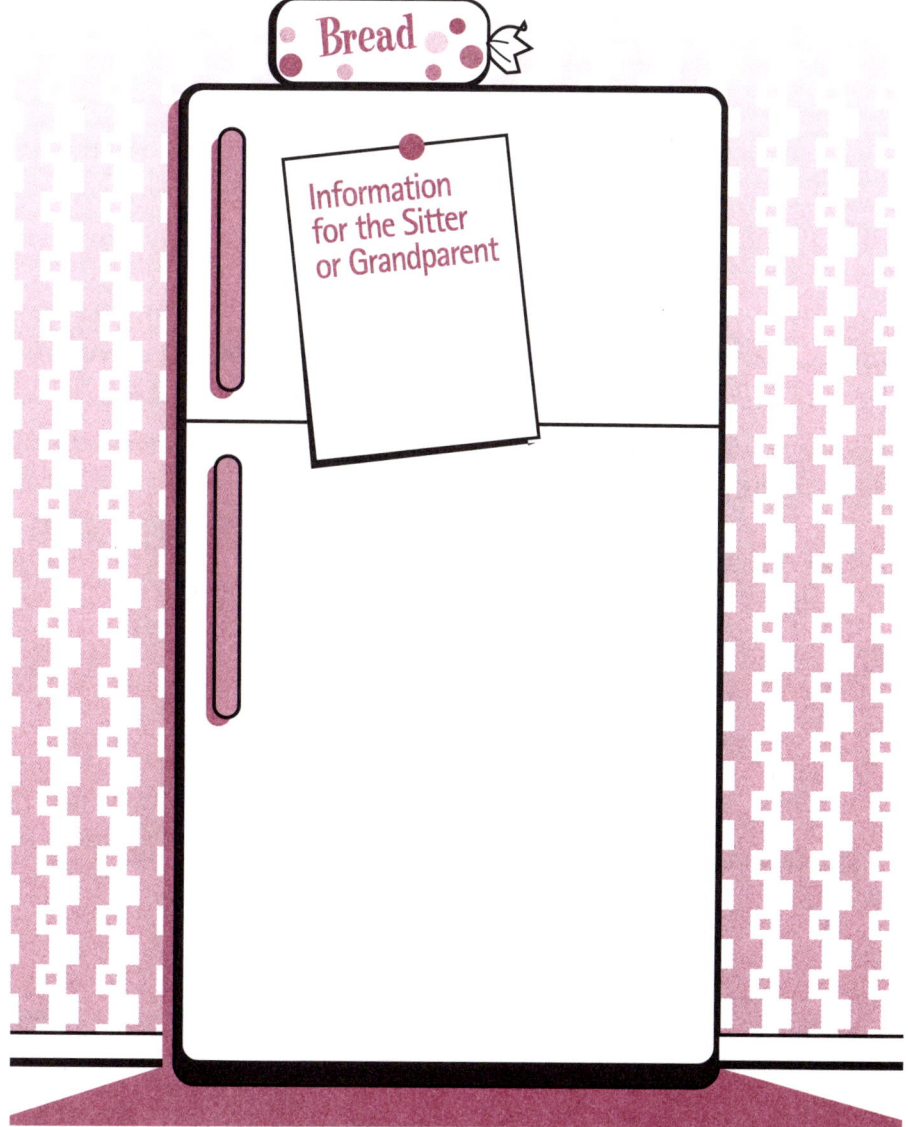

Travel Letter

Name: _____   Date: _____

DOB: _____

To Whom It May Concern:

_____ is a patient at _____. _____ has type 1 diabetes and requires daily insulin injections to remain healthy. To manage diabetes, medical supplies must be carried, including insulin, syringes, blood glucose and ketone checking strips, lancets, a glucose meter, glucagon emergency kit, as well as an emergency food supply and water.

The two most common complications associated with diabetes are hypo- and hyperglycemia events. Hypoglycemia events happen when the patient's blood glucose falls below 70 mg/dL (3.9 mmol/L). When blood glucose levels fall below this value, the patient can become generally confused, lose consciousness and succumb to seizures. If low blood glucose levels are not promptly treated with food, juice or glucagon, death can occur. The other major complication associated with diabetes is hyperglycemia. Hyperglycemia occurs when a patient's blood glucose is above 250 mg/dL (13.9 mmol/L). When hyperglycemia events occur, patients experiences malaise, headaches and generalized poor health. Immediate injections of insulin may be required.

Some people utilize a **continuous insulin infusion pump**, a pager-like device which delivers insulin through tubing (or by a wireless device) beneath the skin. This insulin delivery is constant throughout the 24 hours of the day. The insulin pump requires its own supplies, such as infusion sets with needles, tubing, reservoirs and batteries. Some people also wear a **continuous glucose monitor (CGM)**, which continuously measures glucose levels.

Please note: This patient's insulin infusion pump and CGM cannot be exposed to magnetic x-ray equipment, including a full body scanner or the conveyor belt scanning. Please ensure that these devices be hand-checked by TSA personnel.

Other: _____

_____

_____

_____   _____
Physician   Phone:

CHAPTER 27

Vacations and Camp

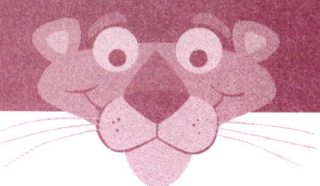

VACATIONS

Diabetes should not interfere with vacations, which are a normal part of life. Some extra "planning ahead" should help prevent problems related to the diabetes.

Planning may include:

✓ discussing your vacation at your clinic visit before leaving

✓ a review of sick day management and the need to have a way to check for ketones

✓ buying Kaopectate and/or ImodiumAD if going to areas where the risk for diarrhea is high (although prevention with frequent handwashing is important).

✓ taking along your doctor's/nurse's phone numbers

TABLE 1:
Packing List

☐ Insulin(s) and/or oral meds
☐ Syringes (and needles for insulin pens)
☐ Test strips
☐ Lancets
☐ Glucagon
☐ Equipment
   (BG meter, CGM and supplies,
   insulin pump [if used] and supplies)
☐ Snacks
☐ Letter from doctor
   (especially if going overseas)

TOPICS:
Psychosocial Adjustment
Physical Activity

TEACHING OBJECTIVES:
The teacher will:
1. Explain the benefits of camps and vacations.
2. Discuss the value of developing independent knowledge and skills.

LEARNING OBJECTIVES:
Learner (parents, child, relative or self) will be able to:
1. List three benefits of attending camps or having vacations.
2. Identify one area of additional knowledge and/or one skill and/or one more area of personal growth needed for the person with diabetes.

AIRPLANE TRAVEL

✓ Share the information with the healthcare team if your travel will be out of the country. *The information should include:*

• both departure and arrival times – going and returning.

• the number of hours traveling.

✓ If going on a plane, carry insulin, glucose meter and strips and glucagon on board in case you need these. If put in checked luggage, they can freeze and spoil or be lost if luggage doesn't arrive.

✓ Insulin should be carried on airplanes and not packed in "check-in" luggage.

289

- ✔ Extras of everything should be carried by a second person when possible, in case one carry-on is lost.
- ✔ Extra snacks (sugar [dextrose] tablets, granola bars, etc.) should be carried, in case food is late or not available.
- ✔ Supplies for measuring ketones.
- ✔ Time changes within the U.S. are usually not a problem, but they must be considered if going overseas. Call your doctor or nurse for help with insulin adjustments if needed. For insulin pumps, the person just resets the time in the pump.

SECURITY MEASURES FOR AIRPLANE TRAVEL

The official security measures since 9/11/01 for flying, especially outside the U.S. (often now not required in the U.S.):

1. Passengers may board with syringes or insulin pumps only if they can show a vial of insulin with a professional pre-printed label which clearly shows the medication. Since the prescription label is on the outside of the box of the vial of insulin, the FAA recommends that passengers come with their vial of insulin in its original labeled box.

2. For passengers who have diabetes and must check their blood sugar levels but do not take insulin, bringing their lancets is all right as long as the lancets are capped. The lancets must be with the glucose meter that has the manufacturer's name on the meter (e.g., One Touch meters say "One Touch," Accu-Chek meters say "Accu-Chek," etc.).

3. People who are traveling with a glucagon kit (intranasal or injectables) should keep it in its original pre-printed labeled container.

4. Travel letters help explain the need for carrying on diabetic supplies (see letter in this chapter), and are often a help.

5. Insulin pump and CGM companies recommend that a pump or CGM not be taken through X-ray (total body scanners or put on the conveyor belt). They state that the electronic components of the pump/CGM may be altered. We suggest explaining to airport security and having them manually check it if there is a problem walking through the usual screening (which does not cause a problem).

FOOD

Concerns regarding food should include:

- ✔ Meals (often best to carry on)
- ✔ Have an ample supply of snacks (e.g., cheese or peanut butter crackers, granola bars, etc.)
- ✔ Have sources of sugar always available (glucose tablets, fruit roll-ups or whatever works best)

EXERCISE

Concerns regarding exercise include:

- ✔ If traveling in a car, plan regular stops to get some exercise.
- ✔ When traveling in a car, **MORE** insulin will probably be needed due to less physical activity. If using an insulin pump, a 120 (or 150?) percent temporary basal rate can be used.
- ✔ On active days (e.g., at beach or at a Disney Park) LESS insulin will probably be needed (THINK AHEAD!). If using an insulin pump, an 80 percent (or less) temporary basal rate can be used.
- ✔ The best way to know the effects of increased or less activity is to do more frequent blood/CGM glucose checks.

INSULIN

A few points to remember:

✓ Pack enough insulin to last the entire trip. Supplies may not be available at your vacation area.

✓ If going by car, keep insulin, glucagon, and glucose meter with strips and CGM sensors in plastic bags in a cooler so they do not get too hot. Do not place directly on ice.

✓ If using an insulin pump, see the list of supplies to take in the Q and A section in the back of Chapter 28.

Make a **check list** ahead of time of things to take. Double-check this list at the last minute. If using an insulin pump, take Lantus (Basaglar)/Levemir/Tresiba insulin and insulin syringes in case the pump breaks down and you need to return to shots. Have a written record of the pump basal rates and times in a secure place. If going overseas, some pump companies will provide a second pump to take along. It is helpful to know the dosage of basal insulin you were on before starting the pump. The basal insulin dose is the same as the pump total basal insulin dose. Remember you can always draw the rapid-acting insulin (Humalog/NovoLog/Apidra) from the pump cartridge into a syringe every three to four hours until you can get other insulins.

Some "Generic Reminders" are:

✓ ALWAYS carry a form of **sugar** with you to treat reactions.

✓ Have enough **snacks** available.

✓ Always wear a diabetes **identification tag**.

✓ Get the name of a **doctor** or emergency room/urgent care in your vacation area so you can call him/her if necessary. Take your own doctor's and nurse's phone number, too. He/she knows your case best, and it may be comforting to make a long-distance phone call when help is needed.

✓ Visit your doctor **a few weeks before** you leave so you have time to work out any problems. Discuss your plans at your visit. Remember to take his/her list of suggestions with you.

✓ If you expect to be **more active** on the vacation (hiking, camping, skiing, etc.), you may need to reduce the insulin dose. Discuss this with your doctor or nurse.

✓ For international travel, remember to check far enough ahead of time to see if you need special immunizations. State health departments can usually give this information. It is also available online (www.cdc.gov/travel).

✓ If international travel is planned, it is wise to carry a travel letter from the doctor (see letter in this chapter) explaining why insulin syringes and other supplies are being taken through customs. As stated earlier, it may be necessary to have prescription labels on the insulin and any other supplies to be carried on board. Check to see if your health insurance covers you in other countries, or if you need supplemental insurance.

✓ The most important advice is to **HAVE FUN!**

HEAT and COLD

All insulins, blood glucose and ketone strips and glucagon may spoil at temperatures above 90°F (>32°C) or if frozen. If kept in an ice chest, do not place in direct contact with the ice. Oral diabetes medicines (e.g., metformin) should also be kept cool (less than 86°F or 30°C).

Insulin pumps can generally withstand greater heat (up to 104°F/40°C) than can insulin. Keeping the pump covered or in a protective case (possibly with a cold gel pack) may help. Some people switch to injection therapy during visits to very hot areas. Having a pump (and tubing) close to the body helps when skiing or at cold temperatures.

CAMP

Children with diabetes are very dependent on their parents for:

- ✓ blood/CGM glucose levels
- ✓ injections, insulin pumps
- ✓ proper nutrition
- ✓ help with avoiding and treating potentially dangerous low blood sugars

These are in addition to their non-diabetic needs. The diabetes care for their child can become one of the main functions in life for a parent. As a result, children with diabetes may become too dependent on their parents.

Advantages of Attending Diabetes Camp

- Diabetes camp often offers the first chance to alter these dependent relationships.
- Most diabetes camps have doctors and nurses at the camp so the parents can feel their children will be safe.
- Camp food is monitored and the amounts calculated by a dietitian. This helps to have the correct content and amounts available for the increased activity.
- Adequate snacks are routinely available and provided.
- It is often a major help for children to meet other friends who take shots and do blood sugar monitoring just like they do. Diabetes is "the norm" at camp.
- It is also a chance for a child to realize that he/she is not the only person in the world who has diabetes.
- Children who are old enough and who do not give their own shots or do their own blood sugar levels may try doing these tasks at camp.
- The children also understand that with proper planning, they can do the same hiking, overnights and other activities that other children do.
- Research has found that after returning from camp, campers felt more confident in caring for their diabetes.
- Other youth with insulin pumps and CGMs will be at camp. This may stimulate an interest in these devices.
- Older teens with diabetes may serve as junior counselors and find that they must take care of themselves in order to set a good example for younger campers.

Other Camp Concerns

It is important for parents not to be upset if they receive the "typical" camp letter from their child asking the parents to come and get them immediately. This type of letter is not unusual and should not cause concern. Most campers are having a wonderful time. If you are overly concerned, call the camp coordinator for support. Whatever you do, don't upset the child by trying to call them at camp, and don't suddenly appear at camp ready to take the child home.

Most diabetes camps also have some educational programs. *These may be:*

- ✓ "rap-sessions"

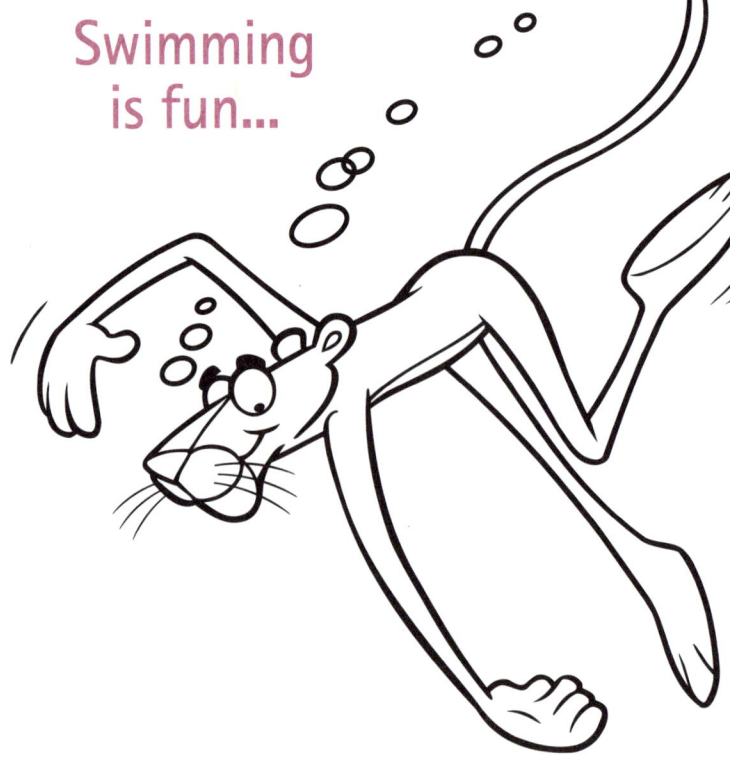

Swimming is fun...

- ✔ problem-solving sessions
- ✔ games to help learning (e.g., carb counting "guesstimates")

The **major** goal of the camp, however, should be to **have fun** and to make new friends. It is not unusual to develop pen pals who can't wait until the next camp when they can meet again.

Insulin doses are generally decreased 20 to 30 percent initially due to increased activity and to avoid hypoglycemia as much as possible.

Scholarship programs are offered for most diabetes camps. If finances are a problem, a request for financial help should be made. Sometimes children can earn part of their own expenses.

After having been at a diabetes camp, the child may decide to try other camps. When this happens, the parents will need to:

- ✔ discuss insulin dose changes with their diabetes care-provider.
- ✔ be in touch with the nurse at the other camp.
- ✔ provide all of the diabetes supplies needed for the camping period.
- ✔ give telephone numbers for emergencies.
- ✔ work out an emergency treatment plan as in the school chapter (Chapter 25).
- ✔ work out a way to have the blood sugars faxed/phoned/emailed to the family or healthcare-provider.

Chapter 7 in Dr. Chase's educational novel, *A Second Cure* (available on Amazon), describes a "real-life" camp for youth with diabetes. Attending a diabetes camp or another camp is often the first step toward independence for the child with diabetes. Encouraging camp attendance can result in a healthy parent-child relationship.

Updated camp information for camps throughout the world can be found at: www.childrenwithdiabetes.com/camps or at www.diabetes.org/in-my-community/diabetes-camp.

... and so is riding an elephant!

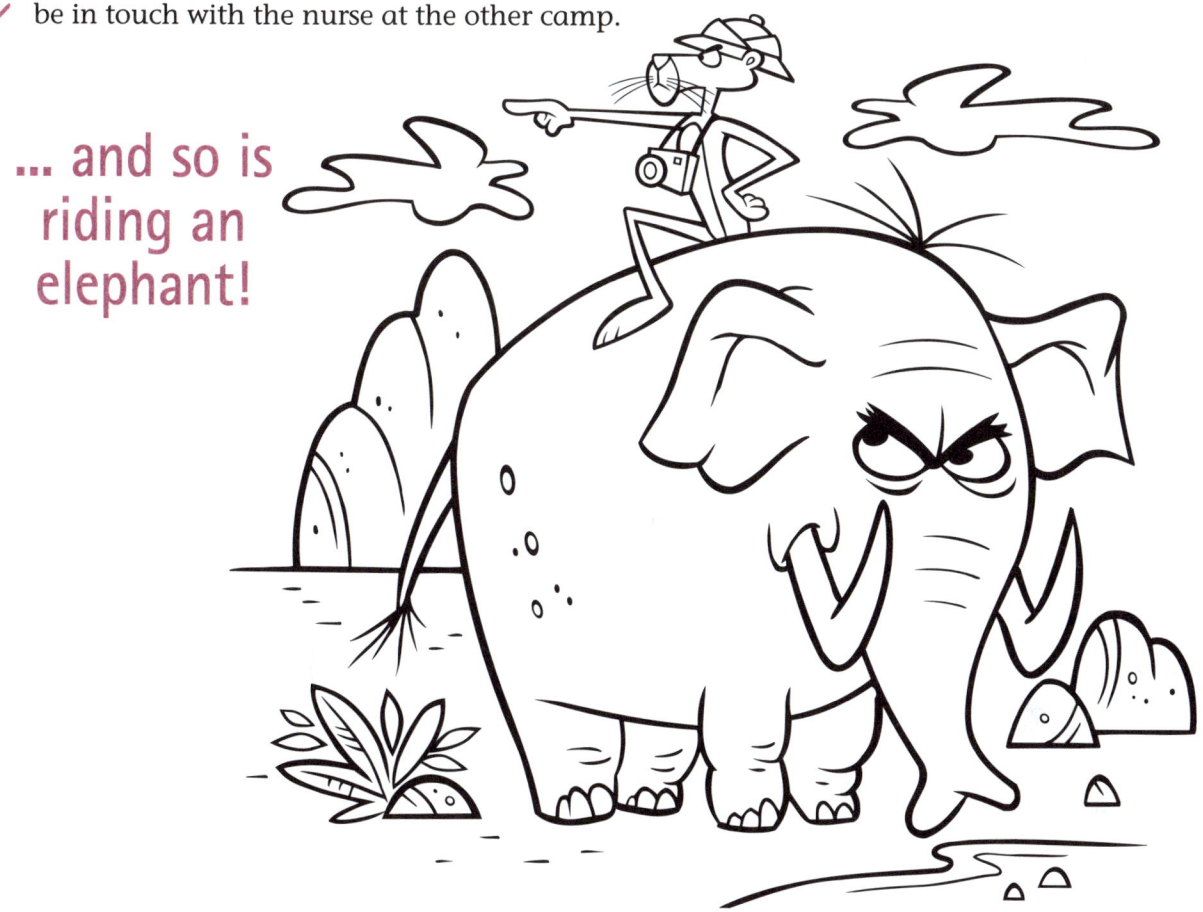

QUESTIONS AND ANSWERS FROM NEWSNOTES

 **Should my child go to diabetes camp?**

We are often asked this question. The lower age limit for the Colorado camp is eight years, although not all eight-year-olds are mature enough to be away from home. Some camps take children at even younger ages. This question was directed to me specifically as it related to a 10-year-old, and I replied without hesitation, "Yes, your child should go to camp."

Camp offers many benefits:

✓ fun (our major emphasis!)
✓ getting to know and live in a cabin with other children the same age who also have diabetes
✓ a great help for children to learn that they are not the only persons their age in the world with diabetes
✓ ten others in the cabin also have to take shots (or wear a pump) and do blood sugars (or use a CGM)
✓ the first chance to break the child-parent inter-dependencies which can develop when diabetes is diagnosed at a young age
✓ a good time for parents to also have a break!

 **We are going to the East Coast on vacation this summer. Will times for giving shots need to be adjusted?**

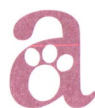 No. A change of one or two hours does not usually make a difference; simply adjust to their time zone.

This is not the case when traveling to Europe, the Far East or even Hawaii. When greater time changes happen, call your diabetes care-provider with the:

✓ time of leaving home and/or the U.S.
✓ number of hours you will be traveling.
✓ time of planned arrival, including a.m. or p.m.
✓ scheduled meals on planes.
✓ same information for your return trip.

Your diabetes care-provider can then help you with the insulin adjustments.

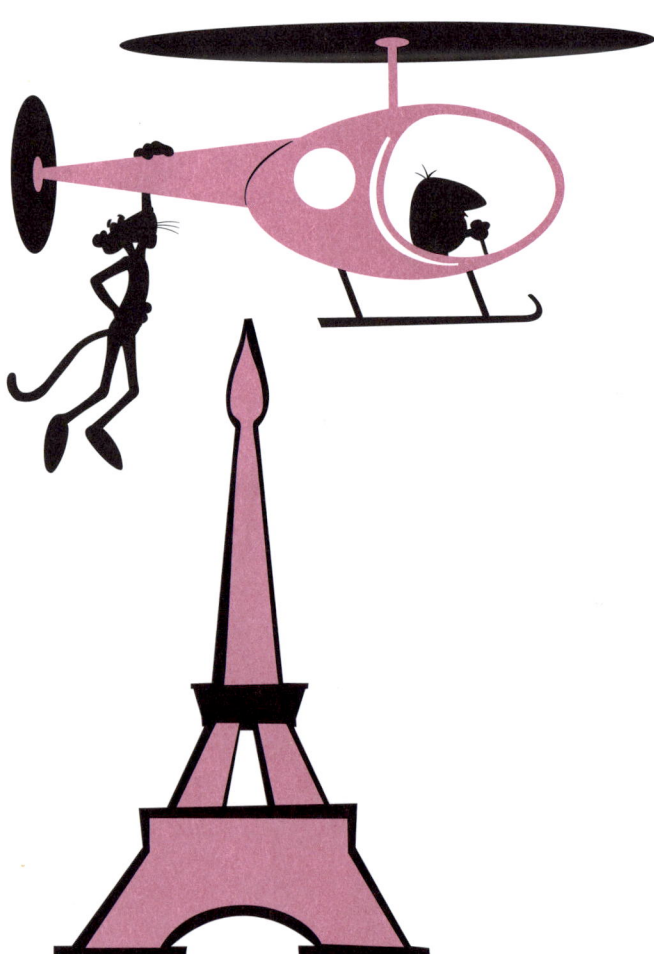

Our son is about to go hiking in a very hot part of the U.S. Is there any way to keep his insulin, blood sugar strips and glucagon cool so they don't spoil?

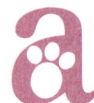 You can order the FRIO Cool Pouch at www.medicool.com. Hopefully all will fit in their larger pack.

VACATIONS AND CAMP

Chapter 28

Insulin Pumps

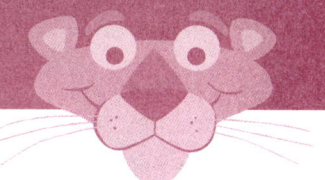

Susie Owen RN, CDE
H. Peter Chase MD
Brigitte I. Frohnert MD, PhD

INTRODUCTION

This chapter is somewhat complex and does not need to be read until the family is ready to consider insulin pump therapy. The chapter is not meant to teach everything one needs to know about insulin pumps. There is a separate book in the Pink Panther series, *Understanding Insulin Pumps, Continuous Glucose Monitors and the Artificial Pancreas,* which goes into more detail (see Other Materials, available in the back of the book). The use of a continuous glucose monitor (CGM, Chapter 29) will be referred to frequently, as these two technologies are now often used together. An insulin pump is a microcomputer (the size of a pager) that constantly provides insulin. When an insulin pump is used, insulin is first put into a special syringe which is then placed within the pump case, or insulin is injected into a pod. A small plastic tube, called a cannula, is then inserted under the skin with a needle. After insertion, the needle is removed, leaving just the plastic tube in place. Insulin is infused through the small plastic tube under the skin (most commonly placed in the abdomen or buttock). Tape may be placed over the cannula set to keep it in place for up to three days.

Pump management involves a high level of diabetes care. It requires a commitment by the entire family to help with the daily management. No matter what age a person begins pump therapy, he/she will need assistance to ensure safety and a positive outcome. Pump management needs to begin during a time when the person with diabetes is ready and when the family can focus on developing new knowledge and skills.

> **TOPICS:**
> **Medications (Insulin Delivery Systems)**
> **Avoid Acute and Chronic Complications Through Risk Reduction**
>
> **TEACHING OBJECTIVES:**
> The teacher will:
> 1. Introduce basic pump concepts, including basal and bolus insulin dosing.
> 2. Discuss advantages and disadvantages of insulin pump therapy.
> 3. Review risk factors resulting in hypo/hyperglycemia in pump users.
> 4. Explain pump options during exercise.
>
> **LEARNING OBJECTIVES:**
> Learner (parents, child, relative or self) will be able to:
> 1. Differentiate between basal and bolus insulin doses.
> 2. Cite two advantages and two disadvantages of insulin pump therapy.
> 3. Identify two causes of low and of high blood sugars in pump users.
> 4. Identify when to use a temporary basal rate.

Insulin pumps do not vary the insulin dose unless used with a CGM in an artificial pancreas (AP) system (see Chapter 30). The pump is programmed to give a pre-set amount of insulin at regular intervals (called the **"basal"** rate). The basal rates do not automatically change as blood sugars change. In addition, each time the person eats, or if the blood sugar is elevated, the user must give a **"bolus"** insulin dose. The bolus calculator (explained below) helps to calculate the amount of insulin the person should give.

There is not a "best age" to begin using an insulin pump. The time is right when the person with diabetes and their family are ready and willing. It must not be just the parents who want and are pushing for the pump. (The situation is obviously different for young children.) The ability to count carbohydrates (**carbs**) and to reliably calculate and give an insulin dose are requirements. Younger children who cannot count carbs or reliably give a bolus insulin dose must be considered on an individual basis. The availability of a parent(s) becomes a major factor when starting a younger child on a pump. A willingness to check blood sugars frequently (or use a CGM) is very important. No matter at what age a person begins pump treatment, assistance will be needed when the person is ill or shows a lack of consistent follow-through with daily tasks.

Some of the possible advantages of insulin pumps include:

✔ improved HbA1c levels
✔ reduced hypoglycemia events
✔ increased flexibility and freedom of insulin management
✔ improved glucose levels after meals
✔ increased safety around management of exercise

Some of the possible disadvantages of insulin pumps include:

✔ forgetting to give insulin boluses prior to food intake
✔ psychological factors
✔ expense
✔ weight gain
✔ skin infections
✔ spoiling of insulin in the reservoir with heat or cold
✔ limitations in "real estate" for site insertions

The advantages (and disadvantages) are discussed in more detail in the book referred to above.

PATHWAY TO THE INSULIN PUMP

1. Initial Pre-pump (Routine Clinic) Visit

✔ The person with diabetes and the family meet with the physician, nurse, dietitian and social worker to discuss the basics and possible advantages and disadvantages of pump therapy.

✔ We request that the person be doing at least four or five blood sugars per day (or use a CGM). This gives us an idea of the commitment of the person and the family, as well as their reliability. The proof of blood sugar checking may also be required by the insurance company.

✔ If the person is not already counting carbs, the dietitian will give instructions in this area. We usually ask that potential pump users or their parents be able to count carbs. Pumps require the user's prescribed insulin-to-carb (**I/C**) ratios be programmed in as part of their basic setup. We may also ask that they bring or send completed blood/CGM glucose level records, food records and insulin dose records. These are then used to help adjust I/C ratios.

✔ Other information is sent home with the family for review or is available online from the pump company. Either the user or an adult must be able to reliably give bolus dosages, and must be able to deal in tenths of units of insulin.

✔ For children, a "dummy" pump may be taped on to see how the child tolerates it.

✔ Further instruction with the dietitian about carb counting is often necessary.

✔ The social worker is available to discuss concerns about using or beginning to use the pump.

In summary, people who are ready for a pump:

- are willing to share with others that they have diabetes
- want the pump themselves and are not being pressured by others
- are willing to do frequent blood sugar monitoring or to wear a CGM
- are either doing carb counting (Chapter 12), are willing to learn, or have a parent who can do it for them
- are willing to use all possible injection sites

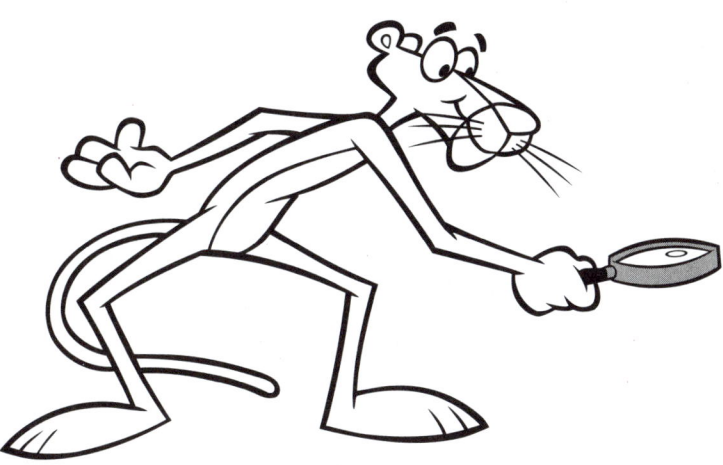

2. Pump Selection

We do not recommend one pump over another. You/your family and your provider must choose the pump type that best fits your needs. Insurance coverage and personal preferences are important. The names and websites (for those who want more information) of some of the pump providers are listed below.

Pump Manufacturer	Website
Medtronic MiniMed	www.minimed.com
OmniPod	www.myomnipod.com
Sooil DANA Diabecare: IIS	www.sooil.com
Tandem Diabetes Care: T-Slim	www.tandemdiabetes.com

3. Pump Preparation Class/ Online Training Module

Families are taught basic pump terminology. The differences in management of high and low blood sugars between injections versus pumps is discussed. Families are shown the various infusion sets. Discussion includes: possible infusion sites, rotation of sites and healthy skin maintenance. Ketone checking and sick day management are reviewed. Families are introduced to pump "uploads" to begin to learn methods for dosage adjustment. They may be asked to complete three days of diet records for evaluation and preparation of initial pump insulin dosing.

An online training module, rather than the Pump Prep Class, is now used at our center. All parent, guardians, and youth (depending on their age) will need to complete the BDC online educational modules prior to scheduling the actual hands-on pump training. The dietitian or provider will ask for your email to have the link sent to you. It will come from bdcpedspumpprep@cuanschutz.edu. You will be given a code upon completion that you will need in order to schedule your pump start. You'll also gain access to your pump-specific homework for completion prior to the saline start.

4. Saline-Start Training Class
(some clinics do not use the saline-start visit)

The person (and family) is trained to wear the pump, program the pump and to do infusion-set changes.

✔ We recommend that the web-based training tutorials be viewed at least two times to become familiar with all of the basic pump functions before the saline training.

✔ The family must bring the pump, case, batteries and supplies for two or three insertions and reservoirs (in case needed) to this class.

TABLE 1:
Pre-Insulin Pump Start Instructions

Name: _____ Saline Start Date: _____ Insulin Start Date: _____

The following instructions should be discussed at the saline pump start:

IF YOU ARE CURRENTLY ON N (NPH), or Lantus (Basaglar), Levemir, or Tresiba at dinner or in the evening, your physician recommends the following for the night before starting to use insulin in your pump (physician to check all that apply):

- ☐ Discontinue Tresiba, preferably 3-5 days before your pump start (because of its long duration) and substitute another insulin.*
- ☐ If you have NPH insulin and use it in the evening, take it as usual.
- ☐ If you take Lantus (Basaglar), Levemir, at dinner or in the evening, take it as usual, and the basal dose will be temporarily withheld in the pump the next day.
- ☐ Withhold any long-acting insulin in the afternoon/evening and supplement with ____ units of rapid-acting insulin every ____ hours through the evening and night or with NPH insulin.*

* If needed, get a prescription from your physician for Humulin or Novolin N (NPH).

If you are currently taking Lantus (Basaglar), Levemir, or Tresiba in the morning, you may take it the morning of the day before your pump start. **(Do not take it the morning of your insulin pump start!)**

The night before the insulin pump start:

- Give the usual insulin dose at dinner of rapid-acting insulin and follow the directions prescribed above for your other insulin. Eat a regular meal.
- Get all of your supplies (see below) organized to take to the clinic.
- Watch the pump instructional video/DVD or use the interactive computer software one more time.
- Read this chapter once again (or the pump sections of the book, *Understanding Insulin Pumps, Continuous Glucose Monitors and the Artificial Pancreas*).

The morning of the insulin pump start:

DO NOT give any N (NPH) or Lantus (Basaglar), Levemir, or Tresiba this a.m.

- Take the usual Humalog or NovoLog insulin dose with breakfast. Do not take any other insulins.
- Bring your pump and pump supplies, Humalog or NovoLog insulin, blood sugar testing equipment, snacks and written materials with you to the clinic.

If you have any questions, please contact your healthcare-provider

_____   _____   _____
Physician   Phone   Date

_____   _____   _____
Nurse   Phone   Date

Remember, you must email, call or fax blood sugar records in frequently for the first 1-2 weeks after your pump start (see Table 4)! Discuss this with your physician or nurse at your insulin start.

TABLE 2: Insulin Doses

Name: _____ Date (for insulin start): _____

Starting Basal Rate(s)

	Start Time	Units per Hour		Start Time	Units per Hour
1.	_____	_____	7.	_____	_____
2.	_____	_____	8.	_____	_____
3.	_____	_____	9.	_____	_____
4.	_____	_____	10.	_____	_____
5.	_____	_____	11.	_____	_____
6.	_____	_____	12.	_____	_____
				Total	_____

Carb Counting

Starting Food Bolus Dosages

	Time	Insulin/Carb Ratios		Time	Insulin/Carb Ratios
1.	_____	_____	3.	_____	_____
2.	_____	_____	4.	_____	_____

Insulin Sensitivity Ratio (Correction Factor); BG = Blood or CGM Glucose Value

	Time	1 unit lowers BG by*:		Time	1 unit lowers BG by*:
1.	_____	_____	3.	_____	_____
2.	_____	_____	4.	_____	_____

Target Blood Glucose Levels

	Time	Target BG*		Time	Target BG*
1.	_____	_____	3.	_____	_____
2.	_____	_____	4.	_____	_____

Duration of Insulin Action: _____ Hours

If you have any questions, please contact your healthcare-provider

_____ _____ _____
Physician   Phone   Date

_____ _____ _____
Nurse   Phone   Date

Remember, you must email, call or fax blood/CGM sugar records in frequently for the first 1-2 weeks after your pump start (see Table 4)! Discuss this with your physician or nurse at your insulin start.

*mg/dL or mmol/L

INSULIN PUMPS

✓ Only sterile saline (salt water) is initially used in the pump. While at home, they learn whether they are able to do the required every-two-or-three-day infusion set changes. It is important to practice using the pump between the saline and the insulin trainings to become comfortable with how it works. The usual syringe insulin injections continue while wearing the pump with saline.

✓ All technical aspects of the pump are taught at the saline start.

✓ The learning objectives from the beginning of this chapter are reviewed with the family(ies) to make sure they are learning the essentials.

✓ The person/family can bring significant others who:
  - may help with future pump programming and/or problems
  - may assist with blood/CGM glucose values (particularly in the middle of the night)
  - may be in charge of child care when the parents are away
  - may need to know how to program an insulin bolus

5. Insulin-Start Visit (See Tables 1 and 2)

a. The morning of the visit:

✓ We ask that NO NPH OR LANTUS (BASAGLAR), LEVEMIR, OR TRESIBA INSULIN be taken on the morning when insulin is started in the pump. The normal dose of rapid-acting insulin can be taken to cover breakfast prior to coming to the visit. If Lantus (Basaglar) or Levemir insulin is usually taken at dinner or in the evening, then the starting of the pump basal insulin can be withheld using a temporary basal rate of zero for 12 hours. Individual instructions are outlined in Table 1.

As instructed in Table 1, we ask that Tresiba insulin not be given for 3-5 days prior to starting insulin in the pump.

✓ The person/family can bring significant others who:
  - might be available to help with possible hypoglycemia or hyperglycemia
  - might be helping with giving insulin boluses
  - will be assisting in the day-to-day maintenance of the pump and infusion sites

The support of the significant other(s) helps with success in pump use.

b. The process:

✓ The care-provider sets the initial basal insulin doses and reviews with the patient and family (see Table 2 in this chapter).

✓ The dietitian again reviews carb counting (Chapter 12) and the food records.

✓ The nurse educator or pump trainer finishes the technical training for the insulin pump and teaches how to troubleshoot and maintain infusion sites.

✓ It is important to review how to reduce the basal doses using the "**Temporary Basal Rate.**" This feature allows the patient/family to temporarily override the usual basal rates (either increasing or decreasing insulin) for a specified length of time. Some pump-users modify their insulin on a daily basis using this feature.

✓ The social worker is available to discuss concerns or fears.

INSULIN DELIVERY

Insulin Infusion Sets (Table 3)

We do not recommend one infusion set over another. Every person is different, and the favored set varies from person to person. Some of the sets most frequently used at present are shown in Table 3. However, new sets are becoming available all the time. For people who have difficulty with needles, it is fine to use EMLA® or L■M■X-4® cream. These are topical anesthetic creams that need to be applied 30 to 60 minutes before doing the insertion. Most

TABLE 3:
Pump Infusion Set Options

Your doctor and your insulin pump trainer can help you choose the infusion set that will work the best for you. The variety has increased greatly, and many new options are appearing on the market every few months. Some of the most widely used infusion sets are listed below:

	Cannula Lengths	Tube Lengths	Inserter or "Sertable"
Medtronic Mini-Med Paradigm Pumps			
Paradigm Mio	6 or 9mm	18", 23" and 32"	yes Paradigm
Quick-Set	6 or 9mm	23" and 43"	yes
Paradigm Silhouette	13 or 17mm	18", 23", 33" and 43"	yes
Paradigm Sure-T	6mm	18", 23" and 32"	no
Other Pumps			
Inset (90° insert)	6 or 9mm	23" and 43"	yes
Inset (30° insert)	6 or 9mm	13" and 23"	yes
Comfort/Comfort Short	13 or 17mm	23" and 43"	no
Contact Detach	6mm	23" or 43"	no
Accu-Chek Ultraflex	6, 8, or 10mm	24", 31" and 43"	yes

All but the Paradigm infusion sets have a luer lock end that will work with all "non-Paradigm" pumps.

people do not need this. Others apply ice briefly to numb the area. Table 3 indicates infusion sets which have an automatic "inserter." These devices push the needle and plastic tube through the skin, usually with the push of a button. The person does not have to use their own strength to push the needle in. The needle is then removed, leaving the tube in the fatty layer under the skin. There are also sets in which the metal needle stays in. These are most helpful when a person has frequent problems with "kinking" of the plastic tube.

For most people, the tape holds the cannula in without difficulty. However, if needed, there are several tips to making infusion sets stick better. The first is to start with clean skin (shaved if necessary). Many people then apply Skin Prep or IV Prep to make the skin sticky (let it dry). Some then place a dressing (Tegaderm™, IV-3000™) directly on the skin and insert the infusion set through the dressing. It is recommended a small hole be cut in the center though which to insert. The IV-3000 infusion set tape comes pre-cut. A second dressing can be placed on top of the infusion set to sandwich it in place. If this is done, a hole must be cut in the top dressing so the set can be connected. Other overlay tapes are the Opsite Flexifix™ (Smith and Nephew), StayPut Medical™, ExpressionMed™ and PumpPeelz™. Some people prefer to just tape the set in place with medical tape (Transpore™, Hypafix™) or standard waterproof athletic tape (e.g., Kinesio Tape™). If the tape is irritating the skin, a wipe-on skin barrier such as Cavilon™ may help. Also, Tincture of Benzoin, Mastisol® or Skin Bond® can be applied to the skin before the tape or set and will work like glue. A medical adhesive remover (Uni-Solve®, Detachol) may then be needed to remove the set and tape. More information about adhesive issues can be found in the book referred to in the introduction; see ordering materials in back.

When possible, it is best to do the set change in the morning. This is because the person may be more sensitive to insulin in the new (non-swollen) site. If the set were changed at night, this might lead to overnight hypoglycemia. Doing the set change in the morning also gives time to make sure the set is working well before going to bed. Many times with the typical busy family schedule, set changes are not possible until later in the day. The second-best time to change the infusion set is after school and activities, but before dinner. Then if the set is not working properly, the family will know before bedtime. If it is necessary to do a set change in the evening or night, it is essential that the blood/CGM glucose value be checked 2-3 hours later, both to make sure the infusion set is working and to make certain the value is not low. Many families use a temporary basal setting (approximately 70 percent) for the next 4-6 hours if the glucose value is not high prior to a nighttime set change. It is generally recommended that set changes be done every two to three days. If blood/CGM glucose values tend to routinely run high on the third day, or if the weather has been hot, it may be necessary to do the set change after two days.

Methods of Delivery

(This section is for people starting an insulin pump that is not part of an artificial pancreas.)

The pump delivers insulin in three ways:

1. Basal Dosages

Basal dosages are programmed into the pump with the direction of the healthcare-provider and remain the same every day unless purposely changed. Table 2 can be used to suggest initial insulin doses. A major goal in the first week is to calculate and fine-tune the optimal basal dosages.

The basal rate:

- ✔ reflects the units of insulin per hour that would be needed to maintain stable blood/CGM glucose values if the person were not eating meals
- ✔ is similar to the small amount of insulin released by the normal pancreas every few minutes
- ✔ usually consists of 40 to 50 percent of the total daily pump insulin dose

Dosing

The insulin dose for the pump is calculated by different doctors in different ways. Sometimes the total insulin dose taken by shots in a day (rapid- and long-acting insulin) is added and 70-100 percent of this total is used for the total daily insulin in the pump.

Approximately half of the pump insulin is given as the basal insulin and half as boluses. If the person is on Lantus (Basaglar), Levemir, or Tresiba insulin, the total basal insulin per 24 hours is about the same as the previous dose of this insulin. Many doctors divide the day into parts (e.g., in three-hour time periods; see Table 2).

Basal doses vary:

- ✔ The number of basal dosages to be used varies between doctors. Some start with one or two basal rates and others with 8-12 basal rates.
- ✔ Many teenagers and young adults need more insulin in the early morning hours to cover the body's normal increase in growth hormone (the "dawn phenomenon").
- ✔ Some toddlers need more basal insulin in the late evening hours.
- ✔ ALL people are different, and the use of different basal doses allows for individual fine-tuning.
- ✔ Once the basal rates are regulated, they tend to stay quite consistent.

Some reasons to change basal rates are:

- puberty (physiologic increase in insulin resistance)
- large changes in body weight
- change of time zones (just change time on pump)
- injuries or illness
- some medications (e.g., steroids)
- periods of inactivity
- temporary reductions for exercise
- temporary increases for menses

Checking accuracy of basal rates:

At a later date, basal rates can be checked by having the person not eat a meal. If the basal rate is correctly set, the person will not have a low (<70 mg/dL [<3.9 mmol/L]) or high (>180 mg/dL [>10.0 mmol/L]) sugar despite not having eaten. Skipping the bedtime snack, fasting overnight and having a late breakfast while measuring the blood sugars every 2-3 hours (or using CGM) is often the first basal test to do. During the day, delaying meals and checking frequently can verify basal rates.

2. Bolus Dosages for Food:

✔ Approximately 50-60 percent of the daily pump insulin doses are given as boluses before meals and snacks and for correction of high glucose levels. At least a part of the bolus (for the correction and for food which will definitely be eaten) should be given 20 minutes prior to the first bite. (Carbs cause blood/CGM glucose values to peak in 60 minutes, whereas Humalog or NovoLog activity peaks in 90 minutes.) People can then give an additional bolus if they decide to eat more.

✔ Everyone is different, and boluses can be chosen to fit individual eating habits.

✔ The dietitian is an important member of the pump team and will need to review and reinforce carb counting. Changes are often suggested in Insulin-to-Carb (I/C) ratios for different meals after reviewing food records, insulin dosages taken, and blood/CGM glucose levels two to four hours after meals.

✔ Many families attend carb counting classes (if not yet counting carbs) prior to starting insulin pump therapy. However, dosages sometimes change after starting the pump. Good record keeping in the period after beginning the pump is essential.

✔ The only way to know if an insulin dose for food is correct is to do blood/CGM glucose levels before and two and four hours after a meal when a correction for glucose levels is not needed. The ADA recommends that the peak blood/CGM glucose levels be less than 180 mg/dL (<10.0 mmol/L) at any time following a meal. Many care-providers recommend the two-hour value after meals be below 140 mg/dL (<7.8 mmol/L). This is often most difficult to achieve following breakfast (due in part to hormones active in the body at this time). To check the I/C ratio, start with the blood sugar in the target range and eat a low-fat (<20 gm) microwavable meal with known carbs. (Excess fat delays stomach emptying and prolongs sugar elevations.) Blood/CGM glucose values must be monitored as described above. Most people use different I/C ratios for different meals and times of the day. Thus, blood/CGM glucose levels should be measured after each meal.

✔ The "rule of 500" is sometimes used to help calculate I/C ratios. The total insulin per day (e.g., 50 units) is divided into 500. For this example (500 ÷ 50 = 10), one unit of insulin would cover 10g of carbohydrate. The I/C ratio would be 1 to 10.

✔ The bolus calculator can be programmed with I/C ratios for different times of the day. Then, when the grams of carbs to be eaten are entered into the pump, the units of insulin to take appear on the screen. The person must activate the suggested insulin dose in order to have it be delivered. This is particularly helpful for people who have different I/C ratios at different times of the day. It is also helpful for people who are not adept at math.

✔ Different types of boluses can be used for different foods (see Advanced Pump Training below).

3. Bolus Dosages for "Corrections"

Extra (unscheduled) insulin boluses are important to use if the blood/CGM glucose level is high. Remember that larger dosages will be required if ketones are present (and should be given by syringe or pen). The healthcare team should be contacted if moderate or large urine ketones or blood ketones >1.0 mmol/L are found. There are several ways to determine correction boluses. The best way is to enter the blood sugar value into the pump and let the pump calculate the dose based on the correction factor for that time of day (as previously entered into the pump). Any "insulin on board" from the previous bolus is automatically subtracted by the bolus calculator built into the pump. Correction factors are also discussed in Chapter 22.

✔ If a person is using a correction factor of one unit of insulin for every 50 mg/dL the glucose is above 150 mg/dL, then 50 mg/dL is the sensitivity factor that says one unit will reduce the blood sugar 50 mg/dL and the 150 mg/dL is the target blood sugar. If the blood sugar level was 300 mg/dL, three units of insulin would be the bolus amount used to bring the blood sugar to 150 mg/dL. (This was determined by subtracting 150 from 300 = 150 and then dividing by 50 = 3 units of insulin.) Most teens and adults correct to 100 mg/dL (5.5 mmol/L) during the daytime hours (e.g., 7 a.m. to 7 p.m.). Younger children often use a target of 120 or 130 mg/dL (6.7 or 7.2 mmol/L). If the blood sugar is lower than the target, and it is time to give a food bolus, most pumps will reduce the insulin bolus. For this reason, it is important not to set the target too high.

✔ For people using mmol/L for glucose values, one unit of insulin for every 2.8 mmol/L above 8.3 mmol/L could be used. For a level of 16.7 mmol/L with a desire to reach 8.3 mmol/L, divide 2.8 into 8.4 (16.7 minus 8.3) and give three units of insulin.

✔ The above calculation and a new bolus can be repeated after two to three hours if the blood/CGM sugar value is still high.

✔ Always utilizing the pump to calculate corrections will allow it to deduct for insulin that has not been utilized from a previous bolus (known as **"active insulin"** or "insulin on board"). This protects the user from accumulating unsafe levels of insulin.

✔ Some people use one target blood/CGM glucose level for the day (e.g., correct to a glucose level of 100 mg/dL [5.5 mmol/L]) and a second, less aggressive target for during the night (e.g., 150 mg/dL [8.3 mmol/L]). Others may choose to use a less aggressive sensitivity setting at bedtime and during the night.

✔ The bolus calculator may suggest a reduced dose when the blood/CGM glucose value is under the target value and some food is being eaten. If the value is below 70 mg/dL (3.9 mmol/L), the pump may suggest not taking any insulin. These adjustments are based on the glucose level, the sensitivity factor, and the target blood sugar level.

✔ If a blood/CGM glucose value during the day is high (>300 mg/dL [16.7 mmol/L]), an extra unit of insulin may be added to the bolus. If moderate or large urine ketones or a blood ketone level >1.0 mmol/L is present, some people double the recommended correction insulin dose. The bolus calculator does not take ketones into account.

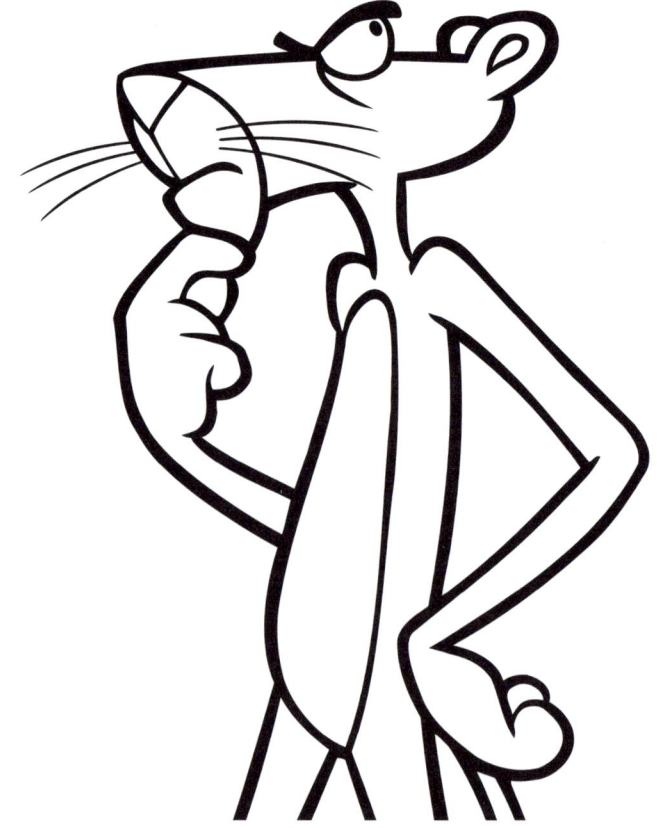

BLOOD/CGM VALUES

More frequent blood/CGM glucose values are required in the first week or two of insulin pump therapy to help set the basal and bolus insulin dosages. The levels to aim for are the same as those shown for different ages in Chapter 7.

At a minimum:

✔ levels should be determined prior to each meal
✔ before bedtime
✔ early in the morning (e.g., 6 a.m.)
✔ two hours after eating each meal
✔ once or twice during the night: e.g., 12 midnight and 3 a.m.
✔ two hours after a correction dose

This amounts to at least eight or ten blood/CGM glucose values per day. This number may be reduced in the second week. It is obvious that parents or a significant other are extremely helpful at this time. The minimum will eventually be six to eight values daily, with occasional checks during the night. Ideally, the family will upload to their particular pump's web-based software. If unable to do this, written records will be needed. The form we like for reporting (faxing or emailing) blood sugar results is shown in Table 4 and may be copied as often as desired. It can also be found on our website (www.barbaradaviscenter.org) for use in emailing results. Many meters (and CGMs) can now be downloaded and emailed to the care-provider.

The person (or family member) uploads, faxes/emails blood/CGM glucose results every other day for the first week, then weekly for several weeks and then every two to four weeks. Good communication at this time is essential. It is important to understand how the basal and bolus insulin doses affect blood/CGM glucose levels at different times of the day. When dose adjustments are needed in the future, this process will be repeated.

ADVANCED PUMP TRAINING

Approximately one month after the insulin pump start, families complete their training with advanced pump training. This may now be done as part of a routine clinic visit.

The following activities and topics may be reviewed:

✔ Any problems the person/family is having with the pump
✔ Programming and application of the advanced features (e.g., special boluses – see below)
✔ How to use the pump to adjust for exercise and how to evaluate the effectiveness of the exercise adjustment. A second set of basal doses may be programmed into the pump to use on heavy exercise days.
✔ If a 90-degree set (e.g., Mio™, Inset™, Quickset™) is primarily being used, an angled set (Comfort™ Short, Silhouette™, Tender™) may be demonstrated. The latter sets often stay in place better with heavy exercise.
✔ Troubleshooting is reviewed for pump and blood/CGM glucose issues.
✔ A food record may be brought to this visit to fine-tune the I/C ratios with the dietitian. Other methods of avoiding high blood/CGM glucose values after meals, such as giving the bolus 20 minutes prior to the meal, are discussed. Special bolus features are introduced called the "square" or "extended" wave, or a "dual" wave. These allow a bolus to be given over a period of time (square and extended boluses) or with a portion of the bolus given in the usual fashion and a portion as a square wave (dual wave). These special features are helpful for meals such as pizza or spaghetti, which are high in carbs and fat and may cause prolonged sugar elevation for some people.
✔ An HbA1c level is checked.
✔ Sick day management, site care and hypoglycemia are reviewed.

Table 4 Weekly Insulin Pump Management Record

Name _____ Week of _____

Day & Date		12M	1A	2A	3A	4A	5A	6A	7A	8A	9A	10A	11A	12N	1P	2P	3P	4P	5P	6P	7P	8P	9P	10P	11P	Notes
	BG																									
	Carbs																									
	Basal*																									
Bolus	Food																									
	Correction																									
	BG																									
	Carbs																									
	Basal*																									
Bolus	Food																									
	Correction																									
	BG																									
	Carbs																									
	Basal*																									
Bolus	Food																									
	Correction																									
	BG																									
	Carbs																									
	Basal*																									
Bolus	Food																									
	Correction																									
	BG																									
	Carbs																									
	Basal*																									
Bolus	Food																									
	Correction																									
	BG																									
	Carbs																									
	Basal*																									
Bolus	Food																									
	Correction																									
	BG																									
	Carbs																									
	Basal*																									
Bolus	Food																									
	Correction																									

Target Range:
Correction:

Time	I/C Ratio

*Basal dosages are only reentered if a change has been made.

This table may be copied as often as desired.

INSULIN PUMPS

TABLE 5:
Keys to Avoiding Lows

- Always monitor AT LEAST four blood/CGM sugar values daily (and occasional checks during the night)
- Estimate grams of carbs to be eaten and give insulin bolus 20 minutes prior to eating (so insulin is not peaking after blood sugar is down)
- Check blood/CGM sugar before, during and after exercise
- Recognize the symptoms of lows and treat promptly
- Think ahead regarding variations in daily schedule which could result in low blood sugars
- If the blood/CGM sugar is below 70 mg/dL (3.9 mmol/L) and it is time for a food bolus dose, subtract one unit from the bolus amount
- Reduce bedtime boluses for the bedtime snack or boluses during the night by half (the reduction may vary for different people)
- Use a temporary (or alternate) basal pattern for heavy exercise and/or during the night after days of heavy exercise
- Try not to do routine set changes in the evening. The new area may be more sensitive to insulin, increasing the chance of hypoglycemia. More frequent blood/CGM glucose values after a set change are essential
- Check active insulin/insulin on board at bedtime to make certain not excessive

HYPOGLYCEMIA

The causes of hypoglycemia are discussed in Chapter 6 and are similar for people using insulin pumps to those of people using insulin injections. *These include:*

✔ too few blood/CGM glucose values

✔ too high basal rates

✔ incorrect insulin bolus doses or timing of insulin

✔ wrong adjustments for exercise

Some keys to avoiding lows are listed in Table 5.

If low, treat as described below and then check the blood/CGM glucose value 15 minutes later to make sure the value is back up (particularly at night). Also think about what was different that day or the previous day (extra exercise, bolus insulin, less food, etc.). This will allow planning ahead to help avoid the low with a similar occurrence in the future. If you have questions, call your doctor or nurse.

Treatment of Hypoglycemia
(see Chapters 6 and 25)

If hypoglycemia is suspected, the person with diabetes should be treated as described in Chapter 6. If the blood sugar is below 70 mg/dL (3.9 mmol/L), we prefer 15g of "quick-acting" carbohydrate first (four ounces of juice or sugar pop or four glucose tablets). If it is still below 70 mg/dL (3.9 mmol/L) after 10-15 minutes, repeat this treatment. When it is above 70 mg/dL (3.9 mmol/L), give solid food. It may be necessary to bolus (or half-bolus) for food given beyond the initial treatment.

If the glucose value is below 50 mg/dL (<2.8 mmol/L) or if the person is "out of it" or unconscious, the pump should be placed on "suspend" or disconnected for a period of at least 30 minutes. (Disconnecting is the most certain way to know insulin is NOT being delivered.) Others will set a temporary basal of 0.0 units per hour for the next hour so that the pump will restart without the person having to

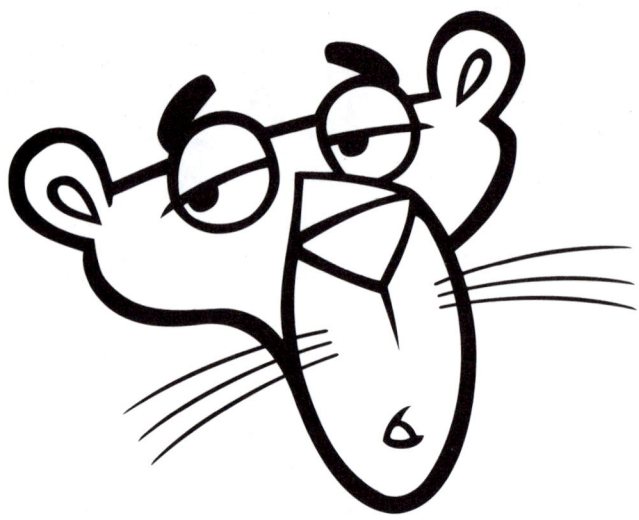

remember. A parent, teacher or significant other must know how to do this, as the person with the low blood sugar may be confused. Treatment with glucagon is discussed in Chapter 6.

It must be remembered that insulin already infused will not yet have peaked, so giving the sugar is essential. Instant Glucose (or cake decorating gel) and glucagon (Chapter 6) must be readily available (as for all people with diabetes).

HIGH BLOOD/CGM GLUCOSE VALUES
Non-Pump-Related Causes
(also see Chapter 25)

Some of the causes of high blood sugars for pump users are the same as for people taking their insulin by shots:

- ✔ insulin dosages are too low
- ✔ extra food intake without an extra bolus
- ✔ lack of exercise
- ✔ forgetting insulin or giving just before or after meals
- ✔ illnesses/infections
- ✔ hormones (stress, menses [many young ladies use a second basal setting which is 0.1 or 0.2 u/hr higher during menses])
- ✔ over-eating with low blood sugars
- ✔ spoiled insulin

In addition, causes of high blood/CGM glucose values related to the pump (see Table 6) include:

- ✔ the reservoir being out of insulin
- ✔ a clogged, kinked or leaking infusion set
- ✔ an infusion set which has come out
- ✔ a malfunctioning pump

If the blood/CGM glucose level has not responded to a correction bolus with the pump or if the value is extremely high or if there are ketones present, the infusion set must be changed and a correction dose given using an insulin syringe. Do not give the correction dose with the pump! If moderate or large urine ketones or a blood ketone level >1.0 mmol/L is present, the correction insulin dose is often doubled. If a syringe correction has been given and the blood sugar does not respond, the insulin used could be spoiled.

In order to prevent running out of insulin, the pump reservoir should be filled every 2-3 days as the set is changed. Table 6 summarizes some possible pump problems. **Remember that all pumps have a 1-800 number on the back to call the pump company for help 24 hours a day.**

TABLE 6:
Possible Pump Problems

Problem	Pump Alarm
• Empty insulin reservoir (syringe)	Yes
• Low pump reservoir	Yes
• Clogged infusion set	Yes
• Partially blocked infusion set	No
• Leaky infusion set	No
• Weak or dead battery	Yes
• Low battery	Yes
• Pump malfunction	Yes
• Cannula has come out	No
• Spoiled Insulin	No

EXERCISE
(see Chapters 13 and 25 for further information)

There are several options for altering the insulin dose with exercise. Different types of exercise will prompt different results. Experience is usually the best teacher to see what works. **Doing more frequent blood sugar (or evaluating CGM) values to determine the effects of the exercise and the changes in insulin dosage is MOST helpful!** Many athletes find pumps are easier to use than injections when exercising. This is because a temporary basal rate can be selected when a time to exercise is suddenly chosen. In contrast, it is not possible to negate insulin activity from a previous basal insulin injection.

✔ If the exercise is mild to moderate (walking, golf, dancing, etc.), reducing the basal dosages by half (50 percent reduction) during the exercise may be sufficient. Some people start the reduction 30 to 60 minutes before the exercise and continue it for 30 minutes or longer after the exercise is over. Every person is different and will need to find what works best. Use of a **"temporary basal"** can be very helpful, and many pumpers use it on a daily basis.

✔ During intense exercise (jogging, football, basketball, etc.), most people just disconnect from the pump. Some disconnect 30 to 60 minutes before the start of the exercise. One can only be disconnected for up to two hours. A blood sugar should then be done and a correction dose of insulin taken (sometimes reduced). This allows another two hours of disconnect time.

There are then several options for insulin adjustments:

Estimate the amount of insulin to be missed while disconnected from the pump and take part of the dose before the exercise (particularly if the blood sugar is high) and the rest of the dose after the exercise. A temporary basal rate after an exercise of long duration and/or high intensity (e.g., an 80 percent basal from 9 p.m. to 3 a.m.) may lower the incidence of delayed hypoglycemia. This is particularly helpful during the night for some people.

Correction boluses given after exercise are frequently reduced by half. This helps to reduce the likelihood of hypoglycemia.

In general, if the pump is to be disconnected for two hours or more, more frequent blood/CGM glucose values must be done (at least each hour). If the value is rising, it is easy to reconnect, take a small bolus and again disconnect.

✔ If it is to be an all-day exercise (e.g., a long hike or all day skiing), it may work best to reduce the basal and the bolus rates (perhaps by half) or possibly to not give any bolus doses. People must determine what works best for them.

✔ With exercise, it is important to remember to stay hydrated and to take extra snacks (see Chapter 13). Drinking water or sports drinks works for some people. The carbohydrates from the sports drinks will provide extra calories and energy. Often a bolus is not given or is reduced to cover the carbohydrate intake. Snacks such as granola bars provide extra carbohydrates and calories. Make sure that coaches or others around at the time know that the person has diabetes and wears an insulin pump.

SCHOOL

If the person using the pump is in school, the school nurse should have some knowledge of the pump. You may wish to copy Chapter 25 for the school nurse.

SUMMARY

Insulin pumps have advantages and disadvantages. It is up to each person and family, working with their healthcare team, to decide if a pump would be appropriate.

DEFINITIONS

Basal dose: A pre-set hourly rate of insulin (for 24 hours) as programmed into an insulin pump.

Bolus dose: An amount of insulin taken prior to a meal or to correct a high blood sugar as entered at any time of the day by the person wearing the insulin pump.

Correction bolus dose: A bolus of insulin used to correct a high blood sugar down to the desired level.

Insulin "on board": A term referring to insulin still remaining active from previous boluses. It is automatically subtracted by the bolus calculator (see smart pump, below) from correction dosages on most pumps.

Insulin pump: A microcomputer with a syringe of insulin within the pager-sized device that can infuse a basal insulin dose at a pre-set hourly rate. Bolus insulin dosages can also be entered and given at any time by the person wearing the pump.

Insulin-to-Carbohydrate (I/C) ratio (see Chapter 12): The number of units of insulin to be taken for a certain number of grams of carbohydrate eaten (e.g., one unit for 15g of carbohydrate).

Smart pump: An insulin pump with a bolus calculator. This is now an outdated term, as all pumps now have bolus calculators. It will recommend units of insulin to give when the number of grams of carbs to be eaten is entered. It also recommends a correction insulin dose when the blood sugar level is entered or transmitted to the pump from the glucose meter/CGM. (The I/C ratios and correction factors must have been pre-entered into the pump by the user.) Any insulin still acting ("insulin on board") from previous boluses will be automatically subtracted from the correction needed (but not from food boluses).

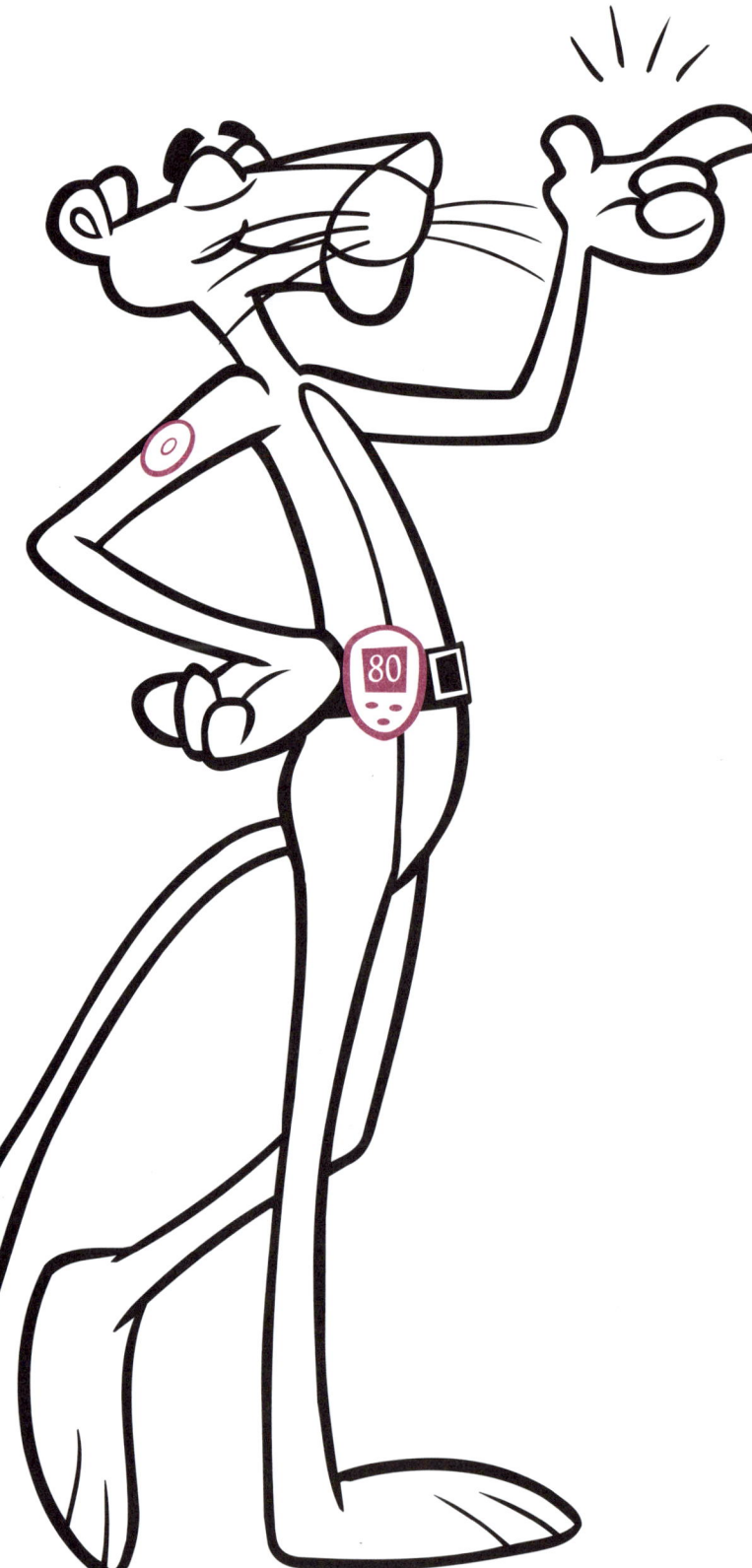

QUESTIONS AND ANSWERS FROM NEWSNOTES

Q: What do you currently recommend for airport screening for people wearing an insulin pump?

A: Pumps (and CGMs) should not be exposed to X-rays or high magnetic fields (amusement park rides may have strong magnetic field braking systems). Pumps, transmitters and sensors must also be removed before MRI, CT or diathermy treatment.

The TSA offers the option of requesting a wand and visual inspection of your medical supplies rather than putting them through an X-ray. This must be requested before the screening process begins. Your medical supplies should be ready in a separate bag when you approach the security officer.

Walking through the metal detector is not usually a problem. It is better to leave the pump on the person and not put it on the conveyer belt. If a body scan is requested, we recommend taking the pump and/or CGM off and handing it to the person doing the screening and getting them to manually check it. Information provided by commercial companies suggests that electronic components of the pump or CGM can potentially be damaged if exposed to ionizing radiation such as x-rays or CT scanner. Again, remember to take your travel letter with you.

Q: My son is going on a trip without other family members. He uses an insulin pump. Could you remind us of supplies he should be taking along?

A: In case of pump malfunction, we generally recommend he take extra syringes and bottles of the long-acting insulin he was on prior to starting the pump. You should also look back in your records to send the dosages as well. It is also important to have him pack his diabetes supplies in his carry-on luggage.

A summary of important items to include are:

1. 24-hour clinic phone number
2. a supply of rapid-acting insulin
3. long-acting (basal) insulin
4. insulin syringes
5. extra pump batteries
6. glucose meter/strips/lancets
7. extra meter battery
8. extra infusion sets and inserter (if used)
9. extra pump syringe (reservoir)
10. alcohol pads
11. dressing, tape
12. glucose tablets/instant glucose
13. urine or blood ketone checking strips
14. glucagon emergency kit

Q: Our teenage daughter is on an insulin pump and seems to forget to take some of her insulin mealtime bolus dosages. Do you have any suggestions?

A: Missing bolus dosages with food is unfortunately fairly common. It is probably the number one cause of elevated HbA1c levels (>9% [>75 mmol/mol]) for people who receive pump or injection insulin therapy.

When teens show signs of forgetting insulin, the parents must again get more involved. They may need to actually observe the breakfast and dinner boluses. Perhaps a friend or teacher can be found to make sure the noon bolus is taken.

Some pumps and meters have alarms to help remind youth to bolus.

One family found a watch with five separate alarms. It could be set as a reminder for bolus dosages. Cell phones and text messaging are other options.

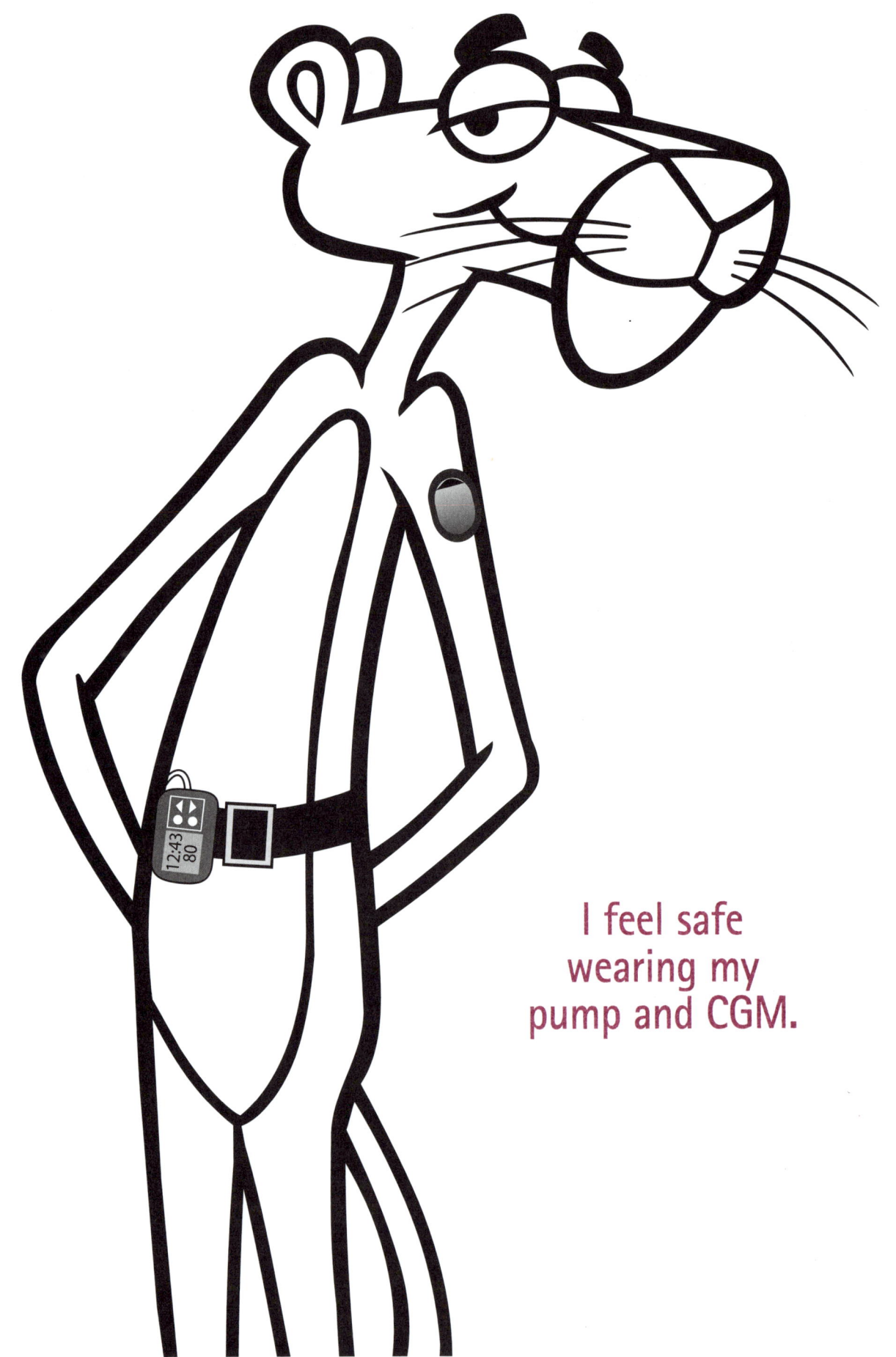

I feel safe wearing my pump and CGM.

CONTINUOUS GLUCOSE MONITORS

CHAPTER 29
Continuous Glucose Monitors (CGM)

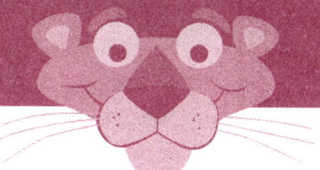

One of the major advances in the treatment of diabetes in recent years has been in the development of continuous glucose monitors (CGM). With the recent advances in CGM accuracy, many doctors now feel use of a CGM is the first priority for introducing diabetes technology. Without CGM, the development of the artificial pancreas (Chapter 30) would not have been possible. The CGM devices give readings of subcutaneous (not blood) glucose levels every five minutes. This compares with finger-stick blood sugar (glucose) readings, which are usually done only four or five times each day.

The use of a CGM with an insulin pump has allowed discontinuing insulin delivery with a low or a predicted low CGM glucose level, greatly reducing the risk of severe hypoglycemia (see Chapter 30). The combination also allows for adjusting insulin delivery for rising CGM glucose levels. Both features result in an increased percentage of time with glucose levels in target range.

The subcutaneous CGM glucose values are approximately five minutes behind the blood sugar values, as the sugar must pass through the blood vessel wall into the subcutaneous space, and then the CGM system must determine the value. This delay is of almost no clinical significance with the frequency of CGM readings.

The purpose of this chapter is to present an overview of CGM. An entire book, *Understanding Insulin Pumps, Continuous Glucose Monitors, and the Artificial Pancreas* is available for people

> **TOPICS:**
> **Monitoring Diabetes (following CGM glucose levels)**
>
> **TEACHING OBJECTIVES:**
> The teacher will:
> 1. Present CGM glucose concepts (rationale, times, frequency and desired ranges for the individual).
> 2. Provide instruction for the CGM of choice.
> 3. Discuss how to troubleshoot problems with their CGM.
> 4. Introduce the concept of following CGM glucose levels and observing trends and time in range.
>
> **LEARNING OBJECTIVES:**
> Learner (parents, child, relative or self) will be able to:
> 1. Describe rationale for monitoring CGM glucose levels and time in range.
> 2. Demonstrate use of real-time and retrospective CGM data.
> 3. Choose and apply a method for following CGM results and recognizing trends.
> 4. Locate and state the 1-800 number listed on the CGM to call for problems.

> **CGMs available in U.S.**
> (listed alphabetically)
> - Abbott FreeStyle Libre
> - Dexcom G5, G6
> - Medtronic Guardian Connect
> - Senseonics Eversense

wanting detailed information (see Ordering Materials in the back of this book). Some essential points to consider are:

✔ In order for CGM to be successful, the person (except for the very young) must want to use CGM, not just the parent or significant other.

✔ Blood sugar levels must still be done at least twice daily to calibrate some CGMs (see below). It is also recommended they be done when: the CGM values do not match clinical symptoms, a low blood sugar is suspected, or the CGM value is in question.

✔ The CGM glucose values have improved in accuracy, and some CGM devices are now approved for insulin dosing without doing a fingerstick blood sugar.

✔ Many studies have shown that use of a CGM will reduce the time spent with low sugars and will increase the time spent with sugars "in-range" (for people using either an insulin pump or injections).

✔ People who wear the CGM at least six days per week are the most likely to have an improved HbA1c value.

✔ Use of a CGM has been shown to reduce the likelihood both of severe hypoglycemia and of diabetic ketoacidosis (DKA).

THE COMPONENTS OF A CONTINUOUS GLUCOSE MONITOR (CGM)

The CGMs currently available in the U.S. all have three basic parts:

1. **Sensor:** As with the insulin pump, a tiny plastic probe is inserted (with the push of a button) under the skin. The sensor then measures glucose values for the next seven to 14 days.

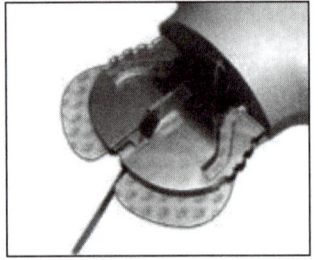

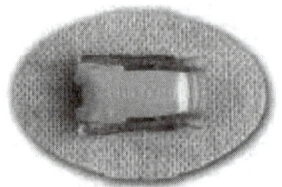

2. **Transmitter:** The transmitter attaches to the sensor and sends the glucose reading from the sensor to the receiver, pump, phone or other device.

3. **Receiver, pump, smartphone, watch or other device (see below).** The receiver receives the subcutaneous glucose readings from the transmitter and converts the signal to a mg/dL or mmol/L value. It is a mini-computer that records and displays much information. Some types of receivers are able to transmit data into the cloud to be shared with others.

TYPES OF CONTINUOUS GLUCOSE MONITORS

Our center does not recommend use of one CGM over another. The various models have different features that may be preferred by different people/families. The diabetes team will review the specific features of the CGM device you select.

Abbott FreeStyle Libre 14-day Flash Glucose Monitoring System and the Navigator (www.abbott.com)

In 2017, the Abbot FreeStyle Libre System was approved by the FDA. The sensor and transmitter are small (~ the size of two quarters) and transmit glucose values to a monitor when it is waved over the sensor. The transmitter stores about 12 hours of data. Therefore, to view complete daily information, the receiver must be swiped over the sensor at least twice a day. As this information can be used for dosing decisions, it is good practice to swipe before every meal, at bedtime and with exercise. It is approved for insulin dosing, and fingerstick blood glucose calibrations are not required. The sensor can be worn for 14 days, and there is no interference from acetaminophen. The monitor shows a graph of scanned glucose values and has rate-of-change arrows. The FreeStyle Libre 2 integrated CGM system was approved by the FDA in June, 2020 for use in adults and in children, ages 4 years and older. In addition to previous FreeStyle Libre features, the Libre 2 provides optional real-time alarms. These use Bluetooth and automatically alert the user to high or low glucose readings without the need to scan the sensor.

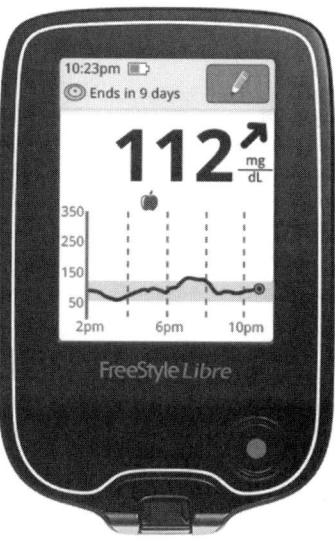

The NightRider BluCon is a reusable Bluetooth transmitter that can be purchased (separately) to transmit the Freestyle Libre sensor values to an iPhone, Android phone, or Apple watch. Alarms for highs and lows, shared readings, and other features can then become available.

Although not available in the U.S., the Navigator CGM has been popular in other countries. It is routinely used for five days, but can often be used longer.

Dexcom CGM Systems (www.dexcom.com)

The FDA has approved insulin dosing using the Dexcom G5 or G6 CGM Systems. Thus, finger-stick blood sugar checks are not required for insulin dosing when wearing these devices. The Dexcom G6 does not require calibration (no finger sticks), can be worn for 10 days, has a simple one-touch sensor insertion and is not affected by acetaminophen (e.g., Tylenol). These devices make care for children, especially in the school setting, much easier. We recommend continuing to use finger-stick blood sugars for verification of low CGM sugar values and for following the rise in blood sugar levels after treatment. Because CGM glucose levels lag behind fingerstick values, using only the CGM to determine treatment for a low can result in overtreatment. We also recommend doing a fingerstick blood sugar in the school setting if the CGM value is below 80 mg/dL (4.5mmol/L) or above 250 mg/dL (13.9 mmol/L).

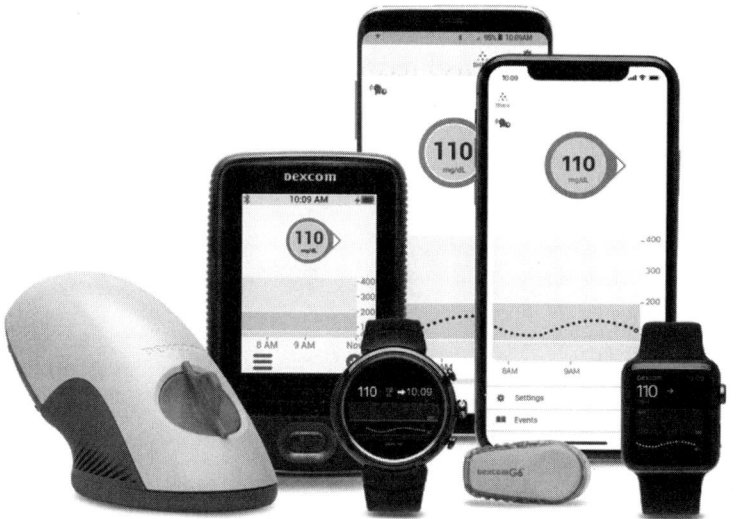

The Dexcom CGM Systems have customizable alerts and alarms. When CGM data is transmitted to a designated smart phone (which a child can carry in a fanny pack), the glucose information can be shared remotely with the devices of family members or friends using internet or cellular connectivity to the cloud. This allows parents or caregivers to monitor a child's glucose data from a remote location, respond to real-time alerts, and gain peace of mind and reassurance when they are apart.

During periods of insulin adjustment, the CGM data can also be continuously shared to Clarity® software linked to a clinic's account. The care team is then able to see daily and summary data via Dexcom's Clarity. Dosing adjustments can be made by phone or email, or during a telemedicine visit.

The Dexcom G6 communicates with the Tandem T:slim X2 insulin pump and artificial pancreas system to help regulate insulin release and to reduce hypoglycemia (see Chapter 30).

Medtronic Minimed CGM and REAL-Time Systems (www.medtronicdiabetes.com)

Medtronic/Minimed currently has two insulin pumps available in the U.S., the 630G and the 670G, both of which connect to a CGM. The 630G system suspends insulin at a preset CGM glucose level. It has alerts for highs and lows, and uses the Enlite™ six-day-wear sensor. The 670G artificial pancreas system is discussed in Chapter 30.

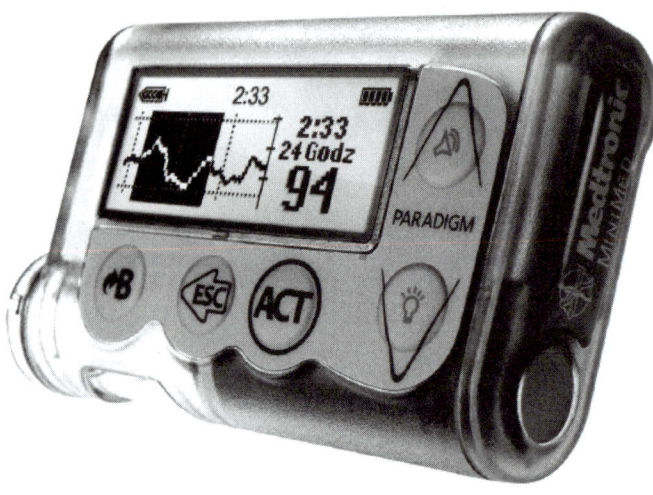

Medtronic also has a "stand-alone" (no connection to a pump) CGM called the Guardian™ Connect smart CGM with sugar IQ. It will transmit CGM glucose levels to an iPhone and Android phone.

Both the Guardian Connect and the 670G systems use the Guardian™ Sensor (3), which is worn for seven days.

Senseonics Eversense Implantable CGM System (www.senseonics.com)

The Eversense CGM System is the first implantable CGM. It has been shown accurate over a period of six months, and after the period of use is then removed. It is similar in size to the birth control implant and is similarly placed under the skin.

INITIATING CGM THERAPY

As with initiation of insulin pump therapy, various clinics will have different protocols. The criteria for deciding who is ready to begin CGM therapy are similar to those discussed in Chapter 28 for starting an insulin pump and include:

- ✔ interest on the part of the person as well as family members (with young children being an exception)
- ✔ willingness to wear the sensor (ideally with commitment to wear it at least six days per week)
- ✔ willingness to evaluate and use a new system/new information
- ✔ adequate financial resources – which may or may not include health insurance coverage. Most CGM systems cost ~ $1000 U.S. dollars, and each sensor (lasting five to 14 days) costs $35 to $70 U.S. dollars.
- ✔ adequate body fat – although everyone has adequate fat on the buttocks, this is sometimes a concern for parents of young children already using an insulin pump.
- ✔ availability of a knowledgeable diabetes care, support, and education system is essential

CALIBRATION of CGMs

As noted above, the Dexcom G6 and the FreeStyle Libre Flash do not require calibrations using finger-stick blood sugars. They are factory-calibrated to remove possible error in user calibration. However, the G6 will allow calibrations if glucose values are not matching finger-stick blood sugars. Other CGMs are calibrated by entering a fingerstick blood sugar value into the receiver. Depending on the CGM, this occurs at least 2 times each day. A difficult issue with CGMs involves calibrating the system so that the CGM values are as accurate as possible and are matching the blood sugar values. Everyone wants their CGM values to match their blood sugar readings. This is most likely to happen if the calibration (entry of the blood sugar value) can be done at a time when blood sugars are relatively stable (e.g., before breakfast, late afternoon). If the person has just eaten and the blood sugar is rising, or if the blood sugar is rapidly falling, the blood sugar value and the CGM value will be further apart, due in part to the five-minute lag. As a result, the CGM values will not match as well until another calibration is performed later in the day. Doing three or four blood sugars during the day and using them for calibrations may result in greater accuracy.

ALARM (vibration) SETTINGS

Most CGM alarm settings are optional. An exception is the Dexcom factory setting of the 55 mg/dL (3.0 mmol/L) for safety. A recent report suggested using a lower level of 75 mg/dL (4.2 mmol/L) in order to attain less than one percent of time in hypoglycemia, and an upper level of 170 mg/dL (9.5 mmol/L) to attain less than five percent of time in hyperglycemia.

SENSOR PLACEMENT AND ADHESION

Placement: Each CGM company has suggestions for where to place their sensors. In general, they can be worn on the back of the arm, the abdomen, hips, or buttocks. The selected area must have enough skin/fat to be able to pinch up a little bit with two fingers. Sensors tend to stick best when inserted while the patient is standing up straight or lying down. This is to make sure that the skin and tissue are relaxed. It is best to avoid areas where the body bends or that are against the pants line. If the skin is hairy, a scissors or a razor can be used to trim the hair short. Finally, it is important to rotate sites so that the skin has time to breathe without tape on it. Using the same site repeatedly can lead to skin irritation and adhesion issues.

Skin preparation: Perhaps the most important tip to ensure a successful sensor insertion is to start with clean and dry skin. Although this sounds simple and obvious, sensors easily fall off skin that is oily, wet, or prone to sweating. Even use of deodorant to reduce sweating is sometimes helpful.

Adhesive use (also see Chapter 28): There are many different adhesive wipes, tapes, and bandages that can help sensors to stick to skin. It is quite common for a person to use an adhesive wipe to treat the skin under the sensor, then place the sensor on the skin, and finally reinforce it with additional tape (Table 1). Some CGM companies recommend that a sensor not be inserted through an adhesive layer, so a small circle can be drawn on the skin to mark where the sensor is to be inserted. Then the adhesive can be applied all around that adhesive-free circle. Every person is different, and what works for one person may not work for others. Some people may need all the help they can get to keep the sets in place, while others may only need reinforcements during particular activities or at specific times of the year. All people need to know the problem is not unique to one product, and there are ways that can help improve the adhesion properties of each set. It may be helpful to review Table 1 with a diabetes nurse educator.

CGM DATA

There are two types of data that can be obtained from CGM usage: **Real Time** data, and **Retrospective** data. This chapter will not go into great detail on how to make insulin adjustments from the data. This is done in the 3rd edition of the book, *Understanding Insulin Pumps, Continuous Glucose Monitors, and the Artificial Pancreas* (see Publications Order Form in the back of this book). Chapter 22 also deals with making insulin adjustments.

The two types of information received from CGMs are discussed below:

A. Real-time CGM Data:

These are the values displayed immediately as the current CGM glucose value is determined. Different people use different aspects of the Real Time CGM data, and three examples will be

TABLE 1:
Adhesive Wipes, Tapes, and Bandages for CGM Sensors (also see Chapter 28)

Adhesive wipes (from least sticky to most sticky) to be used underneath sensor tape

	IV Prep (Smith & Nephew)	✔ Contains alcohol, so may not need to wipe with alcohol first
	Bard wipes® (Bard)	✔ Offers greater protection of skin
	Skin Prep (Smith & Nephew)	✔ Offers proteaction of skin and some additional stickiness. Can be removed with Unisolve (Smith & Nephew)
	Skin Tac™ (Torbot)	✔ Our most commonly used product because of higher degree of stickiness. Can be removed with Tac-Away (Torbot)
	Mastisol (Ferndale)	✔ Most sticky product listed here. Can cause some skin irritation, so only use if other products don't work. Can be used with Detachol (Ferndale)

Adhesive Tapes: To use in addition to the sensor tape

Overbandages	IV3000™ (Smith & Nephew)	✔ Can place directly over the sensor and transmitter
		✔ Can be cut into strips (or cut a hole in the center) and then placed around the sensor/transmitter like a picture frame (best for Navigator and Dexcom). This helps to reinforce the sensor tape and to prevent water from getting into tape creases.
	Tegaderm™ (3M)	✔ If skin is sensitive to the sensor tape, can be used under the sensor mount. Note that a sensor cannot be inserted through tape, so a hole must be cut for the sensor to insert through.
Medical Tapes	Transpore technique (3M)	✔ Use medical grade tapes with the "picture frame" described above.
	Hypafix (Smith & Nephew) Silk Tape	
	Kinesio Sports Tape	
Bandages and additional support	Coban™ (3M) Co-Flex®	✔ Wrap bandages are helpful for securing sensors to the arm.
		✔ We suggest using this technique for people involved in sports or high levels of activity. The bandage can be wrapped around the arm with the sensor/transmitter, and comes in bright colors (which appeals to many children). It is important to unwrap these bandages when not needed and ACE® bandage at night in order to give the skin a chance to breathe. A professional football player wore an ACE bandage over the sensor on his arm during practices!

TABLE 2:
Trend arrows for the three CGM devices

Symbol on CGM	What it means (for all 3)	What to do with insulin
Medtronic*: ↑↑ Abbott**: ↑ Dexcom***: ↑↑	RAPID RISE (Glucose rising >3 mg/dL [>0.17 mmol/L] per minute)	Increase dose by 20% (and possibly more if illness or ketones)
Medtronic: ↑ Abbott: ↗ Dexcom: ↑	MODERATE RISE (Glucose rising 1-2 mg/dL [0.06-0.11 mmol/L] per minute)	Increase dose by 10% (and possibly more if illness or ketones)
Medtronic: none Abbott: → Dexcom: →	STABLE (Glucose level changing <1 mg/dL [<0.06 mmol/L] per minute)	No change in dose of rapid-acting insulin (unless illness or ketones are present)
Medtronic: ↓ Abbott: ↘ Dexcom: ↓	MODERATE FALL (Glucose falling 1-2 mg/dL [0.06-0.11 mmol/L] per minute)	Decrease dose by 10% (and possibly more if post-exercise)
Medtronic: ↓↓ Abbott: ↓ Dexcom: ↓↓	RAPID FALL (Glucose falling >3 mg/dL [>0.17 mmol/L] per minute)	Decrease dose by 20% (and possibly more if post-exercise)

* Medtronic refers to the Guardian REAL-Time CGM system.
** Abbott refers to the Navigator. The Flash has only one arrow up, a horizontal arrow, and one arrow down.
*** Dexcom refers to the Dexcom G5 or G6.

presented here. This is especially useful when the parent is away from the child and can see the glucose values transmitted to their smart phone.

1. **Current CGM Glucose Values:** Knowing this value – for the user, or for the parent of a young child – can be VERY reassuring.
2. **Real Time Trend Graphs:** Trend graphs show the line of previous glucose values (rising, steady, or falling) over recent time. For example, when a blood sugar value of 240 mg/dL (13.3 mmol/L) was detected, the person previously did not know if their values were climbing, falling or staying the same (Figure 1). Trend graphs now enlighten the wearer and make appropriate treatment possible.

FIGURE 1
Illustrated Examples of Real-Time Trend Graphs

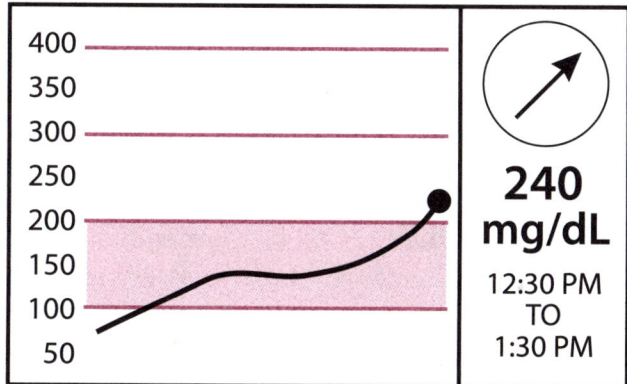
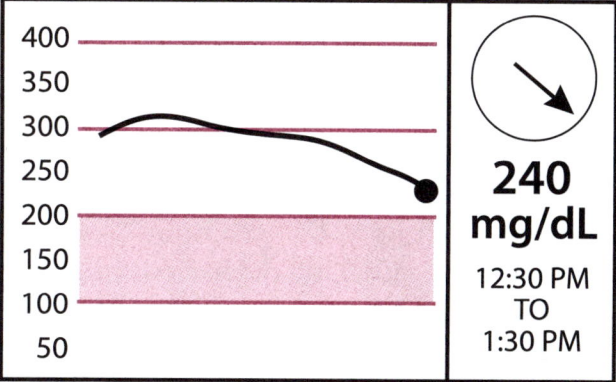

These illustrated graphs show the value of seeing glucose trends prior to getting a CGM glucose value of 240 mg/dL (in both illustrations), in contrast to having a single blood glucose value of 240 mg/dL (13.3 mmol/L).

FIGURE 2
Retrospective CGM Data

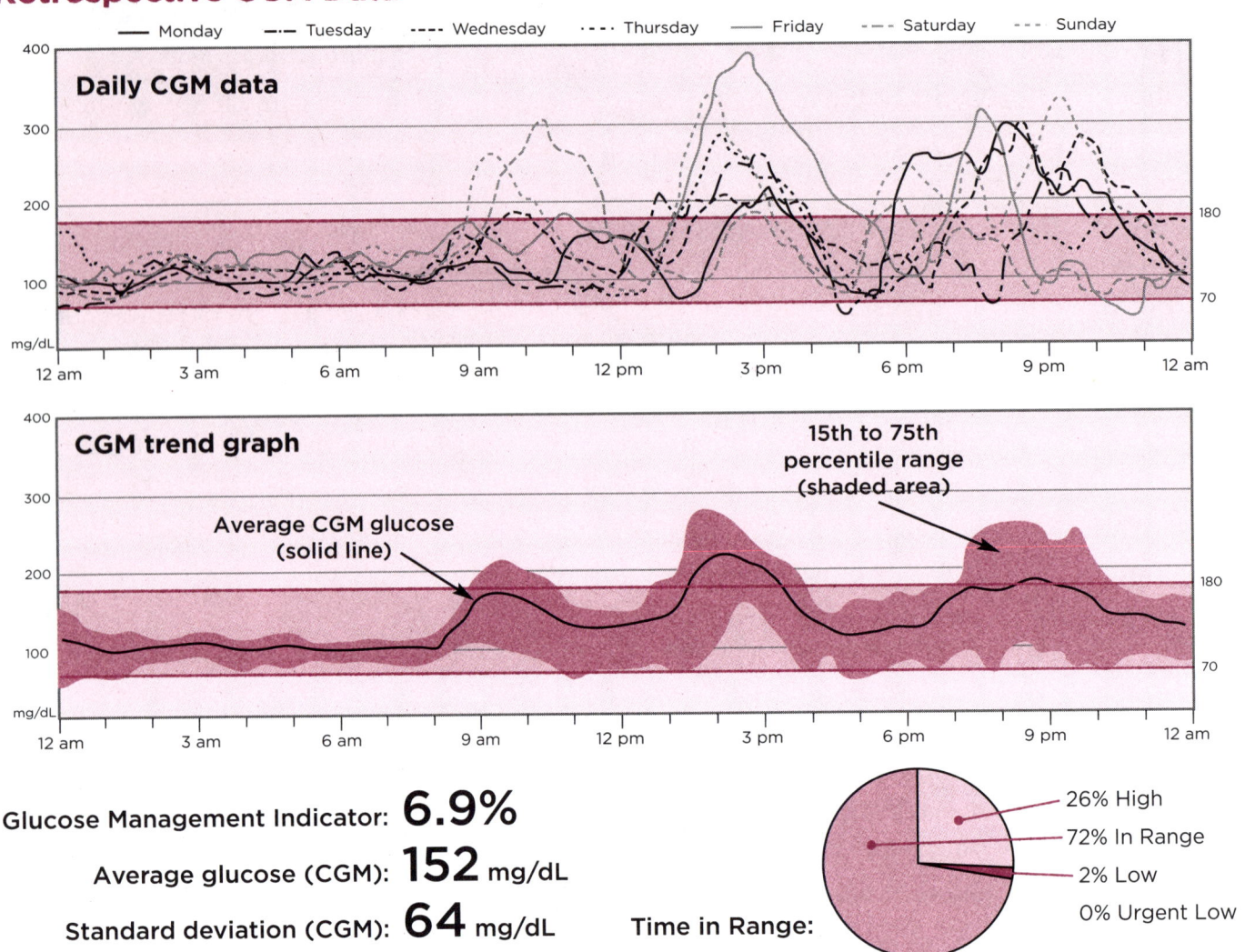

This download shows the estimated HbA1c to be excellent at 6.9%, with an average CGM glucose of 152. Standard deviation is slightly high at 64 (ideally below 50), showing that sugars have had more variability than desired. The time in range is 72%, which is excellent (aim >70%). The daily glucose values are shown in the top graph, and the mean glucose values are shown by the solid line in the second graph. This person tended to have high glucose values after both lunch and dinner. He/she would benefit greatly by giving meal insulin 20 minutes before meals. The alternative, increasing the meal insulin dose, would likely increase post-meal hypoglycemia.

3. **Trend Arrows:** The trend arrows help to show how rapidly the change in glucose levels is occurring. A CGM value of 70 mg/dL (3.9 mmol/L) with trend arrows indicating a rapid rate of fall is more urgent than if a horizontal arrow is indicating a steady glucose level. Table 2 shows the meaning of the trend arrows for the three commonly used CGMs in the U.S. Although suggestions are included in Table 2 for changing insulin dosages, there are now several suggested methods, and the one recommended by the person's diabetes care-provider should be used. Many people gradually learn how to make their adjustment for their body and, using a "thinking" scale (see Chapter 7), make their adjustment accordingly.

B. Retrospective CGM Data:

Retrospective CGM data comes from downloading the data in the receiver to a computer, which then provides further insight into glucose data. The data may be from the previous day, week, month, or whatever is needed. We recommend that the retrospective data be evaluated by the person/family at least once weekly. Three examples of the use of Retrospective data will be presented here.

1. **Trend Graph Reports:** These reports give the CGM glucose values for each day as a continuous line for that day. Several days can be reported on the same graph with each day coded differently (see Figure 2). By comparing multiple days, it can be easy to detect a pattern of high or low glucose levels at specific times of day. The periods of the day, as detailed in Chapter 22, can be evaluated to determine which periods need an adjustment of insulin dose. Missed insulin boluses for meals are also often detectable.

2. **Pie Charts:** The pie charts show the percentage of glucose values that are high, in-range, or low for different periods of the day. Pie charts give rapidly interpretable data for people who like visual presentations.

3. **Tables:** Tables can give much information. Data can include mean glucose values and high and low values for different periods of the day. Standard deviations can be helpful in evaluating fluctuations of glucose levels.

4. **CGM Metrics** (also see p. 162)
   The consistent use of a CGM allows collection of new types of important data. The Time in Range (see below) has been shown to correlate with the HbA1c values. Four metrics to focus on are listed in Table 3.

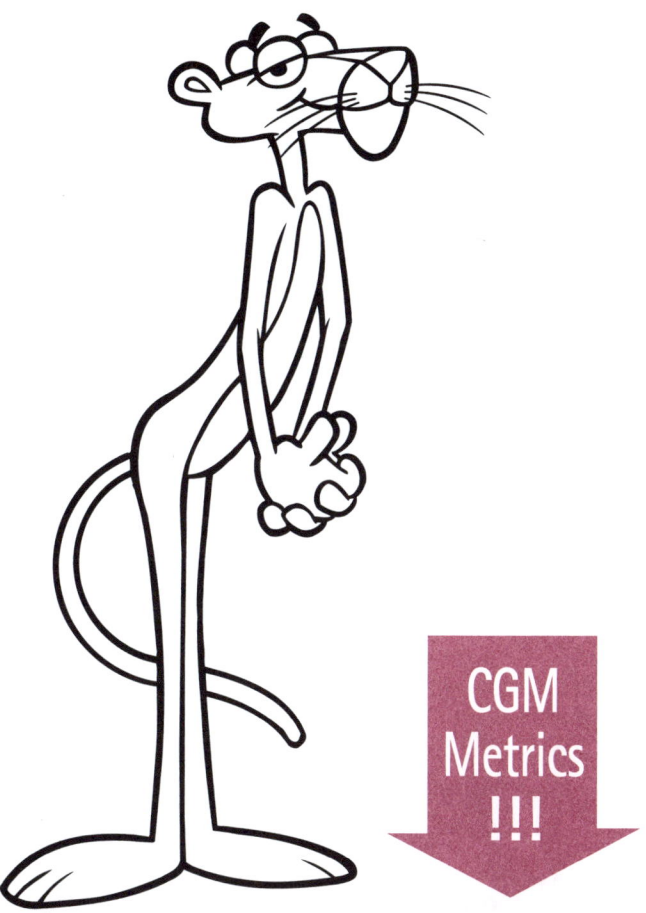

TABLE 3: CGM Metrics*

	Glucose	Aim for 24-hour day	Time
i. Time in Range ** (TIR)	70-180 mg/dL (3.9-10.0 mmol/L)	>70%	16 hr, 48 min
ii. Time above Range (TAR)	>180 mg/dL (>10.0 mmol/L)	<25%	6 hr
iii. Time below Range (TBR)	<70 mg/dL (<3.9 mmol/L)	<4%	58 min
iv. Time below 54 mg/dL	(<3.0 mmol/L)	<1%	14 min

*These metrics will vary for very young or old, with pregnancy, and for high-risk subjects.
**Each 5% increase in TIR is clinically significant.

CONTINUOUS GLUCOSE MONITORS (CGM)

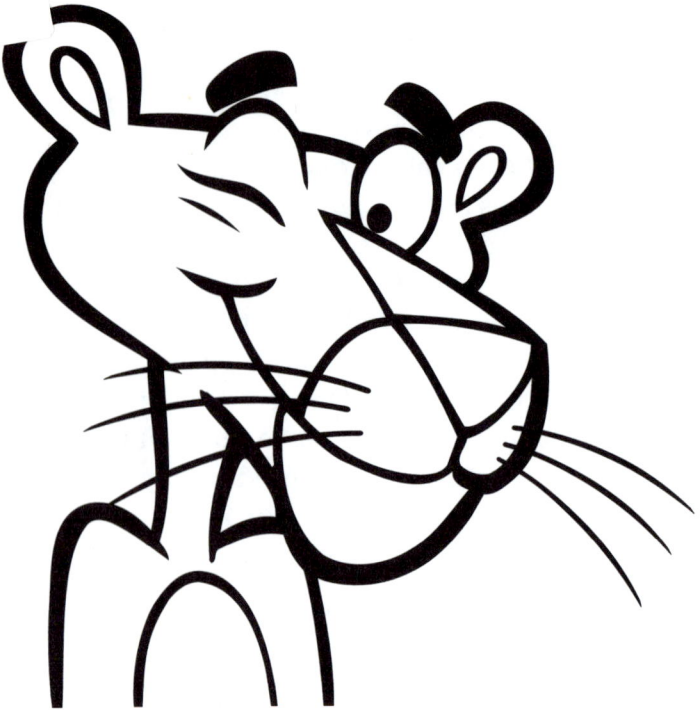

Both Real Time and Retrospective data are important for the user and family. The person using the CGM can glance at the receiver throughout the day and see glucose values and trends (see below). We strongly encourage users/families to download Retrospective data at least weekly. Patterns of high or low glucose levels that occur at consistent times throughout the week can then be recognized. An insulin dose should generally not be changed unless a pattern is seen on two or more days in the week.

In summary, CGM use provides a patient/family with a wealth of information about diabetes management that is not possible with blood sugar checking alone. The use of a CGM can enhance both safety and the collection of information. If used consistently (e.g., at least 6 days/week), diabetes management usually improves. Different people/families will learn to use and favor different aspects of CGM. When CGM use is combined with insulin pump therapy, safety (particularly related to hypoglycemia) is enhanced. In addition, a higher percentage of glucose values are in the desired range, which should reduce the likelihood of acute and chronic diabetes complications. Although it should not be initiated until the person and family are ready, the CGM often becomes the user's "best friend."

DEFINITIONS

Calibration: The entry of a fingerstick blood sugar level into the CGM system to allow the subcutaneous glucose level to be adjusted to match the blood glucose level.

Continuous Glucose Monitor (CGM): A system consisting of a sensor, transmitter and receiver that determines subcutaneous glucose levels every 1 to 5 minutes.

Real Time Glucose Data: Information on the CGM receiver that indicates current glucose levels, direction of glucose change, and if glucose levels are currently too high or too low.

Retrospective Glucose Data: CGM data reviewed from past time periods. This can be shown either on the receiver or from a computer download of the CGM information.

QUESTIONS AND ANSWERS FROM NEWSNOTES

Q We have been doing weekly downloads of our daughter's CGM tracings. She is frequently high after meals. Do you have suggestions?

a The easiest change to make is to give her injections/boluses of rapid-acting insulin (Humalog, NovoLog or Apidra) 15 to 20 minutes prior to the meal. The rapid-acting insulins peak in 90-95 minutes, whereas blood sugars from food peak in 60 minutes. A closer matching of the peaks helps to keep all glucose levels after meals below 180 mg/dL (<10.0 mmol/L), which is the current goal (also see Figure 2 in Chapter 8)

CHAPTER 30

The Artificial Pancreas (AP)

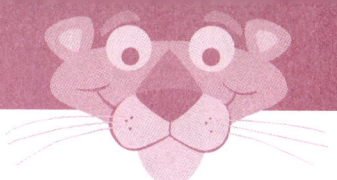

Erin C. Cobry, MD
H. Peter Chase, MD
Brigitte I. Frohnert, MD, PhD

The artificial pancreas (AP) refers to a system that includes a continuous glucose monitor (CGM) and an insulin pump working together to increase, decrease, stop, start or bolus insulin as needed to manage blood glucose levels. The AP systems are sometimes also called closed-loop or automated insulin delivery systems. More detailed information on insulin pumps is provided in Chapter 28 and on CGMs in Chapter 29. In an AP system, the CGM sends the glucose information to the insulin pump, which then uses mathematical formulas (algorithms) to decide how to adjust the insulin. Although a complete AP system is not yet available at the time of this writing, two partial AP systems (or hybrid closed-loop systems) are commercially available in the U.S. (see below for more detailed information): the Medtronic/MiniMed™ 670G system and the Tandem® t:slim X2 Pump with Control-IQ and the Dexcom G6® CGM.

The purpose of this chapter is to provide an overview of current AP systems. Use of an AP system can result in improved glucose management and a reduction in fear of hypoglycemia, particularly for episodes occurring during the night. If a person (family) decides to use an AP system, they will receive detailed instructions on the use of the system they choose from both the diabetes healthcare team and the device manufacturer.

STAGES IN DEVELOPMENT OF THE ARTIFICIAL PANCREAS:

When talking about AP systems, it is helpful to think about what is included in each different stage of automation in insulin delivery:

TOPICS:
Monitoring Diabetes (following CGM glucose levels)
Medications (insulin delivery systems)
Prevention, Detection and Treatment of Acute Complications (hypo- or hyper-glycemia)

TEACHING OBJECTIVES:
The teacher will:
1. Introduce the concept of altering insulin delivery based on CGM glucose trends.
2. Describe how episodes of hypoglycemia or predicted hypoglycemia affect insulin dosing in artificial pancreas (AP) systems.
3. Describe how episodes of hyperglycemia or predicted hyperglycemia affect insulin dosing in AP systems.

LEARNING OBJECTIVES:
Learner (parents, child, relative or self) will be able to:
1. Describe how AP systems alter insulin output based on CGM glucose levels.
2. Explain AP insulin adjustments for high or low glucose levels.

Stage 1: The Low Glucose Suspend (LGS) feature shuts off the delivery of insulin from the pump when the user's CGM glucose level drops below a certain number, such as 70 mg/dL (3.9 mmol/L), to reduce the likelihood of severe low glucose (hypoglycemia). This feature is included in several systems such as the Medtronic/MiniMed 530G (Paradigm Veo outside the U.S.) with the Enlite CGM sensor and the 670G system with the Guardian Sensor 3. It is also found in the Tandem t:slim X2 pump systems (Basal-IQ and Control-IQ) with the Dexcom G6 CGM sensor. The insulin pump may stop insulin delivery for up to two hours if the CGM glucose value is below the set level. Most of the full two-hour insulin suspensions occur during sleep, when alarms are less likely to be noticed by the wearer. This has been shown in multiple research reports to reduce time spent in hypoglycemia, especially at night.

Stage 2: The Predicted Low Glucose Suspend (PLGS) feature predicts when the glucose level is going to be low, for example, below 70mg/dL (3.9 mmol/L), and automatically stops insulin delivery before the low occurs. This feature is present in the Medtronic/MiniMed 670G system and (outside the U.S.) in the MiniMed 640G SmartGuard System. It is also found in the Tandem t:slim X2 Basal- and Control-IQ Systems. Basal- and Control-IQ (in the exercise mode) will stop insulin when the glucose level is predicted to be below 80 mg/dL (4.5 mmol/L) within the next 30 minutes or when the glucose level is already below 70 mg/dL (3.9 mmol/L). These systems will automatically restart delivery when the user's glucose level begins to rise.

It is obviously better to avoid hypoglycemia (by stopping insulin delivery before hypoglycemia occurs) than to have to treat it (by eating sugary foods or drinks). In addition to the person feeling better, the body does not use up its stores of adrenaline (epinephrine) that are normally released when the blood glucose is low. By predicting that the glucose level is going to become low, the pump can decrease or stop insulin delivery to avoid the low or reduce the duration of the low glucose level. Current **overnight** data suggests a glucose level must be below 60 mg/dL (3.3 mmol/L) for over two hours before a hypoglycemic seizure would occur. Use of the PLGS (and the LGS) can greatly reduce the risk of extended hypoglycemia events. Recent research using LGS and PLGS technology in people ages 4-45 years involving ~ 5000 nights showed a 70 percent reduction in time spent below 60 mg/dL (<3.3 mmol/L). This feature may play an important role in improving the sleep quality of users and their family members by decreasing nighttime hypoglycemic episodes.

Stage 3: The Partial AP system (or hybrid closed-loop system) is able to automatically adjust insulin delivery depending on whether the user's glucose is trending up or down. At this stage, the user still has to give meal and high glucose (correction) boluses by entering the carbohydrates and glucose levels into the pump. Meal boluses (ideally 20 minutes before meals) are still required because current insulins do not act quickly enough (see Figure 2 in Chapter 8). The MiniMed 670G and the Tandem Control-IQ systems are the two currently available partial AP systems that include the features listed in all three of these stages. More information on each system is below:

ARTIFICIAL PANCREAS SYSTEMS CURRENTLY AVAILABLE:

Medtronic/MiniMed 670G Hybrid Closed-Loop System:

The MiniMed 670G system includes the 670G insulin pump and the Guardian Sensor 3 CGM. This system automatically adjusts basal insulin delivery every five minutes based on CGM readings, targeting a glucose level of 120 mg/dL

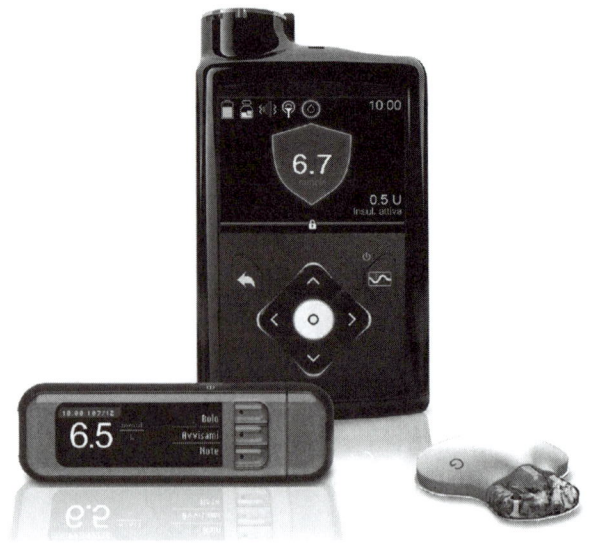

(6.7 mmol/L). The target glucose can also be temporarily raised to 150 mg/dL (8.3 mmol/L) when low blood glucose (hypoglycemia) is more likely to happen, such as during exercise. The Guardian CGM can be worn for up to seven days and requires at least two fingerstick blood glucose calibrations per day (although three to four are recommended). It can operate in Manual Mode (using pre-programed basal and bolus settings and the LGS and PLGS features) or in Auto Mode (using all the features of the partial AP system). Updates are gradually resolving problems that occurred with the initial 670G System.

The MiniMed 780G will be Medtronic's second partial AP system, and a significant upgrade over the MiniMed 670G. The MiniMed 780G will include automatic correction boluses for high glucose levels and an adjustable glucose target down to 100 mg/dL (5.5 mmol/L). The system will also have fewer alarms and be easier to operate than the 670G.

Tandem t:slim X2 Pump with Control-IQ Technology:

The Control-IQ Technology is a free software update for people using Tandem's t:slim X2 pump with Dexcom's G6 CGM sensor. The G6 CGM can be worn for up to ten days and does not require a fingerstick blood glucose for calibration. While both the Basal- and Control-IQ systems will decrease or stop insulin delivery (LGS and PLGS) to reduce the likelihood of low glucose levels, Control-IQ is the first system commercially available to provide automatic correction boluses for high glucose levels. When the system predicts that the glucose level will be above 180 mg/dL (10.0 mmol/L) in 30 minutes, the system will deliver 60 percent of the correction bolus needed to reach a target of 110 mg/dL (6.1 mmol/L). This bolus can occur once per hour if no other insulin bolus has been given. The Control-IQ technology also includes automatic basal rate adjustments and aims to keep glucose values between 112.5 and 160 mg/dL (6.2 and 8.9 mmol/L). Use of this system

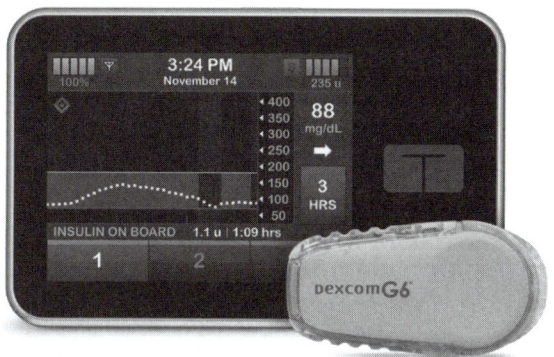

has been shown to increase "time in range" by an average of 2.6 hours per day.

This system has two additional features or modes called Sleep mode and Exercise mode. Sleep mode can be either turned on/off manually or scheduled. When Sleep mode is used, the system tightens the target range to achieve glucose values between 112.5 and 120 mg/dL (6.2 and 6.7 mmol/L); however, the system does not give automatic correction boluses but continues to adjust the basal insulin to reach the target glucose level. The second feature, Exercise mode, is manually set when desired, and during this mode the target glucose range is changed to 140 to 160 mg/dL (7.8 to 8.9 mmol/L). During Exercise mode, the pump still has the predictive low glucose suspension when it predicts a glucose of less than 80 mg/dL (4.5 mmol/L) in 30 minutes to reduce the risk of hypoglycemia. If needed, this mode will also give high glucose boluses to reduce significant hyperglycemia.

If giving the meal bolus after the meal (young, picky eaters), it is important to reduce the insulin dose by half, due to the pump's auto-correction feature already working.

The Dexcom sensor has Bluetooth connectivity to allow data to be transmitted to a designated smart phone. From this phone, the glucose information can be shared remotely with the devices of family members or friends using internet or cellular connectivity (see Chapter 29).

ARTIFICIAL PANCREAS SYSTEMS CURRENTLY IN DEVELOPMENT:

The Beta Bionic iLet™ System will use the Dexcom G6 with the iLet insulin pump. This system is unique in that only body weight is entered at set-up, and the system learns the insulin needs over time. In addition, the iLet system will not require the user to enter carbohydrates for meals; instead, the user gives the system a meal announcement based on the size of the meal. The iLet system is designed to provide both insulin and glucagon, although it likely will be an insulin-only version initially.

The Insulet Omnipod Horizon™ Automated Glucose Control System will use the three-day wear patch pump (Omnipod) combined with the Dexcom G6 CGM. A handheld device, similar to a cell phone, is used to give meal and high glucose boluses. The algorithm that will use the CGM data to make insulin adjustments is included in the patch pump. The Horizon system will include features of all three stages mentioned above. This system is currently undergoing clinical trials, and the data from these will be submitted to the FDA for approval.

Tidepool Loop is an automated insulin-delivery app for iPhones that connects to an insulin pump and CGM, using Bluetooth LE. It is currently under development and is undergoing testing with the goal of submitting to the FDA for official approval. Tidepool is working on an AP algorithm that can be used with available sensors and insulin pumps. The AP algorithm will be available as an app through the Apple store. **Loop** is currently an open-source (free and publicly available), non-FDA-approved AP system that is compatible with the Dexcom sensor and an older Medtronic pump. As it is not approved by the FDA at this time, most health professionals cannot assist in its use. A large virtual study is ongoing for Loop users, and the data will be used to support Tidepool's submission of Loop to the FDA as the Tidepool Loop (or another new name). Tidepool hopes to get Loop approved by the FDA, available in the App Store, and able to work with in-warranty, commercially available insulin pumps and CGMs.

Stage 4: The Complete AP system (fully closed-loop) will have all the features of the first three stages, and will also be able to detect meals and automatically deliver the proper amount of insulin needed to manage blood glucose levels. With elimination of manual boluses, the system will be "fully closed-loop." A faster rapid-acting insulin will be needed to help safely achieve this goal.

The Complete AP system has the potential to improve the quality of life for people with diabetes. Constant glucose monitoring and regulation of food intake will be less of a burden. The main advantages, however, will be in decreasing the frequency of low and high blood glucose levels, resulting in more values in range and a reduced likelihood of immediate and long-term diabetes complications.

CHAPTER 31

Pregnancy and Diabetes

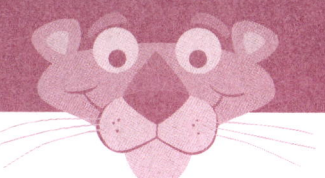

INTRODUCTION

Women with diabetes can have healthy pregnancies and healthy babies. **Pre-pregnancy planning is essential.** We recommend that women with diabetes meet with their diabetes care team at least 3 months in advance of wanting to become pregnant. The purpose of this chapter is to give an overview of diabetes management with pregnancy.

For a woman with diabetes, the most important consideration is having a low HbA1c before and during pregnancy. Normal or near-normal blood sugars reduce the risk of miscarriage and birth defects. **When possible, it is recommended that a continuous glucose monitor (CGM) be used consistently prior to and during pregnancy.**

High blood/CGM sugar levels during pregnancy can:

✔ increase the rate of birth defects (heart, spine, cleft lip and palate, etc.) during the first trimester

✔ result in the birth of large babies

✔ increase the risk for injury to mother or baby during delivery because of a baby's size

✔ increase the risk to the mother of developing high blood pressure, swelling of feet and protein leakage in urine (pre-eclampsia)

Proper planning for pregnancy will result in better HbA1c values before the beginning of pregnancy and thus reduce the risk of birth defects. Pregnancy should be delayed until the HbA1c is <6.5% (<48 mmol/mol) and folic acid

TOPICS:
Preconception Care and Management During Pregnancy
Monitoring
Prevent, Detect and Treat Acute Complications
Prevent, Detect and Treat Chronic Complications Through Risk Reduction

TEACHING OBJECTIVES:
The teacher will:
1. Present the importance of preconception planning.
2. Define key aspects of intensive diabetes management.
3. Discuss the monitoring necessary to prevent complications.

LEARNING OBJECTIVES:
Learner (parents, child, relative or self) will be able to:
1. State the most important consideration when planning a pregnancy.
2. Name the four components of intensive diabetes management.
3. List the additional eye/kidney evaluations, clinic visits and monitoring required during pregnancy.

has been taken for three months (see 3, Close Attention to Nutrition, below).

During pregnancy, the HbA1c value >5.9% (>41 mmol/mol) defines women at greater risk for having infants with birth defects and adverse pregnancy outcomes. HbA1c levels should be checked frequently in women who have diabetes or who are at risk for diabetes.

DIABETES MANAGEMENT

Intensive diabetes management is essential during pregnancy. *As discussed in Chapter 8, this involves:*

1) Insulin pump therapy or multiple daily injections (MDI)
2) Frequent blood/CGM monitoring
3) Close attention to nutrition
4) Frequent contact with the healthcare team

Although all four of these have been discussed in earlier chapters, some details related to pregnancy will be discussed as listed above:

1) Insulin Pump Therapy or Multiple Daily Injections (MDI)

Either of these treatments can be effective for intensive diabetes management:

- **Insulin pump** therapy is discussed in detail in Chapter 28. If an insulin pump is to be used, it is recommended that this be initiated before pregnancy.
- **Multiple daily injections** (MDI – discussed under "Intensive Diabetes Management" in Chapter 8; this may involve ten or more insulin injections daily).

Either method of intensive diabetes management (insulin pump or MDI) is capable of achieving near-normal glucose levels. Less intense diabetes care (two shots a day, etc.) rarely achieves adequate HbA1c levels during pregnancy, and thus should not be used. Insulins often used during pregnancy are as follows:

Humalog/NovoLog/Apidra (rapid onset/short lasting) Insulins

Lower blood/CGM glucose levels after meals and snacks is very important. High blood/CGM glucose levels after meals have been associated with big babies and adverse outcomes. Numerous studies have shown Humalog/NovoLog or Apidra to be more effective for this purpose than Regular insulin. Humalog/NovoLog or Aprida insulin should ideally be taken 20 minutes prior to the time when food is eaten. Use of a pen (Chapter 9) is a convenient way to do this for people choosing MDI. One of these insulins is also used for insulin pump therapy.

Lantus (Basaglar), Levemir and Tresiba (basal) Insulins

Although not well studied, most physicians allow patients to continue using these basal insulins during pregnancy.

NPH Insulin

NPH (N) insulin can be used for the intermediate-acting insulin in MDI. Three or four doses per day (in addition to Humalog or NovoLog) are often used (e.g., breakfast, lunch, bedtime).

Insulin Sensitivity

✓ usually insulin doses go down in the first trimester (insulin-sensitive phase causing a high risk of severe low blood sugars)

✓ insulin doses go up by double or triple in the 2nd and 3rd trimesters (insulin-resistant phase)

✓ insulin needs decrease the most significantly after delivering the baby and placenta to pre-pregnancy doses or less

✓ breast feeding can reduce insulin doses further

TABLE 1:
Target Values for Blood/CGM Sugar and HbA1c Levels Before and During Pregnancy*

Blood Sugars

Time	mg/dL	mmol/L
Fasting and pre-meal	60-99	3.3-5.4
1 hour after meal	<130	<7.2
2 hours after meal	<120	<6.7
2:00 a.m. - 6:00 a.m.	60-99	3.3-5.4
Meter average	100-130	5.5-7.2
HbA1c (%)**	<6.0%	<42 mmol/mol

* Per ADA Consensus Statement: Diabetes Care, 31:1060, 2008.
**A value <6.5% (48 mmol/mol) is advised during pre-pregnancy.

2) Frequent Blood/CGM Glucose Monitoring

Some suggestions:

✓ Blood/CGM sugar and HbA1c goals are given in Table 1.

✓ It is best to do 8 to 10 blood sugars per day as outlined in Table 1 (or use a CGM).

✓ The use of CGM is addressed in Chapter 29 and can be extremely helpful before and during pregnancy.

✓ It has recently been recommended that the blood sugar target range be 63-140 mg/dL (3.5-7.8 mmol/L) with >70% of values in range.

✓ If the HbA1c values are between 5.0 and 5.8%, there is no increased risk of congenital anomalies in the baby.

✓ Blood/CGM glucose values one and two hours after meals (Table 1) are important for optimal glucose management.

✓ Stay in close contact with the healthcare-providers. During pregnancy this may need to be weekly. (Tables for faxing or emailing are included in Chapters 7 and 28.)

✓ Frequent checking of blood/CGM sugar levels will allow the person to adjust their insulin dosages for different times during the pregnancy.

Low Blood Sugars

✓ Low blood sugars are more frequent in the first trimester, due to increased insulin sensitivity. Warning signs and symptoms of hypoglycemia may be diminished.

✓ Frequent blood/CGM sugar checking will help to prevent severe hypoglycemia. A CGM communicating with an insulin pump may allow insulin suspension with a low or predicted low CGM sugar level (see Chapter 30). This can be extremely helpful.

✓ It is well recognized that severe insulin reactions occur more frequently with tight control (Chapter 6), especially at night with sleep.

✓ There has not been evidence that low blood sugars are damaging to the fetus.

✓ Hypoglycemia is not pleasant for the mom, however, and should be avoided if possible.

Ketones

✓ Frequent blood/CGM sugar checking will also help to prevent ketone formation and acidosis (Chapter 15).

✓ Acidosis has been related to miscarriage and is important to avoid.

Ketones should be checked:

- Any time a fasting blood/CGM sugar is above 240 mg/dL (13.3 mmol/L)
- if a random sugar is above 300 mg/dL (16.7 mmol/L)
- every morning during pregnancy (see methods in Chapter 5)

3) Close Attention to Nutrition

Nutrition is important during pregnancy and lactation. Carbohydrate counting and other methods of food management are discussed in Chapter 12.

Special goals:

✔ Provide adequate calories for maternal and fetal weight gain. (This usually involves an additional 300 calories a day during the 2nd and 3rd trimesters and during lactation.) A 25 to 35-pound (11.4-15.9 kg) weight gain is optimal with pregnancy, although this depends on the pre-pregnancy weight. Women who are overweight or obese prior to pregnancy should gain less during the pregnancy.

✔ Provide adequate vitamins and minerals (including iron and calcium). All women wanting to become pregnant should be certain they are taking 800 µg/day of folic acid (preferably for at least three months prior to pregnancy). This helps to prevent birth defects.

✔ Alcohol must be avoided to prevent fetal alcohol syndrome and serious congenital defects.

✔ Not smoking is important in reducing the risk for a premature or low-birth weight infant.

✔ The carbohydrate content of meals should be <33 percent of calories.

✔ Regular meals and snacks are important to prevent hypoglycemia. An evening snack is important to prevent lows during the night and ketone formation.

4) Frequent Contact with the Healthcare Team

✔ The blood/CGM sugar values should be emailed weekly.

✔ Clinic visits will vary but should usually occur at least monthly.

✔ Care from a specialist with knowledge in the areas of diabetes as well as of pregnancy is essential.

✔ Frequent contact with the eye or kidney specialist may also be important (see following).

REDUCING THE LIKELIHOOD OF CHRONIC COMPLICATIONS

A. Kidney (Renal) Damage

✔ Kidney damage does not usually worsen as a result of pregnancy in women who do not already have kidney damage. (This is in contrast to what was presented in the movie *Steel Magnolias*.)

✔ Women planning a pregnancy can do a urine microalbumin screen (and a blood creatinine) prior to pregnancy and after each trimester.

✔ If the person does have some kidney damage already present, it can get worse.

The following are then suggested:

- Urine microalbumin and blood creatinine levels should be done every month.

- **ACE-inhibitors (see Chapter 23) and cholesterol-lowering medicines must be stopped (possible cause of birth defects) in any woman considering pregnancy.** Use of other medications should also be reviewed with your physician.

- If blood pressure increases, other medicines should be used.

- During pregnancies, clinic visits every 2-4 weeks may be advised.

B. Eye (Retinal) Complications

✔ Women who have had diabetes <5 years who do not have eye (retinal) damage already present do not usually get eye damage due to pregnancy. They do need their eyes examined prior to the pregnancy and every three months during pregnancy.

✔ If a person already has moderate eye (retinal) damage from diabetes, this may worsen during pregnancy.

✔ If control (HbA1c) has not been optimal and improves dramatically, there is more risk for eye (retinal) changes due to the rapid change. These women must be followed closely.

PREECLAMPSIA

This involves new-onset or worsening of high blood pressure after 20 weeks gestation and development of one or more of the following:

✔ protein in the urine (>30 mcg/mg creatinine – see Chapter 23).

✔ other maternal organ dysfunction

✔ fetal growth restriction

If preeclampsia is detected, close follow-up is essential.

BIRTH

✔ Large babies are a result of higher blood sugar levels in the mother.

✔ Sugar freely crosses the placenta to the baby, resulting in increased insulin output from the fetal islet cells.

✔ Due to increased fetal islet cell size, babies after birth are at a higher risk for hypoglycemia.

✔ Over 50 percent of deliveries for women with diabetes are vaginal, but many times large babies require a cesarean (C-) section.

✔ Large babies at birth are at greater risk of developing type 2 diabetes in later life.

GESTATIONAL DIABETES

Gestational diabetes is a type of diabetes which occurs in up to 14 percent of pregnancies. It results from insulin resistance and decreased ability to produce insulin. Predisposing factors include genetics, excess body weight, and placental hormones (contributing to insulin resistance). Screening is often at 24-28 weeks gestation, although an HbA1c level above 5.9% (>41 mmol/mol) at an earlier time may indicate the need for an earlier evaluation. The World Health Organization defines gestational diabetes following a 75g oral glucose tolerance test (OGTT) by a fasting glucose level ≥92 mg/dL (≥5.1 mmol/L) or a two-hour value ≥153 mg/dL (>8.5 mmol/L).

After diagnosis, the care becomes similar to the care for the person who had diabetes prior to pregnancy. The target range for glucose levels is the same as in pregnancy (see number 2, above).

Facts:

✔ Regular aerobic exercise and diet may help to lower blood sugars before and after meals.

✔ Insulin treatment may be necessary.

✔ Most women revert to normal glucose metabolism after pregnancy.

✔ Thirty to 50 percent of women will again have gestational diabetes with subsequent pregnancies.

✔ There is an increased risk of the mother developing type 2 diabetes later in life.

DEFINITIONS

ACE-inhibitor: A blood pressure medicine often used to treat people with early diabetic kidney disease (Chapter 23). It must be discontinued if pregnancy is being considered.

Birth defects: Abnormalities in the newborn baby such as heart malformations, spinal cord abnormalities or lip or palate defects. These are more common if glucose control for the mother was suboptimal in the first trimester.

Folic acid: One of the B-vitamins that, when deficient in the pregnant mother, is related to birth defects in the baby.

Gestational diabetes: High glucose levels noted during pregnancy (most frequently in the last trimester). It is treated with diet, exercise and sometimes insulin. It usually reverses after pregnancy is over.

Microgram (μg): A common unit of weight in the metric system. It refers to one thousandth (0.001) of 1g.

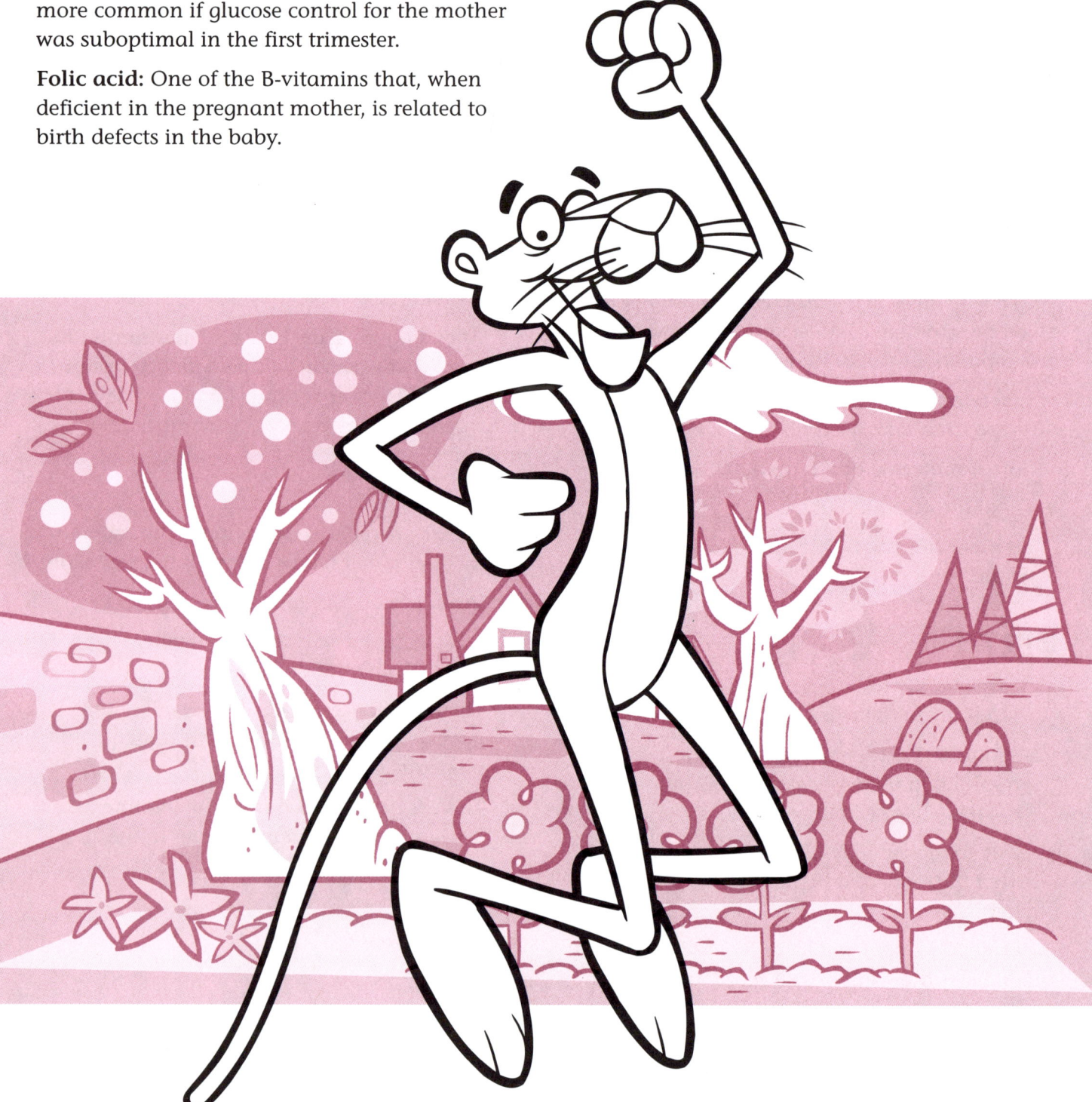

CHAPTER 32

Research and Diabetes

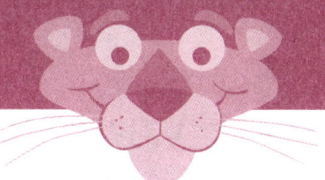

INTRODUCTION

Banting and Best received the Nobel prize for their discovery of insulin in 1921. It was believed that a "cure" for diabetes had been found. Before the discovery of insulin, people with type 1 diabetes lived only about one year after development of symptoms. Insulin was not a "cure," but instead a way to care for diabetes and to save lives. Continued research developments have resulted in great improvements in diabetes care and in lifestyle. These advances will continue in future decades.

Four Common Research Questions

The four questions asked most often about research are listed below:

1. When will there be a cure?
2. Can diabetes be prevented (type 1 or type 2)?
3. Will there be a completely artificial pancreas?
4. Are there advances in avoiding diabetic complications?

There has been wonderful progress in diabetes research over the last ten years. The next ten years will likely show even more progress. The answers to the above four questions are discussed in order below:

> **TOPICS:**
> **Research: A Cure**
> **Prevention**
> **Artificial Pancreas**
> **Delay of Complications**
>
> **TEACHING OBJECTIVES:**
> The teacher will:
> 1. Discuss current research related to type 1 and type 2 diabetes.
> 2. Present available research opportunities to families.
>
> **LEARNING OBJECTIVES:**
> Learner (parents, child, relative or self) will be able to:
> 1. List one current research study related to the individual's type of diabetes.
> 2. Name one research opportunity specific to the family.

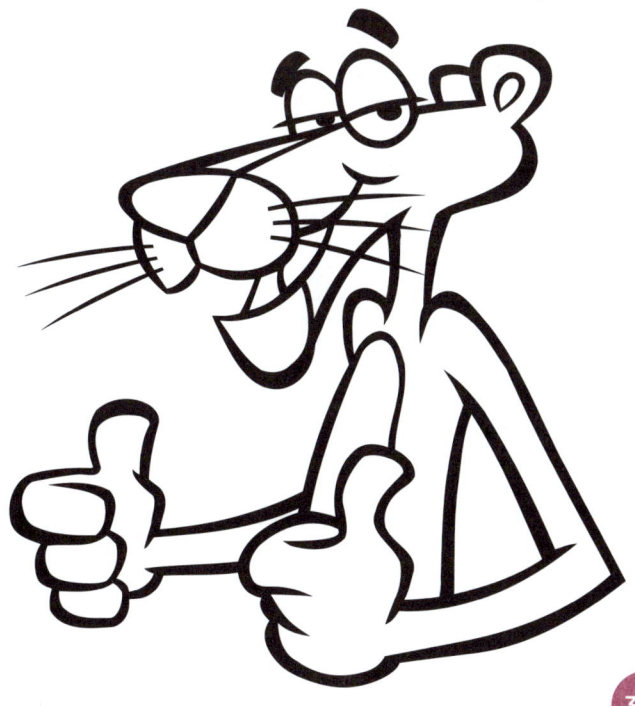

333

1. WHEN WILL THERE BE A CURE?

The following research shows promise:

Islet Transplantation

In 2001, successful islet cell (the cells that make insulin) transplants were done in Edmonton, Alberta, Canada, by Drs. A.M.J. Shapiro, E.A. Ryan, R.V. Rajotte and team.

All patients had "hard to manage" diabetes. Most were having severe insulin reactions (unconscious episodes or seizures) as a result of not recognizing lows ("hypoglycemic unawareness"). For this reason they were willing to take the three potent immunosuppressant medicines needed after receiving the transplant.

A report on the "Edmonton Protocol" described islet transplants in more than 300 adult recipients at many centers, sponsored by NIDDK and JDRF. Three years after their first islet transplant (most had two transplants), 23 percent were insulin injection-free, and 29 percent, although back on insulin injections, were still producing some insulin. A report in 2014 found some insulin production continuing in 80 percent of islet transplants. Most patients, although continuing to have some insulin production, returned to needing additional insulin by the fifth year post-transplant. Similar results were reported from France in 2019. However, other results have been somewhat variable, and some centers have discontinued their programs due to patient complications. Current research is focusing on the use of other anti-rejection medicines, use of other sites for the islets than within the liver (many drawbacks) and improving blood supply to the islet after transplant.

Some of the drawbacks are:

- ✔ there are not enough human-donor islets
- ✔ the medicines used to avoid rejection of the transplants have side effects
- ✔ the medicines must be taken for the person's lifetime
- ✔ the medicines are costly

This procedure is currently used only in adults with diabetes that is "hard to manage." These people often have severe low blood sugars due to "hypoglycemic unawareness." With the advent of continuous glucose monitoring (CGM), it has been our experience that hypoglycemic unawareness can often be reversed.

The main goals for islet transplantation in the future involve:

- ✔ getting islets from an easier source (such as pig islets) or growing and regenerating human islets in the laboratory
- ✔ continued evaluation of new medicines to avoid rejection of transplanted islets
- ✔ investigating new techniques to allow "tolerance" of the new islets so that potent immunosuppressant medicines do not have to be taken indefinitely
- ✔ protecting the transplanted islets from the immune system so diabetes does not reoccur

Whole Pancreas Transplantation

Type 1 diabetes can be cured by a whole pancreas transplant. It is important to remember that in people with type 1 diabetes, the immune system will also attack the transplanted tissue. The medications needed to suppress the immune system are the same as those given after any organ is transplanted (e.g., kidney, liver, heart). The medicines have improved but still have harmful side effects. Some of these are:

- ✔ increased risk for infections
- ✔ low white blood cell counts
- ✔ an increased risk for cancer

If a kidney transplant is needed due to kidney failure, so that the immunosuppressant medicines are needed anyway, a pancreas transplant is often done. This may be done at the time of the kidney transplant or at a later time. Approximately 80 percent of the whole pancreas transplants are still functioning after one year.

Stem-Cell Transplants

Families frequently ask about hope from stem-cell transplants. This involves transforming human stem cells into insulin-producing beta cells. Several groups have had some success when the cells were transplanted into mice. The ViaCyte company has injected immature stem cells into mice and allowed them to mature in the mouse. They are now starting similar research studies in humans. Unfortunately, stem-cell transplants are taking longer to develop than was initially anticipated.

In summary, the most important goal at this time is to maintain optimal diabetes management. This will help avoid complications. Then, if a cure becomes possible, the person will be able to benefit from this miracle.

2. CAN DIABETES BE PREVENTED?

Prevention of Type 1 Diabetes

It is now possible in many people to predict that diabetes will occur. This is done by measuring the following antibodies in the blood (see Chapter 3):

- ✔ insulin autoantibody (IAA)
- ✔ GAD-antibody
- ✔ ICA512 (IA-2) antibody
- ✔ ZnT8 (zinc transport antibody)
- ✔ fluorescent ICA antibody

Type 1 Diabetes/TrialNet (T1D/TrialNet)

The National Institute of Health (NIH), with assistance from the Juvenile Diabetes Research Foundation (JDRF) and the American Diabetes Association (ADA), have wisely decided to support research aimed at preventing diabetes. The assumption is that if you can recognize who is at risk years before disease onset (which is now possible), there must be some way to prevent the disease. A consortium of centers in the U.S. and Canada and five centers in Europe and Australia are working together to identify people at high risk. Family members having a first- or second-degree relative who started insulin treatment prior to age 40 years can receive free screening for the above antibodies. Free screening for antibodies in children who do not have a relative with diabetes is also now occurring in the U.S. (Autoimmunity Screening for Kids, in Denver, CO) and in Germany (Fr1da) and Australia.

Initial data has shown that diabetes can be delayed in relatives with high levels of islet cell antibodies after intravenous therapy with an immunosuppressant medicine. Further research in this area will be important.

The phone number to call (no charge) for the islet cell antibody screening for relatives of people with type 1 diabetes is: 1-800-425-8361. More information is available on the website: www.diabetestrialnet.org.

The T1D/TrialNet consortium is also doing studies in people with recently-diagnosed diabetes to attempt to halt the destruction of the insulin-producing islet cells. It is now known that if a person continues to make some of their own insulin, the course of the diabetes will be easier and the eye and kidney complications, severe low blood sugars (Chapter 6), and ketoacidosis (Chapter 15) will all be less likely. Several immunosuppressive agents have already been found to have a protective effect, and these studies are continuing. The above number can be called for more information (or go to the website above).

A third approach is to try to prevent the initial autoimmune reaction against the islets from occurring (true prevention). As the group in which type 1 diabetes is increasing the most is children under age five years, studies starting early in life are important. The number above (or the website) can be contacted for more information.

Prevention of Type 2 Diabetes

The Diabetes Prevention Program (DPP) is discussed in Chapters 4 and 13. The DPP studied 3,234 people with impaired oral glucose tolerance tests. Although not yet diabetic, this group was close to having type 2 diabetes. The results of the DPP were released in 2002 (N Engl J Med 346:393-403, 2002).

Results:

- ✓ 30 minutes of activity five days per week with a low-fat diet and weight loss **reduced the risk for developing type 2 diabetes by 58 percent**
- ✓ taking metformin (Glucophage) also reduced the chance of getting type 2 diabetes by 31 percent

People with a strong family history of type 2 diabetes now have a clear way to lessen their risk of getting this disease.

3. WILL THERE BE A COMPLETE ARTIFICIAL PANCREAS?

The artificial pancreas (AP) refers to a combination of a continuous glucose monitor (CGM) sending glucose data to an insulin pump, which uses algorhythms (mathematical formulas) to regulate insulin administration based on the CGM glucose values.

The hybrid (or partial) artificial pancreas is already available (see Chapter 30). It is called a "hybrid" artificial pancreas because it is still recommended that pre-meal insulin boluses be administered by the user 20 to 30 minutes before meals. This is necessary because blood sugar levels peak 60 minutes after meals, but insulin activity does not peak until 90 minutes after injection (see Figure 2 in Chapter 8). High blood sugar levels develop after meals if a person/family does not do the pre-meal bolus, and the insulin is only given by the insulin pump after the CGM glucose levels rise. Also, when this happens, low blood sugar levels may be more apt to occur two to four hours after the meal. As better ultra-rapid-acting insulins are developed, pre-meal insulin administration will not be necessary, and the word "hybrid" will no longer be necessary.

4. ARE THERE ADVANCES IN HELPING TO AVOID CHRONIC DIABETIC COMPLICATIONS?

The good news: YES! As a result, the life span for people with type 1 diabetes continues to improve!

- ✓ *The main reasons for this improvement are:*
- **more blood sugar levels in the desired range**
- **blood pressure management is better**
- **fewer smokers among people with diabetes**
- **lessened risk of developing diabetic kidney disease**
- **kidney disease can be diagnosed earlier, and treated with ACE-inhibitors or other high blood pressure medicines**
- **lower blood lipids with lipid-lowering medicines (including statins)**
- **other new medicines**

It is important to have annual screening for the eye and kidney complications of diabetes starting at age 10 years or at puberty, whichever is reached first, for people who have had type 1 diabetes for five or more years (see Chapter 23). People with type 2 diabetes need to be screened at diagnosis and annually thereafter.

Another risk associated with type 1 or type 2 diabetes is cardiovascular disease (particularly heart attacks and stroke). Keeping HbA1c levels in the desired range, not smoking, regular exercise, and maintaining optimal blood pressure, body weight and blood lipids are all important in helping to avoid cardiovascular disease (see Chapter 23). Two new types of medicines, referred to as sodium-glucose cotransporter 2 inhibitors (SGCT2i), or glucagon-like peptide 2 (GLP-2) receptor agonists, have been shown beneficial in avoiding and/or treating diabetic kidney and cardiovascular disease. They are initially being used for people with type 2 diabetes, but will gradually be used in select people with type 1 diabetes.

DEFINITIONS

ADA: American Diabetes Association. This non-profit organization is involved with promoting care, education and research for type 1 and type 2 diabetes.

Artificial pancreas: A man-made device that would fine-tune insulin delivery based on glucose levels.

FDA: Food and Drug Administration.

JDRF: Juvenile Diabetes Research Foundation International. This non-profit organization helps to fund research on type 1 diabetes.

QUESTIONS AND ANSWERS FROM NEWSNOTES

 **When is a cure coming?**

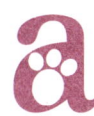 We are asked this question almost daily in clinic. No one knows the answer, other than to say that progress is being made.

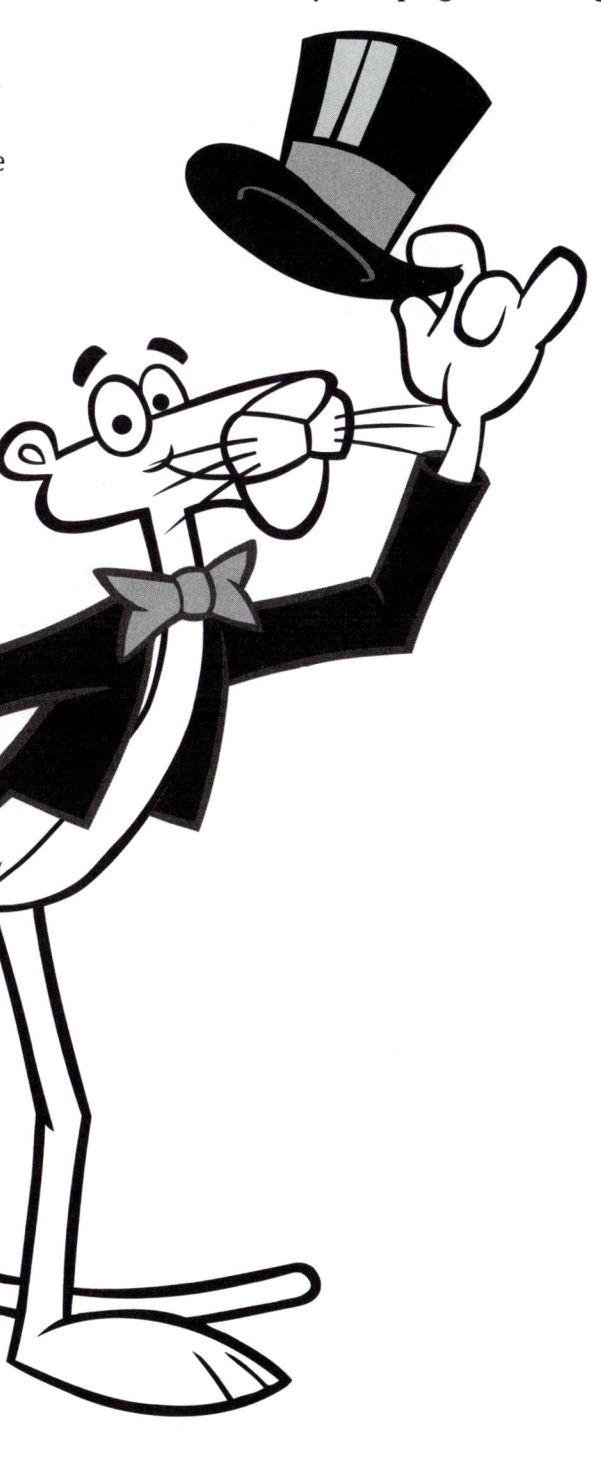

TABLE 1:
Type 1 Diabetes/Trial/Net

People can call 1-800-425-8361 to find out the nearest place to go to obtain the free ICA screening test.

1. **Screening (Phase 1):** Islet cell antibody (ICA) tests

   The five antibodies that can be used in screening (see Chapter 3) are:
   - GAD antibody
   - ICA512
   - IAA (insulin autoantibody)
   - ZnT8 antibody
   - Fluorescent ICA (if one or more of the antibodies listed above are present)

   ✔ If one antibody is found, a second sample will need to be drawn to confirm the result. If the antibody is present in the second sample, then the person can enter Phase 2.

   ✔ If more than one antibody is present, a second sample can be drawn for confirmation OR the person can go directly into Phase 2.

2. **Phase 2:** The following tests are done:
   - Oral glucose tolerance test (OGTT) - to make sure diabetes isn't present
   - Islet cell antibody test (as described above)
   - HLA (looking for the 0602 protective gene)
   - HbA1c

   In a few cases an additional test, the intravenous glucose tolerance test (IVGTT), will be required.

   With all of the test results, the person can be provided with a risk level related to the development of diabetes (within the next five years).

   The risk levels are: less than 25 percent, 25-50 percent and greater than 50 percent.

3. **Phase 3:** The Phase 2 tests (minus the HLA) are repeated every six months.

WEBSITES

Barbara Davis Center for Diabetes
University of Colorado Denver
Mail Stop A140, Building M20
1775 Aurora Court
Aurora, CO 80045
303-724-2323 • Fax 303-724-6779
www.BarbaraDavisCenter.org

Children's Diabetes Foundation
www.ChildrensDiabetesFoundation.org

Children With Diabetes
www.ChildrenwithDiabetes.com

Juvenile Diabetes Research Foundation
www.jdrf.org

American Diabetes Association
www.diabetes.org

GLU TID Exchange
www.myglu.org

Autoimmunity Screening for Kids
www.Askhealth.org

APPENDIX
Glucose Conversion Between mg/dL and mmol/L

Parts of the world use one system, and other parts use the other system. This will allow the book to now be used by both. An easy way to make the conversion from mg/dL to mmol/L is to divide by 18. To convert mmol/L to mg/dL, multiply by 18. The table below may also help.

mg/dL		mmol/L	mg/dL		mmol/L	mg/dL		mmol/L	mg/dL		mmol/L
10	=	.6	125	=	7.0	240	=	13.3	355	=	19.7
15	=	.8	130	=	7.2	245	=	13.6	360	=	20.0
20	=	1.1	135	=	7.5	250	=	13.9	365	=	20.3
25	=	1.4	140	=	7.8	255	=	14.2	370	=	20.6
30	=	1.7	145	=	8.0	260	=	14.5	375	=	20.8
35	=	2.0	150	=	8.3	265	=	14.7	380	=	21.1
40	=	2.3	155	=	8.5	270	=	15.0	385	=	21.4
45	=	2.5	160	=	8.9	275	=	15.3	390	=	21.7
50	=	2.8	165	=	9.2	280	=	15.6	395	=	21.9
55	=	3.0	170	=	9.5	285	=	15.8	400	=	22.2
60	=	3.3	175	=	9.8	290	=	16.1	425	=	23.6
65	=	3.6	180	=	10.0	295	=	16.4	450	=	25.0
70	=	3.9	185	=	10.3	300	=	16.7	475	=	26.4
75	=	4.2	190	=	10.5	305	=	16.9	500	=	27.8
80	=	4.5	195	=	10.8	310	=	17.2	525	=	29.2
85	=	4.7	200	=	11.1	315	=	17.5	550	=	30.5
90	=	5.0	205	=	11.3	320	=	17.8	575	=	31.9
95	=	5.3	210	=	11.6	325	=	18.0	600	=	33.3
100	=	5.5	215	=	11.9	330	=	18.3	625	=	34.7
105	=	5.8	220	=	12.2	335	=	18.6	650	=	36.1
110	=	6.1	225	=	12.5	340	=	18.9	675	=	37.5
115	=	6.4	230	=	12.8	345	=	19.2	700	=	38.9
120	=	6.7	235	=	13.0	350	=	19.4			

Index

(For subjects referenced frequently in a chapter, the chapter number and first page are listed)

Abbott: see FreeStyle Libre

ACE-inhibitor, 248, 262, 336

ACTH, 259

Acesulfame-K, 117

Acidosis, Ch. 15 (p. 167)

Addison's disease, 259

Adhesives, 317, 318

Admelog, 77, 83

Adolescence, 206, Ch. 20 (p 215)

Adrenal problems, 258

Adrenaline (epinephrine), 50

Adult diabetes clinic, 223

Adult-onset diabetes, Ch. 4 (p. 31), Ch. 12 (p. 125), Ch. 13 (p. 141)

Agave Nectar, 116

Age-related responsibilities, Ch. 18 (p. 197)

Airport screening, 289, 290

Alcohol, 119, 219

Alternate site testing, 66, 67

Analog, 83

Anger, 103, 222

Angiotensin Receptor Blocker (ARB), 248

Anorexia, 222

Antibodies, Ch. 3 (p. 25), 338

Anxiety, 104, Ch. 17 (p. 189)

Apidra, Ch. 8 (p. 75)

ARB (angiotensin-receptor blocker), 248

Artificial pancreas, Ch. 30 (p. 323), 338

Aspartame, 117

Atrophy, 95, 100

Autoimmune conditions, Ch. 24 (p. 255)

Autoimmunity (self-allergy), 26, 28

Baby-sitters, Ch. 26 (p. 283)

Baqsimi, 58

Basaglar, Ch. 8 (p. 75), 81, 83

Basal insulin, Ch. 8 (p. 75), Ch. 22 (p. 231), Ch. 28 (p. 295)

Basal IQ, Ch. 30 (p. 323)

Bedtime blood sugar, 69

Beta cells, 83

Binge eating, 222

Birth control pills, 220

Birth defects, 250, Ch. 31 (p. 327)

Blood sugar goals, 69, 321

Blood sugar checking, Ch. 7 (p. 63); at school, 274

Blood sugars (pregnancy), Ch. 31 (p. 327)

Blood sugar record sheet, 70, 306

BMI, 32, 137

Bolus Insulin, Ch. 8 (p. 75), Ch. 28 (p. 295)

Bulimia, 222

C-peptide, 32, 40

Calibration, 303

Calorie needs, 128, 133-134

Camp, Ch. 27 (p. 289)

Carb choice, 109, 134, 140

Carbohydrate, 107, Ch. 11-12 (p. 125)

Carbohydrate counting meal plan, Ch. 12 (p. 125)

Cataract, 245

Causes (type 1 diabetes), Ch. 3 (p.25)

Causes (type 2 diabetes), Ch. 4 (p. 31)

Celiac disease, 256-258

CGM (Continuous glucose monitoring), Ch. 29 (p. 313)

Chemstrip K, 45-47

Child sitters, Ch. 26 (p. 283)

Cholesterol, 111, 249

Cigarettes (tobacco), 219, Ch. 23 (p. 243)

Clinic visits, Ch. 21 (p. 225)

College, 222-223, 228

Coma, diabetic, Ch. 15 (p. 167)

Complications (chronic), Ch. 23 (p. 243)

Constant carbohydrate meal plan, Ch. 12 (p. 133)

Contact lenses, 253

Continuous glucose monitoring (CGM), Ch. 29 (p. 313); at school, 278-279

Correction factor, 239, 242; at school, 271, 273

Control IQ, Ch. 30 (p. 323)

Cure, 334

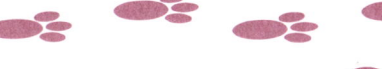

Dawn phenomenon, 302
DCCT (Diabetes Control and Complications Trial), 157
DR3/DR4, Ch. 3 (p. 25)
Delayed hypoglycemia, 51
Denial, 103
Denting, 98, 100
Depression, 194
Dermatitis herpetiformis, 259
Detemir (levemir), Ch. 8 (p. 75)
DexCom G5 & G6, 315, 316, 324-326; at school, 264, 270, 272, 274, 275, 278
Diabetes Medical Management Plan (DMMP), 270, 272
Diabetes prevention program (DPP), 335, 338
Diabetic Ketoacidosis (DKA), Ch. 15 (p. 167); at school, 276, 277, 280
DPP4 inhibitors, 38
Driving (car), 222
Drugs, 220
Dual wave, 303-305
Email, 226, Ch. 29 (p. 313)
Eating disorders, 195, 222
Education, Ch. 1 (p. 9)
Environment, 27
Eversense Senseonics CGM, 313, 316
Exchange meal plan, Ch. 12 (p. 125)
Exercise, Ch. 13 (p. 141); at school, 280
Exercise (pump), 309
Extended wave, 303-305
Eye problems, 245-246

Eye problems (pregnancy), 346
Family concerns, Ch. 17 (p. 189)
Family responsibilities, Ch. 17-20 (p. 189)
Fat, 110
Feelings, Ch. 10 (p. 101)
Fiasp, 78, 83
Fiber, 114
Field days, 52, 233, 275, 285
Flu shots, 209, 221
Foil-wrapped Ketostix, 45
Folic acid, 330
Food record, 120-121
Foot problems, 251
FreeStyle Libre CGM, 313, 314; at school, 264, 270, 272, 274, 275
Fructose, 110
GAD, 19, Ch. 3 (p. 25), 338
Gastroparesis, 249
Genetics, 25, 32
Gestational diabetes, 331
Glucagon, 56-59; at school, 275, 276
Glucagon-like peptide (GLP-1), 38
Glucophage (metformin), 36, 37
Glucose records, 70, 306
Glucose (blood sugar), Ch. 7 (p. 63)
Glucose tolerance test (OGTT), 33
Gluten, 256-258
Grandparents, Ch. 26 (p. 283)
Grief, Ch. 10 (p. 101), Ch. 17 (p. 189)
Growth hormone, 217

Guardian Connect (CGM), 313, 315
Guilt, 104, Ch. 17 (p. 189)
Gym (PE), 51; at school, 275
HbA1c, 158, 163, 164
HDL cholesterol, 111
HLA types, 25, 28
Heart, 111, 249
Heat/Frio cool pouch, 294
Heredity, 25, 32
High blood sugar, 61, Ch. 22 (p. 231); at school, 277
Honeymoon period, 22, 28
Hot tub, 52, 62
Humalog, Ch. 8 (p. 75)
Hypertension, 249
Hypertrophy, 98, 100
Hypoglycemia, Ch. 6 (p. 49); at school, 275
Hypoglycemia (exercise), 147-152
Hypoglycemia (pumps), 307
Hypoglycemic (treatment), 52-56; at school, 275
Hypoglycemic unawareness, 56
I-port, 98
I/C ratios, 134-136, 299, 303, 310
IDEA (Individual Disabilities Education Act), 281, 282
IHP (Individualized Health Plan), 264, 266
Independence, 215
Infusion sets (pumps), 301
Ingrown toenails, 251
Injecting insulin, Ch. 9 (p. 85)
Insuflon, 98

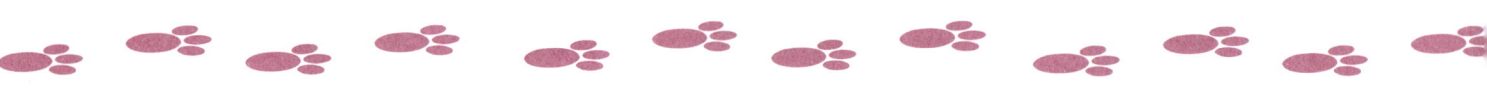

Insulin, Ch. 8 (p. 75)
Insulin autoantibody (IAA), 16, Ch. 3 (p. 25), 338
ICA, 19, 24, Ch. 3 (p. 25), 338
Insulin administration, Ch. 9 (p. 85)
Insulin and exercise, Ch. 13 (p. 141)
Insulin/Carb (IC) ratio, 134-136, 299, 303, 310; at school, 265, 267
Insulin dose adjustment, Ch. 22 (p. 231)
Insulin pens, 95-97
Insulin pumps, Ch. 28 (p. 295); at school, 278
Insulin reaction, Ch. 6 (p. 49); at school, 275
Intensive diabetes management, 81
Islet cell antibody (ICA), 16, 19, Ch. 3 (p. 25), 338
Islet cells, 22, 27
Islet transplantation, 334-335
Joint contractures, 250
Ketoacidosis (DKA), Ch. 15 (p. 167); at school, 276, 277, 280
Ketones, Ch. 5 (p. 43), Ch. 15 (p. 167); at school, 276, 277, 280
Ketostix (ketodiastix), 45
Kidney disease, 247-248, 254
Kidney problems (pregnancy), 330
LDL cholesterol, 111, 249
Label reading, 118
Lactose, 110
Lantus, Ch. 8 (p. 75)

Lantus dosing, Ch. 8 (p. 75), 80, 232
Laser treatment, 246
Leak-back, 92, 100
Legal rights (school), 281
Lens, 245
Levemir (detemir), Ch. 8 (p. 75), 80-81
Levemir dosing, Ch. 8 (p. 75)
Lipids, 111, 249
Loop, 326
Low blood sugar, Ch. 6 (p. 49); at school, 275
Low blood sugar prevention, 51
Low dose glucagon, 58, 184
Lyumjer, 78
Macroalbuminuria, 247-248
Medical identifications, 59, 60
Medicool, 291
Medtronic/MiniMed, 297, 316, 324-325
Meningitis vaccine, 221
Meters (blood glucose), Ch. 7 (p. 63)
Metformin (glucophage), 36
Microalbumin, Ch. 23 (p. 243), 254
MiniMed 670G AP, 324, 325
MiniMed 780G AP, 325
Microaneurysms, 245-246
Mmol/L, 73, 340
MODY diabetes, 17
Navigator, 316
Necrobiosis, 259
Needle fear, 100, 104, 212
Needles (for pens), 97
Neonatal diabetes, 213

Neotame, 117
Nephropathy, 247-248
Neuropathy, 249
Nighttime lows, 51
Non-insulin dependent diabetes (NIDDM), Ch. 4 (p. 31)
NovoLog, Ch. 8 (p. 75)
NPH, Ch. 8 (p. 75)
Nutrition, Ch. 11 (p. 107), Ch. 12 (p. 125)
(Chapters 11 & 12)
Nutrition (pregnancy), 330
OmniPod, 297, 326
Oral medicines, 36-38
Pancreas, 18
Pancreas transplantation, 334-335
Pens, 95-97
Phenergan, 182
Plugged needle, 99
Polycystic ovarian syndrome (PCOS), 39
Precision Xtra meter, 45, 47
Predicted Low Glucose Suspend, Ch. 30 (p. 323)
Preeclampsia, 331
Pregnancy, Ch. 31 (p. 327)
Preschool and toddlers, Ch. 18 (p. 197), Ch. 19 (p. 209)
Prevention (hypoglycemia), 51
Prevention Trial (TrialNet), 335, 338
Proliferative retinopathy, 245-246
Protein, 110
Protein (urine), 247, 248, 254
Psychological disorders, 193

Pump advantages, 296
Pump problems, 296
Pumps, insulin, Ch. 28 (p. 295)
Rapid Acting Insulins, Ch. 8 (p. 75)
Record sheets, 70, 306
Receiver, 314
Regular Insulin, Ch. 8 (p. 75)
Research, Ch. 31 (p. 333)
Retina, 245, 246
Retinal detachment, 245-246
Retinopathy, 245-246
Retrospective CGM data, 317-321
Rule of 500, 303
Saccharin, 117
Sadness, 103
Salt, 114
School, 184, Ch. 25 (p. 261)
School CGM use, 278
School health plans, Ch. 25 (p. 261)
School supplies, 263
Seizure, 54-58
Sensor, 314
Sex hormones, 218, 220
Sexuality, 218, 220
SGL-2 inhibitors, 37
Shower, 50, 62
Sick-day, Ch. 16 (p. 177)
Sick-day medications, 185
Single-parent families, Ch. 17 (p. 189)
Skin problems, 259
Sliding scales, 240
Smoking, 219, Ch. 23 (p. 243)
Snacks, Ch. 12 (p. 125)

Snacks and exercise, 150
Square wave, 303-305
Sprue (celiac), 256-258
Standards of care at school, Ch. 25 (p. 261)
Standards of care management, 228-229
Starch, 109
Stevia, 117
Stress, Ch. 10 (p. 101), Ch. 17 (p. 189)
Sucralose, 117
Sucrose, 110
Supply costs, Ch. 17 (p. 189)
Support groups, 228
Surgery, Ch. 16 (p. 177)
Sweeteners, 117
Symptoms (diabetes), 19
Syringes, Ch. 9 (p. 85)
Tandem insulin pumps, 297, 325
Tapes, 317-318
TSH, 255-256
Teen years, Ch. 18 (p. 201), Ch. 20 (p. 215)
Telephone management, 225
Temporary basal rate, 149, 153, 302
Thinking scales, 240
Three-day food record, 116, 120, 121
Thyroid, 255, 256
Tidepool Loop, 326
Time in Range, 162, 321
Tobacco, 219, Ch. 23 (p. 243)
Toddler, Ch. 18 (p. 197), Ch. 19 (p. 209)
Trans-fat, 111

Transfer, adult clinic, 223
Transition, 223
Transmitter, 314
Transplantation (islet, pancreas), 334, 335
Travel, Ch. 27 (p. 289)
Treatment (hypoglycemia), 52-56
Trend arrows, 319-320
Trend graphs, 319-320
Tresiba, 77, 80, 81
Triglyceride, 111, 249
Type 1 diabetes, Ch. 3 (p. 25)
Type 2 diabetes, Ch. 4 (p. 31)
Urine ketones, 45
Vacations, Ch. 27 (p. 289)
Viagra, 250
Virus, 27
Vitamins, 114
Vitreous, 245-246
Vomiting, 182
Websites, 228
Weight management, 32-35, 115, 137-138, 145
Xylitol, 117
Zinc transport antibody (ZnT8), 16, Ch. 3 (p. 25), 338
Zofran, 182

Publications

Additional copies of *"Understanding Diabetes"* as well as other diabetes publications may be ordered by using this form, by calling the Children's Diabetes Foundation at 303-863-1200, or by visiting www.ChildrensDiabetesFoundation.org

Children's Diabetes Foundation
4380 South Syracuse Street, Suite 430 • Denver, CO 80237

Name: _____

Address: _____

City, State, ZIP: _____

Phone: _____ Email: _____

Item	Price	Qty	Total
Understanding Diabetes, 14th Edition (The Pink Panther Book)	$25		
Understanding Diabetes, 13th Edition Discounted while supplies last	$15		
A First Book for Understanding Diabetes, 14th Edition*	$15		
Un Primer Libro Para Entender La Diabetes, 14th Edition ("First Book" in Spanish)	$15		
Insulin Pumps, Continuous Glucose Monitors and the Artificial Pancreas, 3rd Edition	$18		
Management of Diabetes in Adults, 1st Edition	$15		
DIABETES: A History of a Center and a Patient	$15		
A Cure – A novel about diabetes and the search for a cure*	$20		
A Second Cure – A second novel about diabetes and the search for a cure	Available at amazon.com		
Colorado residents add 8.31% sales tax			
SHIPPING AND HANDLING: $5.00 per book for orders of 1-9 books; $2.00 per book for orders of 10+ books			
*Also available at amazon.com	Total		

Prices subject to change.

☐ Please include me on the Children's Diabetes Foundation mailing list.
☐ Check enclosed payable to: Children's Diabetes Foundation
☐ Visa ☐ MasterCard ☐ Discovery ☐ AmEx

Card #_____ Exp. Date _____

All orders must be paid in full before we can mail. Books are mailed USPS or Ground UPS. Allow one to three weeks for delivery.

Canadian and Foreign Purchasers: Please include sufficient funds to equal U.S. currency exchange rates.

For quantity order pricing and additional information call 303-863-1200 or visit our website at www.ChildrensDiabetesFoundation.org

Notes

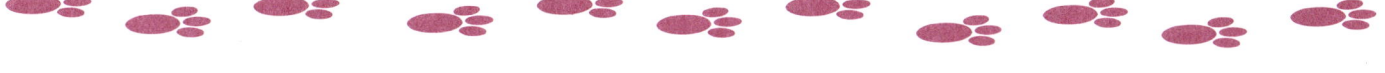

Notes

Notes

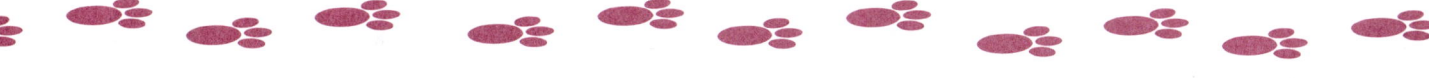

Notes

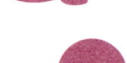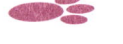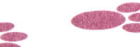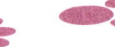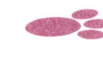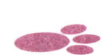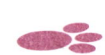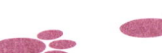

Important Contacts

Contact	Phone
Our Child:	
Parent/Guardian:	
Parent/Guardian:	
Grandparent:	
Grandparent:	
Caregiver:	
Family Friend:	
Diabetes Physician:	
Diabetes Nurse:	
Primary Care Physician:	
Primary Care Nurse:	
School:	
School Nurse:	

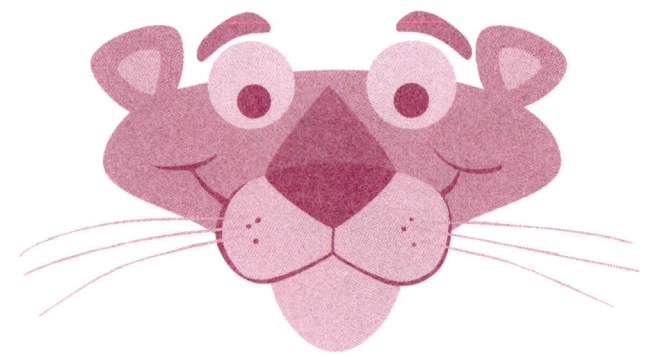